A Coursebook on Aphasia and Other Neurogenic Language Disorders

Third Edition

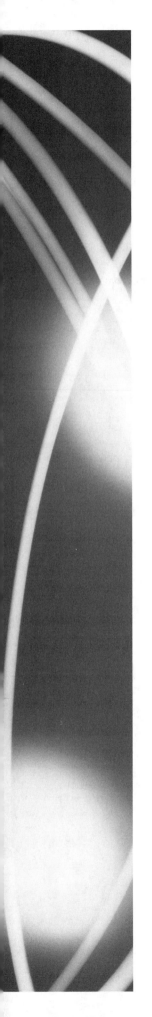

A Coursebook on Aphasia and Other Neurogenic Language Disorders

Third Edition

M. N. Hegde, Ph.D.

DELMAR
CENGAGE Learning™

Australia • Brazil • Japan • Korea • Mexico • Singapore • Spain • United Kingdom • United States

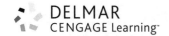

DELMAR
CENGAGE Learning

A Coursebook on Aphasia and Other Neurogenic Language Disorders, Third Edition
M. N. Hegde

Vice President, Health Care Business Unit: William Brottmiller

Editorial Director: Matthew Kane

Acquisitions Editor: Kalen Conerly

Product Manager: Juliet Steiner

Editorial Assistant: Molly Belmont

Marketing Director: Jennifer McAvey

Marketing Coordinator: Christopher Manion

Production Director: Carolyn Miller

Production Manager: Barbara A. Bullock

Production Editor: John Mickelbank

For product information and technology assistance, contact us at
Cengage Learning Customer & Sales Support, 1-800-354-9706

For permission to use material from this text or product,
submit all requests online at **www.cengage.com/permissions**
Further permissions questions can be emailed to
permissionrequest@cengage.com

Library of Congress Control Number: 2005024767

ISBN-13: 978-1-4180-3736-9

ISBN-10: 1-4180-3736-2

Delmar
Executive Woods
5 Maxwell Drive
Clifton Park, NY 12065
USA

Cengage Learning is a leading provider of customized learning solutions with office locations around the globe, including Singapore, the United Kingdom, Australia, Mexico, Brazil, and Japan. Locate your local office at
www.cengage.com/global

Cengage Learning products are represented in Canada by Nelson Education, Ltd.

To learn more about Delmar, visit **www.cengage.com/delmar**

Purchase any of our products at your local bookstore or at our preferred online store **www.CengageBrain.com**

Notice to the Reader

Publisher does not warrant or guarantee any of the products described herein or perform any independent analysis in connection with any of the product information contained herein. Publisher does not assume, and expressly disclaims, any obligation to obtain and include information other than that provided to it by the manufacturer. The reader is expressly warned to consider and adopt all safety precautions that might be indicated by the activities described herein and to avoid all potential hazards. By following the instructions contained herein, the reader willingly assumes all risks in connection with such instructions. The publisher makes no representations or warranties of any kind, including but not limited to, the warranties of fitness for particular purpose or merchantability, nor are any such representations implied with respect to the material set forth herein, and the publisher takes no responsibility with respect to such material. The publisher shall not be liable for any special, consequential, or exemplary damages resulting, in whole or part, from the readers' use of, or reliance upon, this material.

Printed in Canada
3 4 5 6 7 11 10 09

Contents

PART III: TRAUMATIC BRAIN INJURY   351

PART IV: DEMENTIA   421

Preface to the Third Edition

The first edition of this book on aphasia and other neurogenic language disorders was one of the first to be developed as a *coursebook,* a new format for teaching and learning. Instructors and students alike have liked this format, because it makes both teaching and learning easier and efficient.

The *coursebook* format was originally designed as an effective instructional package that reduced the amount of note taking. The coursebook also reduced the variability in the accuracy and completeness of notes students take. The use of this type of book promotes class discussion as the students are not as busy taking notes in the class as they normally are. There is more on the coursebook format of teaching in Appendix A.

My students, who have used this book (and this *type* of book) for the first time in a course on aphasia and related language disorders, have given me much positive feedback. Students have found the coursebook a valuable means of integrating textbook information with class notes they take. They have a single source of information that is easier to study than (literally) a text on the one hand and the class notebook on the other. They have expressed a preference for this type of book for all of their courses. I would like to thank them for their comments and suggestions. I also welcome feedback from instructors who use this coursebook.

The first two editions of this coursebook were written as a supplement to regular textbooks. This third edition is no longer written as a supplemental text. The content of the third edition of this coursebook has been substantially enhanced to make it suitable as a textbook on courses in aphasia and other neurogenic language disorders, whether offered at the undergraduate or graduate level. Nonetheless, this new textbook retains the coursebook format so the instructors can make lecture notes and students can write down instructor's notes on each page of the text.

The third edition, because it contains extensive information on neurogenic language disorders, has been divided into four parts. The first part of the book contains nine chapters and deals with various forms of aphasia, alexia, agraphia, and agnosia, and their neuropathological bases, neurodiagnostic procedures, and assessment and treatment of aphasic communication disorders. The second part contains two chapters that address right hemisphere syndrome and its assessment and treatment. The third part describes traumatic brain injury and its nature, assessment, and treatment in two chapters. Finally, the fourth part of the text is devoted to varieties of dementia and their nature, causes, and associated communication disorders. The final chapter of this section (and that of the text) describes assessment and management of communication deficits in people with dementia. The three chapters on dementia are new for the most part because of extensive research literature that has been published in the last decade.

All chapters have been thoroughly revised and expanded to make them comprehensive, current, and clinically detailed. I have added new information to most chapters to reflect recent developments in the study, assessment, and treatment of language disorders associated with neurologic problems. Furthermore, a glossary, commonly used medical abbreviations and symbols, the World Health Organization's International Classification of Functioning, Disability, and Health (ICF), and Internet resources for clinicians and consumers have been added in separate appendixes.

I trust that instructors and students will continue to find this new tool of teaching and learning useful. I am thankful to many positive comments I have received from instructors across the country. In Appendix A, I have given a brief description of the coursebook method of teaching and learning.

I am grateful to the anonymous reviewers who have given thoughtful suggestions for revising the chapters. Any remaining deficiencies, however, are my own responsibility. My thanks are due to the able editorial and production departments at Delmar, Cengage Learning. Kalen Conerly, the acquisitions editor, has been patient and persistent with this revision. Her periodic and encouraging prompts and support have made it possible to complete the revision on time. Similarly, the continuous and kind support I have received from Juliet Steiner, the product manager, has been valuable in getting this revision published. I thank them both.

About the Author

M. N. (Giri) Hegde, PhD, is Professor of Communication Sciences and Disorders at California State University-Fresno. He holds a master's degree in experimental psychology from the University of Mysore, India, a post master's diploma in Medical (Clinical) Psychology from Bangalore University, India, and a doctoral degree in Speech-Language Pathology from Southern Illinois University at Carbondale.

Dr. Hegde is a specialist in fluency disorders, language disorders, research methods, and treatment procedures in communicative disorders. He has made numerous presentations to national and international audiences on various basic and applied topics in communicative disorders and experimental and applied behavior analysis. With his deep and wide scholarship, Dr. Hegde has authored several highly regarded and widely used scientific and professional books, including *Treatment Procedures in Communicative Disorders, Clinical Research in Communicative Disorders, Introduction to Communicative Disorders, A Coursebook on Scientific and Professional Writing in Speech-Language Pathology, A Coursebook on Language Disorders in Children, PocketGuide to Treatment in Speech-Language Pathology,* and *PocketGuide to Assessment in Speech-Language Pathology.* He has served as editor of the Singular Textbook Series. He also has served on the editorial boards of scientific and professional journals and continues to serve as an editorial consultant to *Journal of Fluency Disorders, American Journal of Speech-Language Pathology, Indian Journal of Communication Disorders,* and *Journal of Speech-Language Pathology and Applied Behavior Analysis.*

Dr. Hegde is a recipient of various honors, including the Outstanding Professor Award from California State University-Fresno, CSU-Fresno Provost's Recognition for Outstanding Scholarship and Publication, Distinguished Alumnus Award from the Southern Illinois University Department of Communication Sciences and Disorders, and Outstanding Professional Achievement Award from District 5 of California Speech-Language-Hearing Association. Dr. Hegde is a Fellow of the American Speech-Language-Hearing Association.

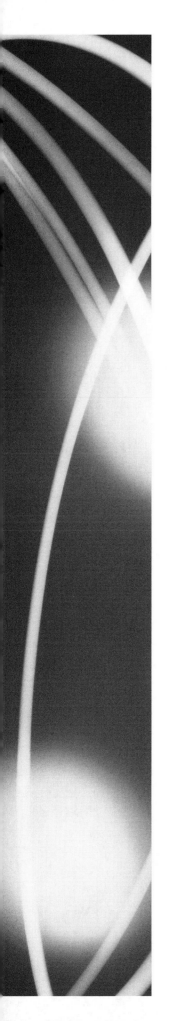

PART I

APHASIA

APHASIA: A HISTORICAL INTRODUCTION

Chapter Outline

- The Importance of Aphasia
- Early Historical Perspectives
- Localizationist and Holistic Approaches
- The Emergence of Cognitivism
- The Modern Period

Learning Objectives

After reading this chapter, the student will:

- Specify the importance of the study of aphasia.
- Give an overview of the historical developments in the study of aphasia.
- Describe the beginnings of the study of aphasia.
- State the differences between the localist and the holist approaches to the study of aphasia.

- Place the contributions of Broca and Wernicke in historic context.
- Describe the differences between the localist, holist, and cognitivist approaches to the study of aphasia.
- Describe the historical trends in the linguistic and speech-language pathology contributions to the study of aphasia.

The Importance of Aphasia

Aphasia is loss or impairment of language skills in adults who have had a history of language skills within the range of normal variations. The loss or impairment is associated with recent cerebral pathology or trauma.

Aphasia is an important syndrome for both clinical and scientific reasons. Clinical and scientific issues surrounding aphasia are intertwined.

Clinical Importance

Although this syndrome has been known for centuries, aphasia was poorly understood for a long time. Many specialists, including neurologists, general medical practitioners, psychologists, and linguists, have studied aphasia.

In recent decades, increased interest in the problems associated with aging has stimulated clinical research on aphasia. Therefore, speech-language pathologists have joined the team of specialists dealing with the study, assessment, and treatment of aphasia.

Demographic changes, too, have spurred further interest in the clinical study of aphasia, which is primarily a problem associated with aging. An increase in the geriatric population, with a concomitant increase in the communicative disorders associated with aging, has created unprecedented demand for clinical services for persons who have such disorders as aphasia and dementia.

We will find out more about demographic and ethnocultural variables associated with aphasia and other neurogenic language disorders in subsequent chapters.

Scientific Importance

Aphasia presents a window on the fascinating and often mysterious relation between brain and language. When various cerebral diseases and trauma cause sudden impairment or loss of language, scientists and clinicians have an opportunity to study that relation. They can correlate affected areas of the brain with lost or impaired language functions.

When cerebral pathology or trauma is systematically and repeatedly correlated with lost language functions, a potential relation between brain and normal language functions is suggested. Clinical data may suggest that specific areas of the brain may control or modulate particular language functions.

Early Historical Perspectives

A review of historical explanations of the etiology of aphasia reveals some of the early misunderstandings associated with it and a slow emergence of more valid observations. An early misconception some physicians held was that ventricles, not the cortical matter, controlled cognitive functions, including language. Another was that aphasia resulted from a paralyzed tongue (Benton & Joynt, 1960).

Valid observations about various functions that are disturbed in aphasia began to be made as early as the 17th century. Some physicians realized that patients could have difficulty talking even though their tongues were not paralyzed. Diseases of the brain began to be suspected (Benton & Joynt, 1960). For example, a few writers gave somewhat detailed descriptions of reading and writing problems associated with stroke, which they called *apoplexy* (Benton & Anderson, 1998). Questionable beliefs and theories continued to be advocated, however.

Some writers of the 17th century used the term *aphonia* to describe symptoms of aphasia (Benton & Anderson, 1998). **Aphonia** technically means lack of voice; the term is now reserved for a type of voice disorder in which the individual cannot phonate but can whisper.

Johann Gesner's 1770 monograph is considered the first major study of aphasia, which he called *speech amnesia,* a term used by some previous investigators (see Benton & Anderson, 1998). Gesner recognized that patients with aphasia do not have dementia. Gesner described a variety of well-established language, reading, and writing disturbances associated with aphasia.

More case studies of aphasic patients were published in the 19th century. Fluent but meaningless speech, paraphasia, jargon, preserved serial speech, and writing problems were all described. The term

agraphia was used to describe writing problems; it currently is used in the same sense. The term *alexia* was also mentioned (Benton & Anderson, 1998).

German anatomist and phrenologist Franz Joseph Gall (1758–1828) was among the first to suggest localization of language and other intellectual functions in the frontal lobes. His views, however, were not accepted, as they were associated with phrenology. A discredited pseudoscience of the day, **phrenology** correlated mental and intellectual functioning to the topographic aspects of a person's skull, including its bumps, shape, and size. Gall believed that a strong behavioral or personality characteristic of an individual would result in an overdeveloped area of brain, which would then produce a bump on the skull. He published detailed maps, or diagrams, of the brain showing specific areas of the brain responsible for many mental functions, including paternal love, self-esteem, benevolence, bravery, and honesty.

Paul Broca (1824–1880)

One of the most enduring names to emerge from the 1800s was that of a French neurosurgeon and physical anthropologist, Paul Broca. He was the first to offer clinical and pathological evidence relating the frontal lobe and left brain to language production, essentially supporting Gall's contention. Through a series of case studies and pathological evidence gathered from autopsies, Broca published two reports in French, the first in 1863 and the second in 1865 (see Berker, Berker, & Smith, 1986, for an English translation of the 1865 Broca report). Broca became convinced that the lesions that lead to language disturbances are typically found in the left hemisphere. Broca has been credited with the famous statement, "We speak with the left hemisphere" (Benton & Anderson, 1998).

The brain damage Broca described was especially evident in the lower, posterior portion of the left frontal lobe at the junction of lateral and central fissures. The area is concerned with motor speech function and soon came to be known as Broca's area (also known as Brodmann's areas 44 and 45).

Broca's term to describe language disorders associated with brain lesions was **aphemia.** He described the following major symptoms:

- Reduced speech fluency
- Agrammatic, telegraphic speech
- Many language production errors
- Only limited impairment of comprehension of spoken language

Experts have debated whether injury to Broca's area is necessary to create symptoms of Broca's aphasia. Some experts question both the syndrome and its localization to Broca's area. We will learn more about Broca's aphasia in Chapter 5.

Other specialists who in the mid- to late 1800s clearly described language disorders associated with brain diseases include the English neurologist John Hughlings Jackson (1835–1911) who wrote about the *affections of speech from diseases of the brain* (Jackson, 1874). We will learn more about Jackson later, in the context of the cognitive school of studies on aphasia.

Carl Wernicke (1848–1905)

Another enduring name in aphasia is that of Carl Wernicke, a German neuropsychiatrist. He was the first to describe a type of aphasia that in many ways contrasted the symptoms of aphasia that Broca described. Based on his clinical studies and autopsies of patients who had had language disturbances, Wernicke published two reports in German, the first in 1874 and the second in 1886 (see Eggert, 1977, and Geshwind, 1967, for details on Wernicke's original reports). His research led Wernicke to conclude that a different kind of aphasia is caused by lesion in the posterior portion of the left superior temporal gyrus. This portion of the brain is now known as Wernicke's area. Wernicke thus strengthened the localist viewpoint (see the next section) of the relation between brain and language.

Wernicke described a case of aphasia with:

- Fluent but meaningless speech
- Grammatically correct speech
- Severe problems in understanding spoken language
- Difficulties in comprehending material read silently or orally

Wernicke called it **sensory aphasia,** now known as *Wernicke's aphasia.* Wernicke also suggested the possibility of several other forms of aphasia, including transcortical motor aphasia (described in Chapter 5), conduction aphasia, and transcortical sensory aphasia (both described in Chapter 6).

Localizationist and Holistic Approaches

The **localizationist** view links specific function to a specific anatomic structure within the brain. The localizationists try to show that lesions in specific areas of the brain affect particular functions (Benton & Anderson, 1998; Goodglass, 1988). Both Broca and Wernicke were localizationists.

Most localizationists are also associationists. The **associationist** view holds that patients who are aphasic have intact intellect but have lost the typical association between words and verbal concepts to the actual objects and events. Lesions in the brain may disassociate different parts of the brain that normally associate events and experiences with words and concepts.

The holistic approach, on the other hand, takes an opposing view. The **holistic approach** advocates that the brain functions as an integrated unit and that a lesion in one area affects functions of most, if not all, areas. In general, the holistic approach denies the existence of specific anatomic structures that control equally specific language functions. Accordingly, in all patients with aphasia, most, if not all, aspects of language are disturbed (Benton & Anderson, 1998; Goodglass, 1988).

John Hughlings Jackson, the previously mentioned English neurologist, was an early opponent of Broca's localization view. As a proponent of the holistic view of brain and language, Jackson suggested that the brain functioned as an integrated unit in formulating and expressing language. Jackson, though not the first to observe that patients with aphasia often retain automatic (emotional) speech in the context of impaired propositional speech, nonetheless emphasized that distinction and pointed out that language is not lost in aphasia but the underlying pathology has made it inaccessible in certain contexts (Basso, 2003). As we will see in a later section, Jackson also laid the foundation for a cognitive approach to the study of aphasia.

Another early opponent of Broca's who argued against localization of brain function was the Frenchman Pierre Marie (1853–1940). Marie's position was that aphasia is a single disorder, not a collection of multiple disorders distinguished on the basis of the site of lesion. Marie also published evidence that a lesion in Broca's area may not produce Broca's aphasia and that patients with symptoms of Broca's aphasia may have lesions elsewhere in their brains (see Cole & Cole, 1971, for a historical account of Marie's contributions). Furthermore, Marie argued that auditory comprehension deficits (generally not considered significant in Broca's aphasia) exist in all aphasia patients. Marie believed that only Wernicke's aphasia was "true" aphasia and that other varieties clinicians may describe are due to additional lesions in other parts of the brain. Finally, Marie believed that intellect is affected in aphasia. Because of his clearly argued position and the clinical evidence he often marshaled, Marie was the most influential early proponent of the holistic approach to aphasia (Basso, 2003; Benton & Anderson, 1998).

Henry Head (1861–1940), an English neurologist whose books are classics, gave further support to Marie's claim. Dubbing associationists as "diagram makers," Head rejected the associationist idea of aphasia. Head proposed, just as Marie had, that some level of intellectual impairment is a part of aphasia. He believed that aphasia is a disturbance in symbolic formulation and expression. According to Head (1926), aphasia affects both verbal and non-verbal symbolic behavior.

Kurt Goldstein (1878–1965), a German neuropsychologist of the gestalt school, also opposed the idea of strict anatomic localization of brain functions. He insisted that abstract thinking ability is impaired in aphasia (Basso, 2003; Benton & Anderson, 1998; Goodglass, 1988). Goldstein's work on language and brain was originally published in German in 1924 and in English in 1948 (Goldstein, 1948). Goldstein and other gestalt psychologists advocated that each higher mental function is organized into a unitary whole, called *gestalt,* whose total meaning cannot be derived from its part. Applied to the study of aphasia, this approach implied that language functions were organized in the brain as a unitary activity and that lesions in one anatomic region affected functions in all other regions. Paradoxically, Goldstein also believed that disturbances in specific aspects of language may be associated with specific lesion sites (Basso, 2003).

The Emergence of Cognitivism

The cognitive school emerged when clinicians began to demonstrate that aphasic patients do have intellectual or cognitive impairments. **Cognition** is the complex of intellectual functions, including knowledge, memory, and the presumed modes of information processing in the brain.

The French clinician Armand Trousseau (1801–1867) argued against a purely linguistic-associationist view of aphasia, which asserted that problems found in aphasia are limited to impaired language function. According to the linguistic-associationist theory, there is a loss in aphasia of association between words and experiences the words help express. Contrary to this view, Trousseau claimed that intelligence (cognition) is *always* impaired in aphasia. In his view, aphasia was not limited to impaired language functions.

The founder of the cognitive school is thought to be the holistic approach advocate John Hughlings Jackson (Benton & Anderson, 1998). As noted earlier, Jackson held that speech has an automatic (emotional) component and a propositional component (meaningful, voluntary speech and speech produced when demanded).

Meaningful, purposive speech and speech considered appropriate to given situations and produced when demanded (stimulated) is called **propositional speech.** Most aphasic patients may have difficulty answering specific questions with appropriate words (purposive, propositional speech) but may say the same words without any difficulty when they are not asked to say them. According to Jackson, aphasia is the loss of ability to use propositional speech. Because speech is a part of thought, aphasic patients with disturbed speech (language) are also disturbed in thought processes.

Benton and Anderson (1998) report that the two other neurologists who contributed heavily to the cognitive school of thought include the previously mentioned French neurologist Pierre Marie and the English neurologist Henry Head.

The modern period saw additional contributions to the cognitive view of aphasia. Currently, many disciplines, including neuropsychology, cognitive psychology, and linguistics, contribute to the cognitive approach.

The Modern Period

Modern interest in the study and treatment of aphasia intensified after World War II. The Russian neuropsychologist Aleksandr Luria (1902–1977) was an important post-war investigator of aphasia. In his extensive study of patients with aphasia who suffered war injuries, Luria avoided the extremes of the strict localizationist or strict holistic approaches (Luria, 1963, 1970). He emphasized the more moderate view that each brain structure may be primarily responsible for a function and yet the brain works as a whole in the comprehension and production of language (Benson & Ardila, 1996).

Hildred Schuell, an early and influential speech-language pathologist believed that aphasia is a unitary language disorder without general cognitive involvement (Schuell, Jenkins, & Jimenez-Pabon, 1964). Schuell even questioned the distinction between expressive and receptive aphasia (Schuell, Jenkins, & Carroll, 1962). She also developed an early diagnostic test, the Minnesota Test for Differential Diagnosis of Aphasia (Schuell, 1955). Other pioneering speech-language pathologists specializing in aphasia, including Joseph Wepman (1951), Jon Eisenson (1954), Martha Taylor Sarno (1969), and Frederick Darley (1982), also took a more holistic view of aphasia.

American neurologist Norman Geshwind (1926–1984) is credited with the 1960s resurgence of interest in the anatomic localization of aphasic symptoms (Basso, 2003; Benson & Ardila, 1996). Challenging the then popular holistic view, Geshwind supported the early localizationist view of aphasia with new clinical and anatomic evidence.

He claimed that aphasia could result either from a localized lesion in the language areas or from lesions in the fibers that connect different language areas. He considered aphasia a cortical disconnection syndrome (Geshwind, 1965).

Clinical assessment of aphasia advanced in the modern period. Psychologists Weisenburg and McBride (1964) developed one of the earliest quantitative assessment procedures. Their assessment included both verbal and nonverbal communication skills. Weisenburg and McBride were among the first to publish comparative assessment data obtained on aphasic patients, nonaphasic patients, and normal controls.

Linguists Enter the Scene

Because aphasia is a language disturbance, linguists soon entered the scene and created a new term for their activity, *neurolinguistics.* Roman Jakobson's 1956 work on the phonological aspects of aphasia generated a new trend of neurolinguistic research that has been popular in recent years. As linguistic research of aphasia flourished, new clinical descriptions and theoretical models emerged. Some of the language disturbances of aphasic patients came to be described as *agrammatism, paragrammatism,* and *word retrieval problems.* Even terms like *syntactic aphasia* were introduced to the literature.

Darley (1982), who was not impressed with the neurolinguistic approach to aphasia, nonetheless has superbly summarized most of the neurolinguistic research that has tried to find out if patients with aphasia respond differently to linguistic units that are *shorter* or *longer, subjects* or *objects, present* or *past, simple* or *complex, direct* or *indirect, active* or *passive, abstract* or *concrete, salient* or *nonsalient, redundant* or *nonredundant, singular* or *plural, embedded* or *unembedded, marked* or *unmarked, stressed* or *unstressed, affirmative* or *negative, interrogative* or *declarative, expository* or *narrative,* and so on.

The Contribution of Speech-Language Pathologists

Language therapy for patients with aphasia was initiated mostly because of World War II. A great number of individuals who suffered brain injuries and, as a consequence, aphasia needed communication rehabilitation. As speech-language pathologists began to make important contributions in the post World War II years, the study and treatment of aphasia became well established in the 1950s and 1960s and gained momentum in subsequent years. Currently, many speech-language pathologists are among the renowned aphasiologists in the world. They are intensely involved in clinical research on aphasia.

In the subsequent chapters, we study in greater detail information on the assessment and treatment of communication disorders found in patients with aphasia. This information is largely the contribution of experts in speech-language pathology.

The Question of Handedness

In 1936, the California neurologist Joannes Nielsen (1890–1969) revived the hypothesis of the 1860s that handedness and cerebral dominance for language were symmetrical: Language was in the hemisphere that was on the opposite side of the preferred hand.

Subsequent research has shown that handedness is not a reliable indicator of hemispheric language dominance (Benson & Ardila, 1966; Calvin & Ojemann, 1980; Davis, 2000). Left hemisphere lesions in many left-handed persons produce aphasia.

Recent research, as summarized in various sources (Calvin & Ojemann, 1980; Davis, 2000), suggests that:

- About 85 percent of the general population are right-handed. Most, but not all, right-handed persons have language in their left hemisphere.

- About 15 percent of the population are left-handed. A majority of the left-handed individuals (up to 70 percent) have language in their left hemisphere; therefore, most left-handed patients with aphasia will have lesions in their left hemisphere. About 15 percent of the remaining 30 percent have bilateral representation of language. Only 15 percent of the left-handed persons have language in their right hemisphere; thus only a very small percentage of the general population has language in the right hemisphere.

- When the hemispheric dominance for language is analyzed without regard to handedness, about 95 percent of the general population have left dominance for language. Therefore, most patients with aphasia will have left dominance for language and, hence, will have a left hemispheric lesion. Fewer than 4 percent of right-handed persons with aphasia have a lesion in the right hemisphere.

- The right hemisphere shares the language function with the left in individuals who have bilateral representation, which is a small number of people.

- Clinical data suggest that the right hemisphere mediates some aspects of language. For example, patients with right hemisphere lesions may exhibit difficulty in using certain kinds of words, especially collective nouns (*fruit* instead of *apple* or *banana*); difficulty in comprehending narratives and conversation; and difficulty in formulating appropriately connected speech.

Chapters 10 and 11 offer more information on right hemisphere syndrome and its assessment and treatment.

The Debate Goes On

Whether aphasia is one disorder or a collection of different disorders depending on the site of lesion continues to be debated. Although recognizing some of the difficulties of the strict localization viewpoint, most aphasiologists now view aphasia as a syndrome whose specific and complex manifestations depend on the site of lesion. Even then, the clinical literature is replete with case studies that contradict the localizationist view. Although, by and large, lesions in certain areas tend to cause certain patterns of communication deficits, there is hardly a one-to-one relationship between the site of lesion and a specific pattern of language deficits. A lesion in a particular area may not produce the expected results, and a symptom complex that predicts a site of lesion may not be associated with that predicted site of lesion. For example, Broca's aphasia may not always mean a lesion in the Broca's area; the lesion may be elsewhere. A lesion in Broca's area may or may not produce Broca's aphasia.

The current debate on aphasia classification is not as intense as it once was, and for good reasons. Most clinicians and researchers subscribe to a moderate localizationist view and loathe tendencies to invent brain centers for specific functions with little or no evidence. Such clinicians readily admit diversity in both the symptom complex and the underlying sites of lesion. Perhaps the localizationist view is grossly correct but lacks precision. Although contradicted by many exceptions, the view may be true in just enough cases that it is acceptable to many clinicians. Nonetheless, whether the generally accepted classification system based on the site of cerebral lesion or lesions is more convenient than scientifically valid is still an unresolved question. We will find out more about the classification systems and arguments for and against them in Chapter 4.

Suggested Readings

Read the following for an excellent historical account of the study of aphasia:

Basso, A. (2003). *Aphasia and its therapy.* New York: Oxford University Press.

Benton, A., & Anderson, S. W. (1998). Aphasia: Historical perspectives. In M. T. Sarno (Ed.), *Acquired aphasia* (3rd ed., pp. 1–24). New York: Academic Press.

Cole, M. F., & Cole, M. (1971). *Pierre Marie's papers on speech disorders.* New York: Hafner Press.

Eggert, G. H. (1977). *Wernicke's work on aphasia.* The Hague: Mouton.

Geshwind, N. (1967). Wernicke's contributions to the study of aphasia. *Cortex, 3,* 449–463.

Goldstein, K. (1948). *Language and language disturbances.* New York: Grune & Stratton.

Goodglass, H. (1988). Historical perspectives on concepts of aphasia. In F. Boller & J. Grafman (Eds.), *Handbook of neuropsychology* (Vol. 1, pp. 51–63). Amsterdam: Elsevier.

Head, H. (1926). *Aphasia and kindred disorders.* London: Cambridge University Press.

Jackson, J. H. (1874). On affections of speech from diseases of the brain. *Brain, 1,* 304–330.

Luria, A. R. (1970). *Traumatic aphasia.* The Hague: Mouton.

Schuell, H. M., Jenkins, J. J., & Jimenez-Pabon, E. (1964). *Aphasia in adults: Diagnosis, prognosis and treatment.* New York: Hoeber Medical Division, Harper & Row Publishers.

Weisenburg, T. S., & McBride, K. L. (1964). *Aphasia.* New York: Hafner.

Wepman, J. M. (1951). *Recovery from aphasia.* New York: Ronald Press.

NEUROANATOMIC AND NEUROPHYSIOLOGIC CONSIDERATIONS

Chapter Outline

- Terminological Orientation
- Anatomic Orientation
- Overview
- Neurohistology
- Neural Transmission
- The Divisions of the Nervous System
- The Protective Layers of the Brain
- Cerebral Blood Supply
- Blood Supply and the Watershed Area of the Brain
- The Veins and Venous Sinus System
- The Blood-Brain Barrier

Learning Objectives

After reading this chapter, the student will:

- Define the terms of anatomic orientation.
- Distinguish *neuroanatomy, neurophysiology,* and *neurohistology.*
- Describe the central and the peripheral nervous system.
- Describe and distinguish the various types of neural cells.
- Distinguish cranial and spinal nerves, both structurally and functionally.
- Describe the surface structure of the cerebral cortex.

- Describe the cerebral locations of language, motor, and auditory areas.
- Describe the relevant subcortical structures of the brain.
- Describe the arteries that supply the particular regions of the brain.
- Distinguish the different protective layers of the brain.

Terminological Orientation

Aphasia is a language disorder based on recent brain trauma or pathology. **Neurology,** which is the study of neurological diseases and disorders and their diagnosis and treatment, is the medical discipline concerned with aphasia. Therefore, to appreciate the physical basis of aphasia and other neurogenic language disorders, a basic understanding of the branches of neurology is essential. Four main branches of neurology are important for a student of aphasia: neuroanatomy, neurophysiology, neuropathology, and neurodiagnostics.

As a branch of neurology, **neuroanatomy** is the study of structures of the nervous system. **Neurophysiology,** also a branch of neurology, is the study of the function of the nervous system. In this chapter, neuroanatomic and neurophysiologic aspects of aphasia are briefly reviewed. Chapter 3 reviews neuropathology associated with aphasia and neurodiagnostic methods used in assessing those pathologies.

The information presented in this chapter is meant only as a review for students who have had detailed coursework in neurology of speech, language, and hearing. Students are urged to review other sources, including books on anatomy and physiology of speech and hearing, neuroanatomy, neuroscience, and neurology (Bear, Connors, & Paradiso, 2001; Bhatnagar, 2002; Castro, Merchut, Neafsey, & Wurster, 2002; Haines, 2004; Haines & Lancon, 2003; Kierman, 2005; Love & Web, 2001; Nolte, 2002; Seikel, King, & Drumright, 2005; Webster, 1999; Zemlin, 1998).

Anatomic Orientation

Study of anatomic structures begins with an understanding of terms used to refer to anatomic positions, planes, directions, and viewpoints. Such an understanding is essential to grasp the relationship between anatomic structures and their absolute and relative spatial positions within the body. The brain has to be cut (sectioned) to view its deeper layers or structures. The brain may be sectioned from different angles, giving rise to different terms. See Figure 2-1 for a graphic orientation to anatomic planes. Remembering the following brief descriptions and the definitions of technical terms will facilitate an understanding of neuroanatomy:

- The human brain has evolved along two axes: a *vertical axis* on which the spinal cord has evolved and the *horizontal axis* on which the brain has evolved. A **horizontal**

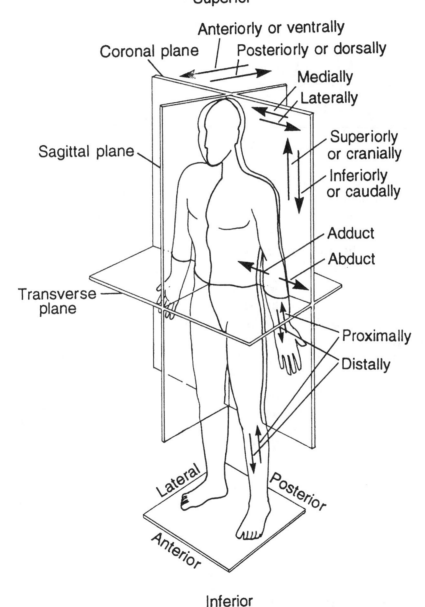

Figure 2-1. Anatomic planes and orientations.

From *Anatomy and physiology for speech, language, and hearing* (3rd ed., p. 9, Figure 2.1), by J. A. Seikel, D. W. King, & D. G. Drumright, 2005. Albany, NY: Thomson Delmar Learning. Reprinted with permission.

plane of the brain sections it into two halves: an upper half and a lower half.

- **Coronal plane** requires a vertical cut, resulting in an equal frontal and a back portion.

- **Median** or **midsagittal plane** requires a longitudinal (vertical) section that divides the brain into a right half and a left half. A **sagittal plane** also sections the brain with a longitudinal cut into unequal left and right portions.

- **Lateral plane** refers to structures away from the median plane. A side view of the brain is its *lateral* view.

- **Anterior (rostral)** brain is the portion of the brain in the frontal part of the head.

- **Superior** brain refers to the top portion of the brain.

- **Posterior** brain refers to the back portion of the brain.

- **Dorsal** brain also refers to the back portion, but specifically to the portion that lies between the superior and posterior portions. Therefore, in some sources, dorsal is defined as the top of the brain. Referring to the whole body, dorsal means the back side.

- **Ventral** brain refers to the lower portion of the brain. The ventral portion of the brain also may be called *inferior*. Both *ventral* and *inferior* contrast with *superior*. Referring to the whole body, ventral means the frontal or belly side.

- **Caudal** portion typically refers to the lower or tail section of the spinal cord; it may also refer to the back part of the brain.

- **Proximal** structures are those that are relatively close to a reference structure.

- **Distal** structures are those that are farther from a reference structure.

Overview

Much neurophysiological research and writing related to aphasia deals with specific regions of the brain that may control particular language functions. From Chapter 1, we already know that the left hemisphere in most individuals is dominant for language. We also know that two specific areas—

Broca's for language production and Wernicke's for language comprehension—are important in the study of aphasia.

To understand the brain structures involved in language formulation, production, and comprehension, we should start with the basic building blocks of the nervous system. We will then consider the divisions of the nervous system and concentrate more on structures that are important for speech and language. We will take note of the functions of the structures being discussed. Gaining a basic understanding of the nervous system with an emphasis on the central nervous system will be our main concern.

Neurohistology

Neurohistology is the study of the basic structures of neural cells, tissue, and organs in relation to their function. Neurohistology is an extensive discipline. What follows is a brief review of the basic neural cell structure in relation to neural function. We will review the structure and function of neurons and glial cells and describe neural transmission.

Neurons

Neurons, also known as nerve cells, are the basic building blocks of the nervous system. A neuron is a functional unit of the nervous system in that it receives information from other neurons through its dendrites, processes that information in its cell body, and transmits the information through its axon to other neurons.

The size and shape of neurons vary a great deal. Figure 2-2 shows a typical neuron and some variations. Neurons have three parts: soma (cell body), dendrites, and axon. Collectively, dendrites and axons are called *neurites.*

The *cell body* (soma; *somata,* plural) contains the nucleus and cytoplasm. Cytoplasm includes everything the soma contains except for the nucleus. The term *protoplasm* includes both the nucleus and cytoplasm. The chromosomes, which contain the genetic material called *deoxyribonucleic acid* (*DNA*) are contained within the nucleus.

The cytoplasm is enclosed with *neuronal membrane.* The membrane is important in understanding the cell function because it regulates the flow of chemicals (and chemically transmitted information) to and from the cell.

Dendrites and axons are two kinds of nerve fibers. **Dendrites** (*tree* in Greek) are short, unmyelinated fibers that extend from the cell body. Each neuron may contain several dendrites. Neurons that project

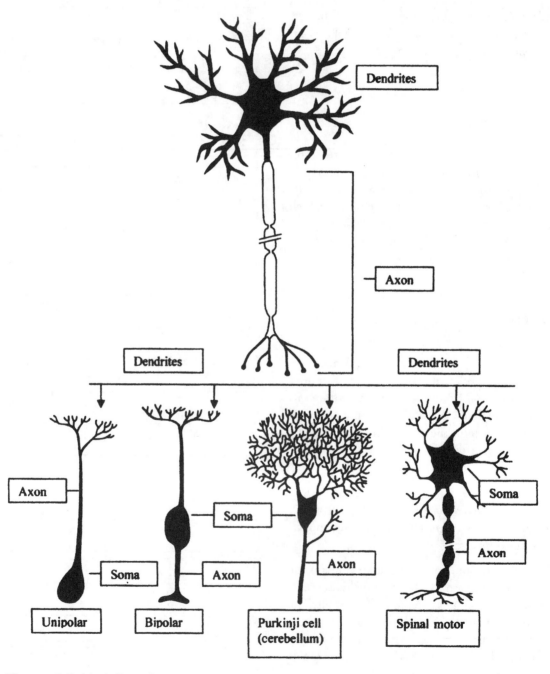

Figure 2-2. *Varieties of neurons.*

out to several dendrites are called *multipolar.* When only one dendrite extends from the cell body, the cell is called *unipolar*; when two dendrites extend from it, the cell is *bipolar.*

Dendrites receive information from axons of other cells. Hence, they are classified as *afferent* (receptive). Dendrites transmit information thus received to the cell body.

While cells may have multiple dendrites, they only have a single axon (*axle* in Greek). An **axon** is the nerve fiber that is longer than dendrites and originates from the soma in its cone-shaped region called the *axon hillock.* Looking like a string of sausages, the tubular axon is thinner at its origin and becomes thicker as it becomes longer. Axons are not structurally intact; there are structural gaps in the axon (Nolte, 2002).

Axons may be myelinated or unmyelinated, although the thicker, longer axons are *myelinated,* or wrapped in a thin layer of white, protective, and fatty material called **myelin.** An axon finally branches into many small filaments called **telodendria.** The terminal points of an axon are capped with small structures called **terminal buttons.** The terminal buttons are the functional contact points between neurons.

Functionally, axons are efferent in that they transmit messages to other neurons, away from the cell body. They transmit messages either to another neuron or to muscles.

To communicate with each other, an axon of one neuron makes contact with another neuron in multiple methods. An axon may make a contact (synapse) with (a) a dendrite of another neuron (*axodendritic synapse*), (b) the soma of another neuron (*axosomatic synapse*), (c) another axon of a neuron (*axoaxonic synapse*), or (d) an effector cell such as a skeletal muscle. The point at which two neurons come in contact with each other is called a **synapse,** a neural junction. The several smaller branches of an axon at its end form synaptic terminals that come in contact with a dendrite, the soma, or axon of another neuron or motor muscle. The contact, however, is not physically continuous as the neural junction has a small space, or a gap, called the **synaptic cleft.** The synaptic cleft is a structural gap, not a chemical gap. The cleft is filled with a specialized form of protein.

Once injured or destroyed by disease processes, axons of the central nervous system do not regenerate to the extent that the function is recovered. This is why in cases of severe brain injury or tissue loss due to disease, the cognitive functions may not be recovered fully. Incapable of rejuvenation, dead neural cells only leave a clump of debris.

Glial Cells

The **glial cells** (also known as *glia,* meaning glue) are the nonneural cells of the nervous system. Also called *neuroglia,* these nonneural cells provide a structural framework for the neural cells. Outnumbering neural cells by at least 5:1 and occupying half the volume of the brain, glial cells are essential for normal functioning of the nervous system.

Glial cells in the central nervous system (CNS) are classified into three types: *astrocytes, oligodendrocytes,* and *microglia.* Important glial cells of the peripheral nervous system (PNS) include the *satellite cells* that myelinate peripheral axons and the *Schwann cells* that surround certain neuronal cell bodies.

Glial cells do not receive or send messages. In addition to providing a structural framework, glial cells help maintain neural metabolic activity. They also regulate concentrations of neurotransmitters (described in the next section). See Figure 2-3 for a representation of the three types of glia.

An astrocyte

Blood vessel

An oligodendrocyte

Nerve cell

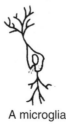

A microglia

Figure 2-3. Common types of glia cells that surround nerve cells in the brain.

Astrocytes—the glial cells of the CNS—are small cells with varied branches that occupy the space between neurons. The branches of astrocytes end in structures called *end-feet.* The most common of the glial cells, astrocytes are found in all parts of the CNS, including the gray and white matters of the brain. Functioning like connective tissue, some astrocytes extend to the brain surface to provide structural support to neural cells. The various end-feet of astrocytes cover cerebral blood vessels and separate them from neural tissue.

Functionally, astrocytes are involved in neuro-transmitter metabolism. They also help create the *blood-brain barrier* by forming tight endothelial vessel junctions with their end-feet. This barrier, though helpful in keeping harmful chemicals from reaching the neural tissue, also can prevent life-saving medicine from reaching that tissue.

Astrocytes are the most common site of malig-nant tumors within the brain. This is because the astrocytes, unlike the neural cells, can proliferate even in the mature brain. The two most common types of tumors are called *astrocytomas* and *glioblas-tomas* (see Chapter 3 for details). Any injury to the brain (e.g., strokes) resulting in cell loss will trigger proliferation of astrocytes that then migrate and fill the space of lost cells. This results in *astrocytic scar,* which impedes transmission of messages.

Oligodendrocytes, another form of glial cells, are found in both the gray and white matters of the CNS. Smaller than astrocytes, oligodendrocytes are dark staining round nuclei that provide myelination of some axons in the CNS. **Myelination** is an elec-trochemical insulation around some axons in the white matter; the gray matter is unmyelinated. The *myelin sheath* that provides this insulation is a white, fatty wrapping material. The peripheral nerves also are wrapped in myelin sheath, but this sheath is pro-vided by **Schwann cells.**

The myelin sheath helps increase the speed of con-duction of neural impulses across the axon. The speed is increased because the action potential (neu-ral impulse) jumps from one axonal node to the other. Demyelinating diseases degrade or destroy oligodendrocytes and the myelin sheath, resulting in slow or disrupted conduction of neural messages, causing motor, visual, sensory, or cognitive dysfunc-tions. A prominent demyelinating disease is multiple sclerosis. It is thought that the body's immune system attacks the myelination of nerve fibers. Consequently, the brain functions are disrupted.

Microglia

A third type of glial cells, **microglia,** are elongated and dark staining, with long and branched cytoplasmic processes (thin projections). Constituting only 10 percent of the glial cells, microglia are considered quiescent (at rest) during health and become active upon brain injury. Subsequent to brain injury, microglia transform themselves into *phagocytes,* which are scavenger cells that ingest dead cells, bacteria, and foreign bodies. Phagocytic microglia migrate to the cite of lesion or brain injury to digest cell debris.

The human immunodeficiency virus is known to invade the CNS microglia, causing neuronal damage. Especially when activated, microglia secrete a variety of chemical substances, some of which may be cytotoxic (harmful to cells) and may lead to cerebral inflammation and opening of the blood-brain barrier.

Neural Transmission

Such communicative disorders as aphasia and dementia are associated with impaired transmission of messages within the neural network. Normal transmission of messages within the neural network is essential for both normal communication and cognitive functions. Various neuropathologies disrupt the efficient and speedy neural transmission of messages, giving rise to various communication and general behavioral deficits. Therefore, speech-language pathologists need to have a basic understanding of neural transmission and neurotransmitters that make this possible.

Neurotransmitters

The human nervous system, for the most part, is not a physically and completely connected network of fibers. Instead, it is a collection of individual neurons (Nolte, 2002). There are structural gaps within this network. As noted earlier, individual axons have structural gaps, as do the connecting points between neurons (the synaptic cleft). Therefore, neural transmission of information is not strictly like the physical flow of messages in an intact telephone network. It is more an electrochemical reaction than a pure physical transmission over uninterrupted lines of fibers.

Axons conduct electrical impulses (messages) across their length. The message, however, need to be transferred to the next neuron. As we know, the connecting points between neurons have a gap (the synaptic cleft). The message, therefore, cannot be directly transmitted through electrical means of conductance. The message is transmitted as a chemical reaction at the synaptic level. Neural transmission across synaptic connections, more precisely the synaptic gaps, is an electrochemical process of information exchange. Chemical compounds known as **neurotransmitters** contained within the axon terminal buttons help make contact between two cells by diffusing across the synaptic space. This diffused neurotransmitter becomes bound to receptors in the postsynaptic membrane (neuron receiving the impulse). The diffused neurotransmitter may either excite or inhibit the next neuron in a chain.

The several varieties of neurotransmitter chemical compounds are classified into three main types: (a) amino acids, (b) amines, and (c) peptides. Amino acids and amines are sometimes grouped because their molecules are small. Peptides are a class unto themselves because their molecules are large. Generally, while smaller molecules produce effects that are short-lived, the larger ones produce longer-lasting effects.

Amino acids include gamma-aminobutyric acid (GABA), glutamate (Glu), and glycine (Gly). **Amines** include acetylcholine (Ach), dopamine, epinephrine, histamine, norepinephrine, and serotonin. There are several varieties of **peptides,** including cholecystokinin (CCK), dynorphin, neuropeptide y, and somatostatin. Each neuron specializes in releasing a certain kind of neurotransmitter. For instance, most *CNS synapses* release amino acids (glutamate, GABA, and glycine) to accomplish fast transmission of messages. At *neuromuscular junctions* and throughout the peripheral nervous system, acetylcholine (Ach) mediates fast message transmission; its action in the CNS is somewhat slower. Ach primarily mediates voluntary movement. All varieties of neurotransmitters are involved in slower forms of message transmission.

Various neurological diseases and trauma affect neurotransmission, giving rise to many neurological and psychiatric disorders. Neurotransmitters are involved in both motor and cognitive deficits associated with many such disorders. For instance, dopamine deficiency due to the death of dopamine-producing cells in the brainstem are related to tremor and poor control of movements in Parkinson's disease, described in Chapter 15.

There is evidence that Alzheimer's disease, described in Chapter 14, may be associated with deficiencies in acetylcholine in the hippocampus and frontal cortex. In Parkinson's disease, dopamine deficiency in the basal ganglia (especially in substantia negra) is linked to tremor and other movement disorders along with dysarthria. On the other hand, excessive production of dopamine in the forebrain may be involved in schizophrenia.

GABA, an amino acid and a derivative of glutamate, is the main neurotransmitter in the brain. While glutamate is excitatory, GABA is inhibitory. Death or degradation of neurons that produce GABA in basal ganglia, especially in the caudate and putamen, causes involuntary movements of Huntington's chorea, described in Chapter 15.

Afferent and Efferent Nerves

Bundles of axons, dendrites, or both, often specializing in certain functions, are called **nerves.** Two major kinds of nerves of interest to us are motor nerves and sensory nerves.

Motor nerves, or **motor neurons,** are those that cause muscle contractions (movement) or glandular secretions. Because the motor nerves transmit impulses away from the central nervous system, they also are called **efferent nerves.** Efferent nerves terminate at an effector, which leads to glandular secretion or muscle movement. Motor or efferent neurons have their origins in the brain and terminate in a gland or muscle. In essence, it is through the efferent neurons that the brain issues commands to the glands or muscles.

Sensory nerves are those that carry sensory impulses from the peripheral sense organs toward the brain. Because they carry information toward the center, sensory nerves also are known as **afferent nerves.** Afferent nerves help the brain gather information about the body's internal (visceral) environment as well as its external, physical environment. Sensory organs (e.g., eyes and ears) send the information they gather to the brain through afferent nerves. Information thus brought to the brain may generate efferent impulses that lead to some action dictated by the received sensory information.

The Divisions of the Nervous System

Anatomically, the nervous system is divided into the central nervous system and the peripheral nervous system. The **central nervous system** includes the brain and the spinal cord, both encased in bone. The brain is encased within the cranial structure (skull) and the spinal cord is encased within the bony vertebral column (spinal column). For a study of aphasia and other language disorders associated with cerebral disease or trauma, the central nervous system is more important than the peripheral system. See Figure 2-4 for the division of the nervous system.

The **peripheral nervous system** includes all of the nervous system except for the brain and the spinal cord. It is a *peripheral* system because it connects the brain and the spinal cord with the structures that are away from the brain. This system includes the cranial and spinal nerves and the visceral (autonomic) system.

The Peripheral Nervous System (PNS)

As noted, the nervous system located outside the skull and the vertebral column is called the peripheral nervous system (PNS). Cranial nerves, spinal nerves, and parts of the autonomic system are included in the peripheral nervous system.

Cranial nerves are those that emerge from the brainstem; they are attached to the base of the brain (see the section on the brainstem for a

A

B

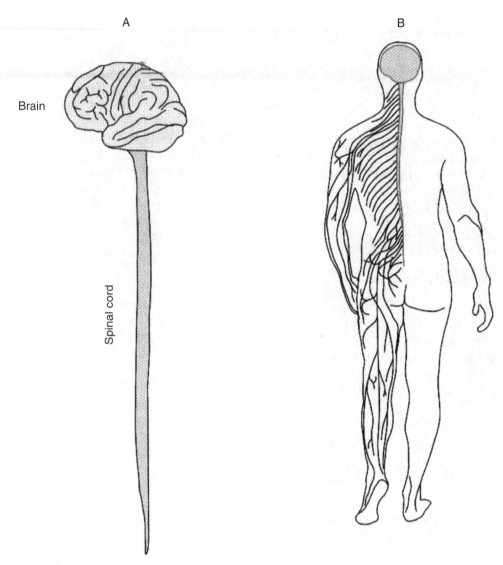

Brain

Spinal cord

Figure 2-4. The two main divisions of the nervous system: A. The central nervous system. B. The peripheral nervous system, which includes the cranial and spinal nerves.

graphic representation of the brainstem and the cranial nerves that emerge from it). Cranial nerves innervate (supply and stimulate) the larynx, tongue, pharynx, and muscles of the face, neck, and head. Because of their innervation, cranial nerves are important for phonation, voice, and speech. There are 12 pairs of cranial nerves:

  I. Olfactory: Sense of smell (sensory)
 II. Optic: Vision (motor)
III. Oculomotor: Eye movement (motor)
 IV. Trochlear: Eye movement (motor)

V. Trigeminal: Face (sensory); jaw (motor)

VI. Abducens: Eye movement (motor)

VII. Facial: Tongue (sensory); face (motor)

VIII. Vestibular acoustic: Hearing and balance (sensory)

IX. Glossopharyngeal: Tongue and pharynx (sensory); pharynx only (motor)

X. Vagus: Larynx, respiratory, cardiac, and gastrointestinal systems (sensory and motor)

XI. Accessory: Shoulder, arm, and throat movements (motor)

XII. Hypoglossal: Mostly tongue movements (motor)

Some cranial nerves carry sensory or motor messages while others carry both. Those that carry both sensory and motor messages are called *mixed nerves*. Cranial nerves are not important in understanding language comprehension, formulation, and expression. Because they innervate speech mechanisms, cranial nerves are important in understanding speech production, hence effective communication. Cranial nerve damage is associated with dysarthria, a motor speech disorder. Some patients who have aphasia and those with traumatic brain injury may have associated speech production problems.

Spinal nerves are those that arise from the spinal cord. There are 31 pairs of spinal nerves. There are 8 pairs of cervical nerves, 12 pairs of thoracic nerves, 5 pairs of lumbar nerves, 5 pairs of sacral nerves, and a single pair of coccygeal nerves. The nerves are named after the specific portions of the spinal cord to which they are attached (cervical, thoracic, lumbar, sacral, and coccygeal). Being mixed in function, spinal nerves carry sensory information to the CNS and motor information to the muscles.

Spinal nerves are not important in language comprehension, formulation, and expression. Those nerves are important, however, in speech production because certain spinal nerves control respiration, which is essential for normal speech production. Damage to spinal nerves may impair the functioning of the muscles of breathing. Such an impairment may be associated with dysarthria.

The **autonomic nervous system** is concerned mostly with the internal environment of the body.

The system supplies the smooth muscles (e.g., blood vessels and the intestine) and glands within the body and controls such involuntary functions as the heartbeat, blood pressure, and diameter of the blood vessels. The system is further divided into a *sympathetic branch,* which mobilizes the body functions under stressful, fearful conditions, or emergency conditions to meet the demands of such conditions. The system will then heighten certain physiological responses by increasing the heart rate and blood pressure, suppressing digestive functions, and activating the glucose reserves. When the stressful, fearful, or emergency situation is over, the *parasympathetic branch* becomes active and calms the body by returning the mobilized physiological processes to normal levels.

We will not be concerned with the details of PNS in this chapter as it is not directly involved in language disorders associated with cerebral pathology or trauma. As noted earlier, the student should understand this system (especially the cranial nerves) for a full understanding of speech production and motor speech disorders.

The Central Nervous System (CNS)

The discoveries of Broca and Wernicke, as described in Chapter 1, made it clear that the brain is the most important organ for language comprehension, formulation, and expression. Other clinical evidence, including the knowledge generated by brain mapping in patients with epilepsy, firmly established the connection between the brain and verbal behavior and that between brain pathology and communication disorders.

The CNS includes the brain and the spinal cord. Structures within the CNS that are especially relevant to a study of neurogenic language disorders include the following:

- Spinal cord
- Brainstem
- Cerebellum
- Cerebrum

See Figure 2-5 for a gross representation of the major parts of the CNS.

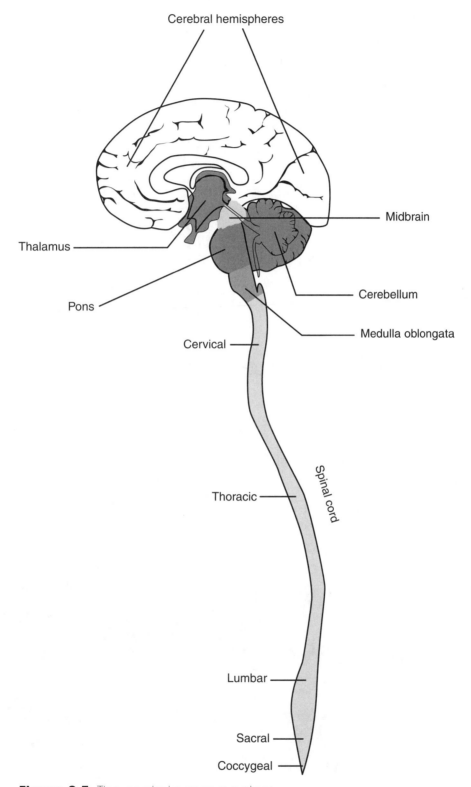

Figure 2-5. The central nervous system.

The Spinal Cord

The spinal cord is a part of the CNS, although spinal nerves are a part of the PNS. The **spinal cord,** a bundle of nerve fibers within the vertebral column, is a cylindrical and caudal (lower) continuation of the medulla oblongata, which is the lowest structure of the brainstem. See Figure 2-6 for a

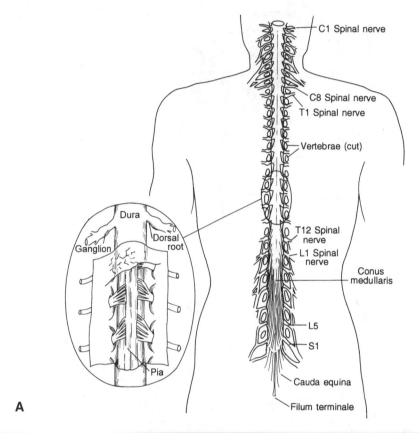

A

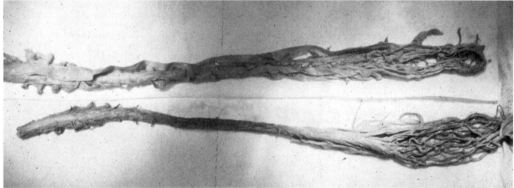

B

Figure 2-6. The spinal cord.

From Anatomy and physiology for speech, language, and hearing (3rd ed., p. 517, Figure 12.8), by J. A. Seikel, D. W. King, & D. G. Drumright, 2005. Albany, NY: Thomson Delmar Learning. Reprinted with permission.

drawing of the spinal cord and photographs of excised spinal cords.

As noted earlier, the nerve fibers of the spinal cord (spinal nerves) carry motor impulses to various organs, including muscles and glands. Spinal nerves carry such sensory impulses as pain, touch, temperature, and pressure from peripheral organs to the brain. The spinal cord is also responsible for all reflexive activity. Therefore, the spinal cord is the main structure with which the brain keeps in touch with the rest of the body.

The Brainstem

The upper end of the spinal cord is continuous with the lower end of the brainstem. The **brainstem,** illustrated in Figure 2-7, includes the medulla, pons,

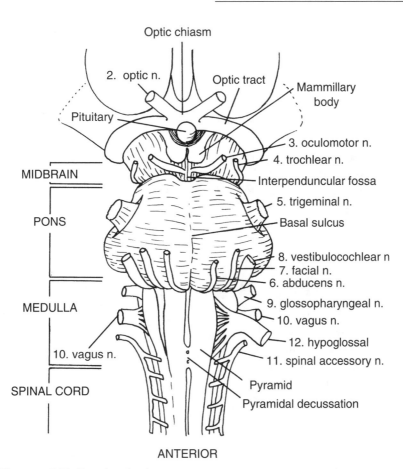

Figure 2-7. The brainstem.

From *Anatomy and physiology for speech, language, and hearing* (3rd ed., p. 554, Figure 12.26), by J. A. Seikel, D. W. King, & D. G. Drumright, 2005. Albany, NY: Thomson Delmar Learning. Reprinted with permission.

and midbrain. The medulla is the lowest (caudal) part of the brainstem and the midbrain is the highest; the pons is in the middle. Note that Figure 2-7 shows the cranial nerves that are attached to the brainstem.

The **medulla,** or medulla oblongata, also called *myelencephalon,* is the upward extension of the spinal cord as it passes through the foramen magnum at the base of the skull. Descriptively, the spinal cord ends at the beginning of the medulla. The medulla contains all the fibers that originate in the brain and cerebellum and move down to form the spinal cord. The medulla includes several centers that control such autonomic functions as digestion, breathing (affecting speech), blood pressure, and heart rate.

The **pons,** a part of *metencephalon* (which includes the cerebellum, not a part of the brainstem), is a bridge to the hemispheres of the cerebellum (not cerebrum). The pons is concerned with hearing and balance; some cranial nerves (trigeminal, facial) originate here. The pons transmits information relative to movement from the cerebral hemispheres to the cerebellum.

The **midbrain,** also called *mesencephalon,* lies above the pons. Cranial nerves III and IV originate in the midbrain. The midbrain controls many sensory and motor functions, including eye movements, postural reflexes, and coordination of visual and auditory reflexes. Structures at the midbrain-diencephalon junction provide transition from midbrain to thalamus.

Cerebellum

The **cerebellum** is the major portion of the hindbrain. The cerebellum covers most of the posterior (back) side of the brainstem. It is located at the base of the brain (dorsal to the pons and medulla). The cerebellum may be aptly named the "little brain," because it contains as many neurons as the rest of the CNS. Like the cerebrum, the cerebellum has two hemispheres called *cerebellar hemispheres* (not to be confused with *cerebral hemispheres*). See Figure 2-8 for an inferior and a lateral view of the cerebellum.

Each cerebellar hemisphere also has *lobes* like the cerebrum. Anterior, posterior, and flocculonodular lobes are found in each hemisphere. The cerebellum

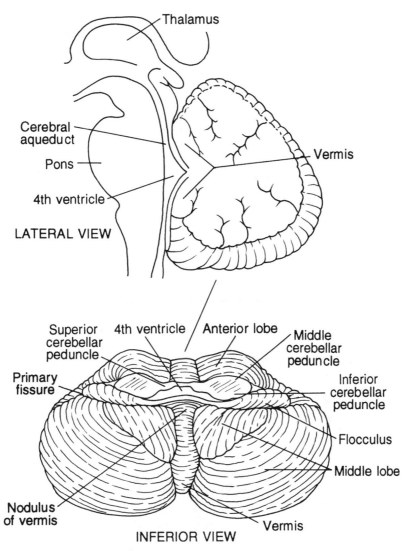

Figure 2-8. The cerebellum.

From *Anatomy and physiology for speech, language, and hearing* (3rd ed., p. 548, Figure 12.23), by J. A. Seikel, D. W. King, & D. G. Drumright, 2005. Albany, NY: Thomson Delmar Learning. Reprinted with permission.

has fissures like the cortex, and its surface is full of small ridges called *folia*. The cerebellum has gray matter on the surface and white matter on the inside. The core white matter contains important nerve fibers that connect to the cerebellar cortex.

The cerebellum is a part of the motor system. It coordinates and modulates the force and range of body movement. Although it does not initiate movement, the cerebellum coordinates actions to produce smooth and rhythmic movements, including those involved in speech. Damage to the cerebellum is associated with a type of dysarthria called *ataxic dysarthria,* characterized by dominant articulatory and prosodic problems. In addition, damage to the cerebellum results in uncoordinated movements, impaired postural control, and abnormal voluntary movements.

Diencephalon

The **diencephalon** is a structure in between the brainstem and the cerebral hemispheres. The diencephalon lies above the midbrain and below the cerebral cortex. Within it is the third ventricle, a narrow and tall space filled with the cerebrospinal fluid. Among its four major structures—the thalamus, epithalamus, subthalamus, and hypothalamus—the thalamus is especially relevant for our purposes and is shown in Figure 2-9. Note that the figure also shows structures of the basal ganglia, described in the next section.

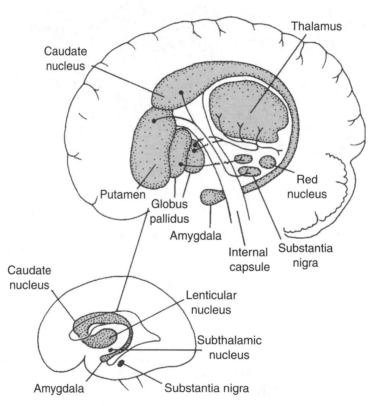

Figure 2-9. The thalamus in relation to the structures of the basal ganglia.

From *Anatomy and physiology for speech, language, and hearing* (3rd ed., p. 539, Figure 12.19), by J. A. Seikel, D. W. King, & D. G. Drumright, 2005. Albany, NY: Thomson Delmar Learning. Reprinted with permission.

The **thalamus** is the largest of the diencephalon structures. Portions of corpus callosum lie above the thalamus; the hypothalamus lies below the thalamus. The thalamus integrates sensory experiences and relays them to cortical areas. The thalamus also receives information about motor impulses from the basal ganglia and cerebellum and relays these to motor areas of the cortex. The thalamus plays a major role in maintaining consciousness and alertness.

There is increasing evidence that the thalamus plays some role in speech and language, although the details need further research. Recent research suggests the possibility of a thalamic aphasia. In addition, stimulation of left thalamic areas improved acquired stuttering (Bhatnagar, 2002). We will learn more about thalamic aphasia in Chapter 7.

Basal Ganglia

Found deep within the brain, the **basal ganglia** are structures located near the thalamus. These subcortical structures are important in understanding certain neurogenic communication disorders. Dementia associated with Parkinson's disease, for example, is related (among other neuropathological conditions) to neurochemical disorders of basal ganglia.

While a few experts include basal ganglia in their discussion of the diencephalon, most consider them separately. Still, experts differ on their description of the basal ganglia, but most include the caudate nucleus, the putamen, and the globus pallidus. In addition, substantia nigra and subthalamic nucleus—essentially brainstem structures—are considered a part of basal ganglia because of their functional relationship. The putamen and the globus pallidus are collectively known as the *lenticular nucleus,* because they are placed closed to each other. On the other hand, the caudate nucleus and the putamen are collectively called the *striatum,* because of their striped appearance. Please refer back to Figure 2-9, which shows the structures of the basal ganglia in relation to the thalamus.

The caudate nucleus (*caudate* means *tail* in Latin) lies around the lateral ventricle. It has a C-shape with a thin tail that ends in the amygdaloid nucleus, a body that forms the wall of the lateral ventricle, and a relatively massive head that is continuous with the anterior part of the putamen.

Because of its connection to the caudate nucleus, the putamen lies caudal and lateral to it. The globus pallidus lies medial to the putamen. The substantia nigra—although some do not consider it a part of basal ganglia—projects its fibers to the putamen and caudate nucleus. Finally, the subthalamic nucleus is below the thalamus as its name implies.

Basal ganglia receive input mostly from the frontal lobe and send information back to the higher centers in the brain through the thalamus. Basal ganglia play an important role in modulating movement because they produce important neurotransmitters, including dopamine, GABA, and acetylcholine. Being inhibitory in their effects, these neurotransmitters help regulate and control movements.

Damage to or diseases of the basal ganglia result in depleted neurotransmitters. As a result, the patient experiences various movement disorders. Both Parkinson's disease and Huntington's disease are associated with basal ganglia damage or pathological conditions. The motor disorders associated with impaired functioning of basal ganglia include dyskinesias (such involuntary movements as tremors), hypokinesia (restricted range of movement), and bradykinesia (slowness of movement). In addition, the patients may show unusual postures and impaired muscle tone. The patients also may exhibit a form of dysarthria, a motor speech disorder.

Eventually, some patients with Parkinson's or Huntington's disease may develop dementia and associated cognitive and communicative deficits. In addition, these patients may have such psychiatric disorders as depression (especially with Parkinson's disease) and mood disorders (especially with Huntington's disease). See Chapter 15 for a description of Parkinson's disease and Huntington's disease.

White Matter and the Connecting Fibers in the CNS

Extensive networks of fibers found deep within the white matters of the brain connect cerebral structures to each other. Also, any information coming into or going out of the brain has to pass through the subcortical white matter. Various bundles of connecting fibers keep the information flowing throughout the brain, so that information about sensory stimuli received and actions planned and performed are coordinated within various brain structures.

Some connecting fibers are short and others are long. Shorter fibers connect adjacent areas, and longer fibers connect distant areas. The longer fibers also are known as *fasciculi* (*fasciculus*, singular). The connecting fibers found in the white matter core of the brain are classified as projection fibers, commissural fibers, and association fibers.

Projection fibers are a band of fibers that transmit sensory information to the brain and motor information to the muscles and glands. These fibers form a connection between the cortical structures at the top and the brainstem and spinal cord at the lower level. The projection fibers are compact and concentrated as they pass through the internal capsule near the brainstem. As they move toward the upper regions of the brain, projection fibers fan out in a structure called the *corona radiata,* through which information is transmitted to other regions of the brain. See Figure 2-10 for an illustration of the corona radiata.

Efferent projection fibers pass through the thalamus and basal ganglia. These fibers transmit motor

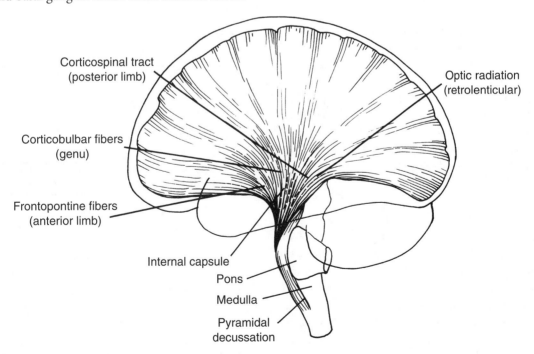

Corticospinal tract (posterior limb)

Optic radiation (retrolenticular)

Corticobulbar fibers (genu)

Frontopontine fibers (anterior limb)

Internal capsule

Pons

Medulla

Pyramidal decussation

Figure 2-10. Corona radiata.

From *Anatomy and physiology for speech, language, and hearing* (3rd ed., p. 537, Figure 12.18), by J. A. Seikel, D. W. King, & D. G. Drumright, 2005. Albany, NY: Thomson Delmar Learning. Reprinted with permission.

commands to muscles and glands. Afferent projection fibers transmit sensory information from the peripheral sense organs to the brain.

Association fibers may be short or long, but both connect areas within a hemisphere. Thus they are *intrahemispheric* in their connections. Shorter association fibers connect adjacent structures. Longer fibers connect more distant areas within the hemisphere. Longer association fibers, or fasciculi, connect more distant parts of the brain. For example, the longer *inferior longitudinal fasciculus* connects temporal and occipital lobes, and the similarly long *uncinate fasciculus* connects frontal and temporal lobes. These and other fibers help maintain communication among structures within a hemisphere.

From the standpoint of speech and language, the most important of the longer association fibers are the *superior longitudinal,* also known as the *arcuate fasciculus.* Some consider the arcuate fasciculus to be a branch of the superior longitudinal fasciculus. This bundle of fibers arches backward from the lower part of the frontal lobe to the posterior superior part of the temporal lobe. It is just below the cortical surface; hence it is superior longitudinal.

The superior longitudinal fibers (especially the arcuate fasciculus branch) connect the motor speech area (Broca's) with the sensory speech area (Wernicke's). These fibers are important for language acquisition, propositional (meaningful, purposeful) language production, and verbal memory. The rest of the superior longitudinal fasciculus connects frontal, parietal, and occipital cortexes.

The various fasciculi that connect the different parts of the brain are shown in Figure 2-11.

The **commissural fibers** connect the corresponding areas of the two hemispheres, which are divided by the median longitudinal fissure. Thus, the commissural fibers are interhemispheric connectors, whereas association fibers are intrahemispheric. The corpus callosum is the most important of the commissural fibers. Found at the base of the hemispheres and forming the roof of most of the lateral ventricles, the **corpus callosum** is a broad and thick band of 300 million to 400 million fibers that connects the two hemispheres. The corpus callosum is shown in Figure 2-12.

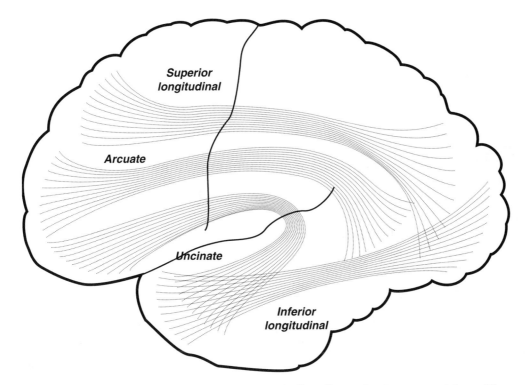

Figure 2-11. Fasciculi, the longer association fibers that connect the different parts of the same hemisphere.

From *The speech sciences* (p. 248, Figure 7.17), by R. Kent, 1998. Albany, NY: Thomson Delmar Learning. Reprinted with permission.

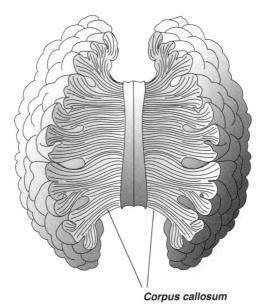

Figure 2-12. Corpus callosum that connects the two hemispheres.

From *The speech sciences* (p. 249, Figure 7.18), by R. Kent, 1998. Albany, NY: Thomson Delmar Learning. Reprinted with permission.

Damage to the corpus callosum disconnects the two hemispheres. The resulting problems in movement, reading, and naming are known as **disconnection syndromes.**

The Corpus Callosum and the Split Brain Controversy

In some severe cases of epilepsy, the corpus callosum has been cut in a surgical procedure called **commissurotomy** to prevent the spread of seizures from one hemisphere to the other. The result of this procedure is that the two hemispheres are independent of each other. Experiments on patients with such *split brains* have suggested that what the right brain knows may be unknown to the left brain. Such experiments also have suggested that the left brain is more concerned with logical, analytical, and verbal skills, whereas the right brain is more concerned with intuitive, holistic, spatial-perceptual skills. Based on some of these observations, individuals have been characterized as being left-brain or right-brain people.

More recent research has suggested that the left-brain, right-brain distinction in individuals with a normally functioning brain is overblown. The two hemispheres often work as an integrated unit, although one side may be more active than the other while certain tasks are performed.

Cerebral Cortex

The **cerebral cortex,** or **cerebrum,** is the final integrative and executive structure of the nervous system. It is responsible for all higher brain functions, including everyday thinking; logical, abstract, and mathematical reasoning; remembering (memory); speaking, including production of language; creative activities, including all artistic and scientific achievements; judgment; and emotional experience. The cerebral cortex is the outer layer of the brain. It is a thin layer (2 to 4 mm in thickness) with an area of about 2.5 square feet. In the evolutionary scale, it is a more recently evolved structure than the rest of the brain; therefore, the cerebrum is also known as the *neocortex* (*new* cortex). Some basic facts of the human brain include the following:

- The brain contains about 10 to 14 billion neurons. Two-thirds of this massive number are buried in the various fissures.
- An average human brain weighs about 3 pounds.
- Most regions of the cortex are structured in six layers; the outermost surface is gray.
- The cerebral cortex is organized into two hemispheres connected by thick bands of long fibers (*corpus callosum* and *anterior commissure*).
- The regions within a hemisphere are connected by shorter association fibers.
- The term *cortex* means the bark of a tree because the cortex does resemble the bark.
- The surface is a folded mass of rolling "hills" and "valleys."

The hills, folds, convolutions, or elevated masses are called **gyri** (*gyrus,* singular). The various gyri help distinguish different landmarks on the cortex. The grooves, or valleys, are called **sulci** (*sulcus,* singular), or fissures. Figure 2-13 shows the major gyri and sulci on the right hemisphere.

The **longitudinal cerebral fissure** separates the left and the right hemisphere of the cerebrum. This fissure is a groove in the middle of the brain, running from front to back. One can see this fissure in a superior view of the cortex (viewed from above).

At the top of the brain, a major fissure that runs laterally (from one side to the other), downward, and forward is called the **fissure of Rolando,** or the **central sulcus.** The central sulcus arbitrarily and roughly divides the anterior half of the brain from the posterior half of the brain. In a top view of the brain, one can see four portions of the brain divided by the longitudinal and central fissures. The longitudinal fissure and central sulcus are shown in Figure 2-14.

At the lower (inferior) frontal lobe at the base of the brain, a deep fissure starts and moves laterally and upward. This is the **lateral cerebral fissure (sulcus),** also known as the *sylvian fissure.* The regions surrounding the sylvian fissure are especially involved in speech, language, and hearing. The central and lateral cerebral fissures are shown in Figure 2-15.

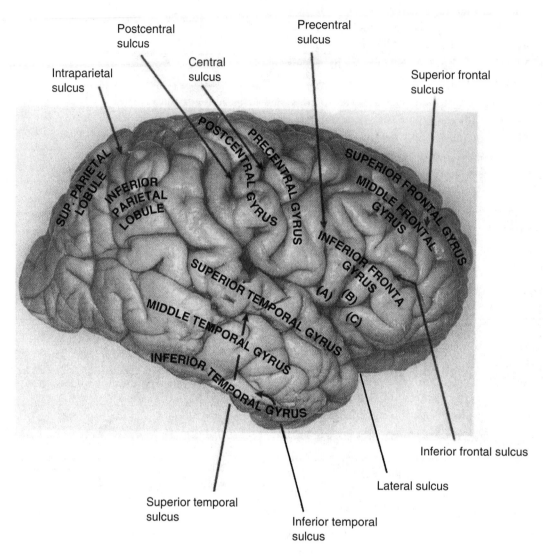

Postcentral
sulcus

Precentral
sulcus

Central
sulcus

Intraparietal
sulcus

Superior frontal
sulcus

Inferior frontal sulcus

Lateral sulcus

Inferior temporal
sulcus

Superior temporal
sulcus

Figure 2-13. Major gyri and sulci of the brain.

Each cerebral hemisphere is divided into four primary lobes: the frontal, parietal, occipital, and temporal. (A secondary lobe is described as the *insular lobe,* a small oval region buried in the depths of the lateral fissure.) Each lobe is associated with a predominant function. Therefore, to understand the different functions of the brain, one needs to study these four lobes. The four lobes of the cortex are shown in Figure 2-16.

The Frontal Lobe

The frontal lobe is extremely important for speech and language. This lobe is in front of the central fissure and above the lateral fissure. The frontal lobe is

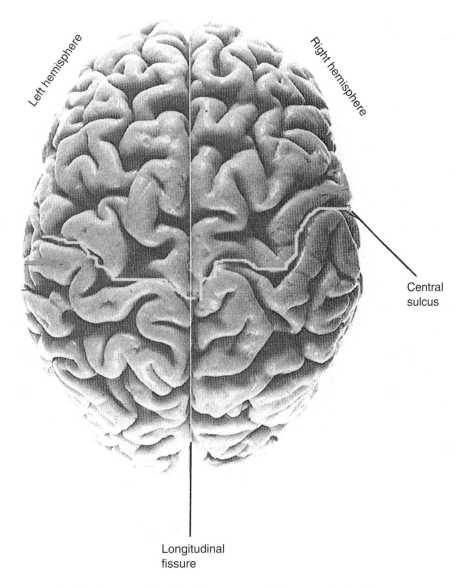

Left hemisphere

Right hemisphere

Central
sulcus

Longitudinal
fissure

Figure 2-14. The longitudinal fissure and the central sulcus.

all of the cortex in front of the central fissure; being the largest of the lobes, it makes up about one-third of the surface area of the cortex. The frontal lobe is identified in Figure 2-16, which shows the four lobes of the brain.

In front of the central fissure in the frontal lobe, there is a large bulge called the *precentral gyrus*. The precentral gyrus is the major portion of the **primary motor cortex** (motor strip) controlling voluntary movements of skeletal muscles on the opposite (contralateral) side of the body (see Figure 2-13). The precentral gyrus controls the movements of the arms, hands, fingers, face, lips, legs, and feet. The mouth, lips, hands, and fingers are controlled by relatively large areas, suggesting the importance of fine motor movements (including speech) at the human level. The motor strip controls movements through a neural pathway called the *pyramidal system.* The motor impulses are modified by another system, called the *extrapyramidal system,* with a complex set of indirect relay stations.

Just anterior to the primary motor cortex lie two areas that specialize in complex and fine motor skills. These are called the *premotor area* and the *supplementary motor area* (Brodmann area 6). The rest

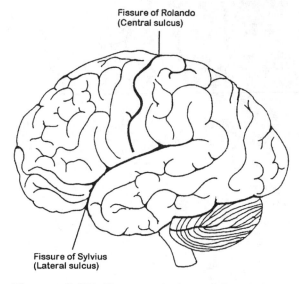

Figure 2-15. The central and the lateral fissures.

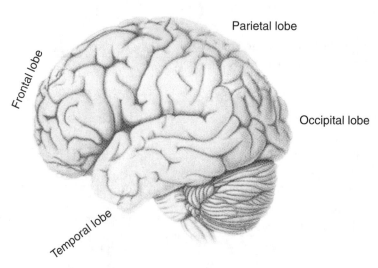

Figure 2-16. The four lobes of the brain.

of the large anterior section of the frontal lobe is called the *prefrontal cortex* (Brodmann areas 10–12), thought to be involved in such intellectual tasks as thinking, reasoning, decision making, and planning. Additional functions the prefrontal area controls include a sense of purpose, social responsibility or propriety, and foresight.

Whereas the precentral gyrus is vertical, the other important gyri in the frontal lobe are horizontal. Three such gyri are the superior frontal gyrus, middle frontal gyrus, and the inferior frontal gyrus. Of these three, the *inferior frontal gyrus* in the dominant hemisphere (the left in most individuals) is of special significance to speech production. It contains the famous **Broca's area,** shown in Figure 2-17. It is in the left, lower, and posterior portion of the frontal lobe on the inferior frontal gyrus at the juncture of the lateral and central fissures. Broca's area corresponds to Brodmann's area 44 (and may extend to parts of area 45). Broca's area is also known as the *motor speech area,* because this area controls motor movements involved in the production of speech. In Chapter 5, we learn more about Broca's aphasia, which is thought to be caused by lesion or lesions in Broca's area.

The Temporal Lobe

The *temporal lobe* is the lowest one-third of the brain. The lobe lies under the temporal (*tempus* in Latin for time) bone. Because the hair of the temples

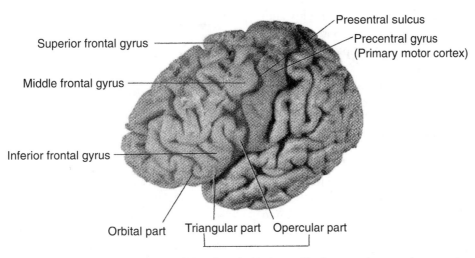

Figure 2-17. Lateral view of the frontal lobe with the motor cortex and Broca's area in the inferior frontal gyrus.

first turn gray due to age, the temporal bone is essentially called the *time bone*. The temporal lobe starts at the lateral fissure and ends at the imaginary boundary of the anterior portion of the occipital lobe. The temporal lobe is under the frontal and parietal lobes and in front of the occipital lobe. There is no natural demarcation between the temporal lobe and the occipital lobe. The lateral fissure gives a partial demarcation between the temporal lobe and the parietal lobe. The temporal lobe looks like an extended thumb.

The three important gyri of functional significance are the (1) superior (upper) temporal gyrus, (2) the middle temporal gyrus, and (3) the inferior (lower) temporal gyrus. The two areas of interest are the primary auditory cortex and Wernicke's area.

The superior, middle, and inferior temporal gyri are all found on the lateral surface of the temporal lobe. The *superior temporal gyrus* lies parallel to the lateral fissure; posteriorly, it turns upward in the region of the angular gyrus of the parietal lobe. As the name indicates, the *middle temporal gyrus* is located between the other two temporal gyri. The *superior temporal sulcus* separates the superior and the middle temporal gyri. The *inferior temporal gyrus* lies at the undersurface of the middle temporal gyrus.

The **primary auditory cortex** (area), concerned with hearing, is at the border of the superior temporal gyrus and the lateral fissure. The primary auditory cortex, also known as *Heschl's gyrus,* corresponds to Brodmann areas 41 and 42 and is buried within the lateral sulcus. (See Figure 2-25 in a later section for the location of the primary auditory cortex.) This area is found in both the hemispheres, but in a majority of people it is typically larger in the left hemisphere. This suggests the left-dominance of receptive language functions. An area adjacent to the primary auditory area is called the *secondary auditory area (cortex)* and is the same as the Brodmann area 42.

While the left temporal lobe is significant for language comprehension, the right temporal lobe may be mostly silent. Surgical removal or sectioning of the right temporal lobe produces only minor deficits. Nonetheless, evidence suggests that the right temporal lobe may be involved in nonverbal memory and the appreciation of musical experience, especially rhythm.

Located posterior to the primary auditory area, **Wernicke's area** is the posterior two-thirds of the superior temporal gyrus in the left (or dominant) hemisphere. Wernicke's area in the left hemisphere may be up to seven times larger than the corresponding area in the right hemisphere. It is close to the intersection of the temporal, parietal, and occipital lobes. This is important in comprehension of written and spoken language. As noted earlier, this area is connected to the frontal (motor speech) area through the arcuate fasciculus. A lesion in the posterior portion of the superior temporal gyrus causes Wernicke's aphasia with significant language comprehension problems but fluent if meaningless speech. We learn more about Wernicke's aphasia in Chapter 6. Figure 2-18 shows a lateral view of the temporal lobe with Wernicke's area.

The medial part of the temporal lobe contains the *hippocampus,* which forms the medial wall of the lateral ventricle. The medial temporal lobe and hippocampus mediate memory and learning. If this part of the brain is damaged or surgically removed (as in cases of intractable epilepsy), the patient fails to retain any new learning. In one well-known case, a therapist worked for more than 40 years with a man who had a portion of his medial temporal lobe removed. Unfortunately, she had to introduce herself each time she met her patient as he would not remember having ever met her (Bear, Connors, & Paradiso, 2001). He could not remember anything

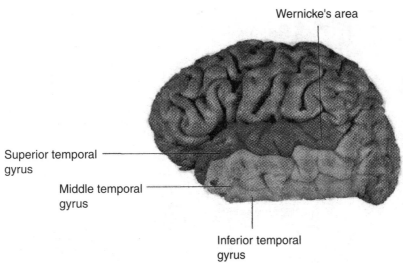

Figure 2-18. Lateral view of the temporal lobe with Wernicke's area in the posterior portion of the superior temporal gyrus.

encountered recently, and his memory was generally poor for events since the operation.

The temporal lobe is the site of auditory reception and interpretation and auditory-visual association. The temporal lobe also is the site of receptive language functions, including comprehension of spoken and written material, processing of semantic and syntactic information, and comprehension of nonverbal sounds, including music.

The Occipital Lobe

The smallest of the lobes, the occipital is behind the parietal lobe, forming a caudal end of the hemisphere. Its boundaries are mostly imaginary (no sulci separate it from the other lobes). The major structure of the occipital lobe is the *primary visual cortex* (Brodmann area 17) and *secondary visual cortex* (Brodmann area 18), because the lobe is concerned with vision. The primary visual cortex is also known as the *striate cortex* and *V1*. The occipital lobe is illustrated in Figure 2-19.

The visual cortex in each hemisphere receives visual information from the contralateral visual fields of each eye. The right visual cortex receives information from the left visual fields of each eye. The left visual cortex receives information from the right visual fields of each eye.

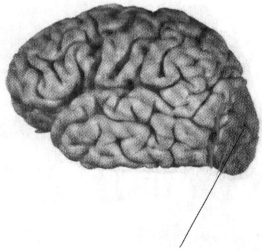

Occipital lobe

Figure 2-19. The occipital lobe, which is mostly concerned with vision.

The Parietal Lobe

The parietal lobe lies just behind the central fissure and just above the lateral fissure, with an imaginary posterior boundary that separates it from the occipital lobe. The parietal lobe lies at the back of the frontal lobe, above the temporal lobe, and in front of the occipital lobe. Just behind the central sulcus is the *post central gyrus,* better known as the *sensory cortex* (sensory strip). This narrow vertical strip of the parietal lobe is the *primary sensory area* controlling and integrating somesthetic sensory impulses. The parietal lobe is illustrated in Figure 2-20.

The parietal lobe is concerned with perception, somesthetic sensation (sensations of touch, pressure, position in space, and body awareness), and integration of sensory experiences. This lobe, especially in the nondominant (often the right) hemisphere controls understanding of spatial relations and selective attention. Damage to right parietal lobe may cause **left neglect,** a condition in which the patient is unaware of objects and persons on the left side. Left neglect and related problems associated with right hemisphere injury are described in Chapters 10 and 11.

The two gyri in the parietal lobe that are significant for language are the supramarginal gyrus and

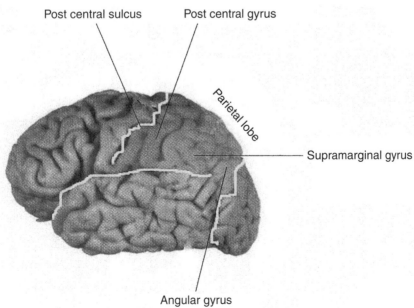

Post central sulcus   Post central gyrus

Parietal lobe

Supramarginal gyrus

Angular gyrus

Figure 2-20. The parietal lobe, which lies above the temporal lobe and behind the frontal lobe.

the angular gyrus. The *supramarginal gyrus* lies above the lateral fissure in the inferior portion of the parietal lobe, and its posterior portion curves around the latter fissure. Damage to this gyrus may cause *agraphia* (writing problems, described in Chapter 7) or a type of aphasia called *conduction aphasia* (described in Chapter 6).

The **angular gyrus** lies posterior to the supramarginal gyrus. Damage to the angular gyrus can cause naming, reading, and writing difficulties and, in some cases, a type of aphasia known as *transcortical sensory aphasia* (described in Chapter 6).

The Ventricles

A system of cavities deep within the brain is called the **cerebral ventricles.** These interconnected cavities are filled with the cerebrospinal fluid. The cerebral ventricles are illustrated in Figure 2-21.

There are four cerebral ventricles: the two lateral ventricles along with the third and the fourth ventricle. The four ventricles are interconnected through small ducts and canals.

The two *lateral ventricles,* one in each hemisphere, are the largest of the four. They are found

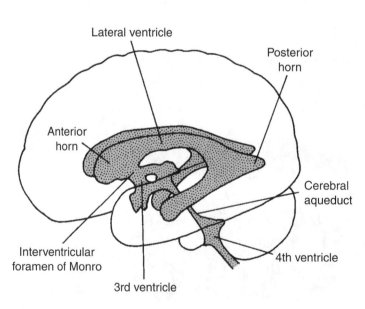

Figure 2-21. The ventricles.

From *Anatomy and physiology for speech, language, and hearing* (3rd ed., p. 519, Figure 12.9), by J.A. Seikel, D. W. King, & D. G. Drumright, 2005. Albany, NY: Thomson Delmar Learning. Reprinted with permission.

just below the corpus callosum. They are C-shaped and course through the lobes of the cortex. Its four landmarks include the body, the anterior horn, the posterior horn, and the inferior horn. Each horn is a small extension in its structure.

The *third ventricle* is at the top of the brainstem, below the lateral ventricles. The floor of the third ventricle is the hypothalamic nuclei. The third ventricle looks somewhat like a broad disk. The foramen of Munro connects the third ventricle with the lateral ventricles.

The *fourth ventricle* is between the pons and cerebellum. The pons and medulla are its floor and the cerebellum is its roof. It is continuous with the central canal of the spinal cord below and above with the *cerebral aqueduct,* which connects it to the third ventricle.

Ventricles contain the *choroid plexus*—vascular membranous materials—that produce the **cerebrospinal fluid (CSF).** This fluid circulates throughout the central nervous system. The cerebrospinal fluid cushions the brain, regulates intracranial pressure, nourishes the neural tissues, and removes waste products. When the CSF movement within the ventricles is blocked or its absorption is impaired, the result is a clinical condition called **hydrocephalus,** in which the accumulation of CSF causes a dilation of the cerebral ventricles. In children, the condition is associated with mental retardation.

The Protective Layers of the Brain

The brain is well protected by a layer of skin, bones of the skull, and layers of tissue called the meninges (from the Greek word *meninx* for membrane). The CSF adds a cushioning structure to this protective system. The spinal cord is protected by the bony vertebral column. Only because of these protective structures, the brain retains its shape and stays stable when the body and the head move around. The shape of a brain removed from the skull would soon be distorted because of gravitational forces. The three meninges of the brain are shown in Figure 2-22.

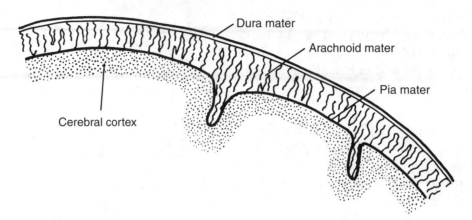

Figure 2-22. The meninges of the brain.

From *Anatomy and physiology for speech, language, and hearing* (3rd ed., p. 515, Figure 12.6), by J. A. Seikel, D. W. King, & D. G. Drumright, 2005. Albany, NY: Thomson Delmar Learning. Reprinted with permission.

The meninges are three layers of membranes covering the brain and the spinal cord: (1) an outermost membrane called the *dura mater* ("tough mother"), (2) a middle membrane called the *arachnoid* ("spider web")[1], and (3) an innermost membrane called the *pia mater* ("tender mother").

The cranial **dura mater** is a tough and thick, leatherlike membrane with one side adhering to the skull and the other side to the arachnoid, the second meninx (Greek; singular of *meninges*). This outermost membrane of dense connective tissue covers the brain and the spinal cord and protects them from external shock. The dura has two layers, the outer *periosteal* layer adhering to the skull and an inner *meningeal* layer attached to the arachnoid. There are sinuses between the two layers of the dura to absorb blood and to let the cerebrospinal fluid circulate. Normally, there is only a potential but no actual space between the dura mater and the skull (*epidural* space) or the dura and the arachnoid (*subdural* space). In some pathological conditions, fluid may form in those potential spaces.

---

[1] Arachnoid is the zoological class including spiders. The name comes from Arachne, a girl in Greek mythology who was turned into a spider because she challenged the goddess Athena in a weaving contest and lost. Arachne continued to weave beautiful things but also tried to commit suicide.

The **arachnoid** is a thin, semitransparent, non-vascular, delicate, and weblike membrane with the dura mater above and the pia mater below. The arachnoid normally adheres to the dura without space in between. However, it is separated from pia with a *subarachnoid space.* The cerebrospinal fluid fills the subarachnoid space.

The **pia mater** is also a thin, delicate, and transparent membrane that adheres to the brain surface, closely following the surface sulci and gyri. The pia also covers the blood vessels. Many blood vessels enter the brain by penetrating the pia mater.

The meninges may be damaged in cases of traumatic brain injury, tumors that grow within them, and infections and inflammations (e.g., viral or bacterial meningitis). Tumors that grow within the cerebral meninges are called **meningiomas,** requiring their surgical removal. Head (brain) injuries may cause subdural hemorrhages. Clinical conditions associated with brain injury are described in Chapter 12.

Cerebral Blood Supply

Many neurological problems arise from disrupted blood supply to the brain. In adults, disrupted blood flow within the cortical regions is a major cause of neurogenic language disorders, especially aphasia. Different types of aphasia result, often depending on the area in which the blood supply is disrupted. Vascular pathologies may either restrict blood flow to a region or may result in hemorrhage within the brain. Therefore, a basic understanding of the cerebral vascular system that supplies blood to the brain is essential to a clear understanding of aphasia and its varieties.

The brain is a big eater.

- Though it only is 2 percent of a typical human adult's body weight, the brain receives 17 percent of the body's blood.
- It consumes 25 percent of the body's oxygen.

The brain is totally dependent and vulnerable.

- It depends on the supply of blood for nourishment and normal functioning.

- A person loses consciousness within 10 seconds of blood interruption.
- Electrical activity of the brain ceases after 20 seconds of blood interruption.
- The brain will be permanently damaged within 4 to 6 minutes of interruption of blood supply.

Essentially, the brain receives blood from the heart through a network of arteries. The brain sends deoxygenated blood back to the heart through a network of veins and sinuses. The heart again sends the reoxygenated blood (through the lungs) to the brain. To gain a basic understanding of the blood supply of the brain, we need to look at the following major structures:

- Vascular network
- The aorta
- Two common and internal carotid arteries and their branches
- Two subclavian and vertebral arteries and their branches
- The circle of Willis
- The venous system
- Blood-brain barrier

The main structures of the cerebral blood supply are shown in Figure 2-23.

Vascular Network

The vascular network includes arteries and veins. While a network of arteries carry oxygenated blood to the brain from the heart, a similar network of veins carry deoxygenated blood from the brain back to the heart for reoxygenation through lungs. Both arteries and veins have three muscular layers, but arteries are generally thicker than veins.

Arteries may be large or small. **Arterioles** are smaller branches of larger arteries. Arterioles branch out into a minute hairlike network called *capillaries* from which the oxygen and other nutrients in the blood filter into tissue. Metabolic waste from the tissue filters back into the capillaries, which connect

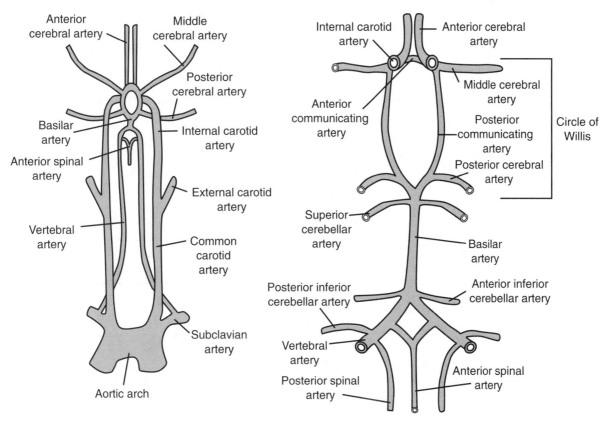

Figure 2-23. The main structures of the cerebral blood supply.

to **venules,** minute branches of veins. Veins thus receive blood low in oxygen and carry it to the heart.

The Aorta

The main artery of the heart, the **aorta** carries the blood from the left ventricle to all parts of the body, except the lungs. Just above the heart, the aortic arch divides into four branches: the two common carotid arteries (one on each side of the neck) and the two subclavian arteries (one on each side of the neck).

From the two subclavian arteries, two vertebral basilar arteries branch out and ascend to the base of the brain. Several other branches of the subclavian artery supply the thoracic wall, upper arm, and shoulder. In essence, then, the arterial systems that supply the brain are the two carotid arteries and the two vertebral basilar arteries.

The Carotid Arteries

As they enter the neck, the left and the right common carotid arteries branch into an internal carotid artery and an external carotid artery. Through the base of the skull, the arteries enter the brain through the dura mater and the subarachnoid space. The **external carotid** moves toward the face and branches into smaller arteries. The external carotid supplies blood to muscles of the face and neck, nasal and oral cavities, sides of the head, skull, and dura mater.

The major blood supplier to the brain is the **internal carotid artery,** which branches into several smaller blood vessels supplying various portions of the brain. Its two main branches of special interest are the anterior cerebral artery and the middle cerebral artery.

The **anterior cerebral artery** supplies mostly the middle portion of the frontal and parietal lobes. In addition, it supplies blood to such structures as the basal ganglia and corpus callosum. Branches of the anterior cerebral artery anastomose (join) with the posterior cerebral artery in the posterior medial areas of the brain. Figure 2-24 shows the distribution

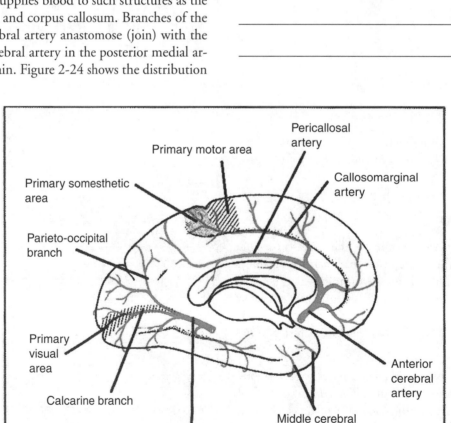

Figure 2-24. The distribution of the anterior and posterior cerebral arteries.

of the anterior cerebral artery and the posterior cerebral artery, described later.

Damage to the anterior cerebral artery can cause disruption of the blood to the midsagittal portions of the motor cortex. The motor symptoms of this disruption include paralysis of the legs and feet. Associated cognitive deficits include impaired reasoning, judgment, and concentration, often described as *prefrontal lobe symptoms.*

The **middle cerebral artery,** the biggest branch of the internal carotid, supplies the entire lateral surface of the cortex, including the major regions of the frontal lobe. With its several branches, including lateral, frontal, parietal, and temporal, the middle cerebral supplies blood to major areas concerned with sensory and motor functions and speech, language, and hearing functions. The areas it supplies include the somatosensory cortex, motor cortex in the precentral gyrus, Broca's area, primary auditory cortex, Wernicke's area, the angular gyrus, and the supramarginal gyrus. Furthermore, its smaller branches serve the putamen, caudate nucleus, globus pallidus, and portions of thalamus. Figure 2-25 shows the distribution of the middle cerebral artery.

Damage to the middle cerebral artery is a frequent cause of stroke and aphasia. Contralateral

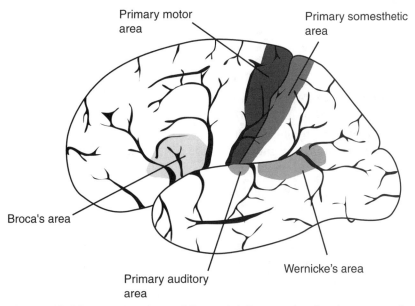

Figure 2-25. Distribution of the middle cerebral artery, supplying blood to Broca's and Wernicke's areas as well as the primary auditory area.

hemiplegia, plus impaired sense of touch, position, pain, and temperature, may also result. Reading and writing deficits may be a part of the symptom complex.

The Vertebral Arteries

The left and the right **vertebral arteries** are branches of the two subclavian arteries that emerge from the aortic arch (see Figure 2-23). As noted previously, the other branches of the subclavian supply mostly the upper extremity. The vertebral arteries enter the skull and branch to supply many organs, including the spinal cord. As they move up to the lower level of the pons, the two vertebral arteries join together to form a single **basilar artery.**

As the single basilar artery moves toward the upper portion of the pons, it divides again into two **posterior cerebral arteries.** These arteries supply the lower and lateral portions of the temporal lobes and the middle and lateral portions of the occipital lobes (please refer to Figure 2-24 for the distribution of the posterior cerebral artery). Several other branches of the basilar artery supply such other structures as the pons, cerebellum, and the inner ear.

The Circle of Willis

At the base of the brain, the two carotid and two vertebral arteries ascending from the heart *anastomose* (join together) to form the **circle of Willis** (*circulus arteriosus*). This circle is completed by the two communicating arteries (*anterior communicating* and the *posterior communicating*). The anterior cerebral, the posterior cerebral, and the middle cerebral arteries branch out from the circle. Figure 2-26 shows the circle of Willis.

The circle of Willis provides a common (redundant) blood supply to various cerebral branches. If an artery is blocked below the circle, the damage to the brain is minimal, because an alternate channel of blood flow may be maintained. But if the blockage occurs after or above the circle, the brain will not receive the blood, because of lack of a common source.

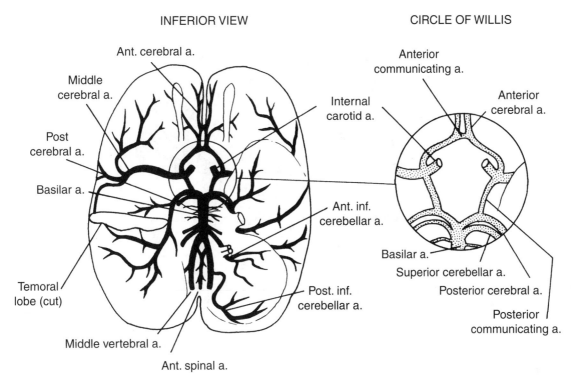

INFERIOR VIEW

Ant. cerebral a.

Middle cerebral a.

Post cerebral a.

Basilar a.

Temoral lobe (cut)

Middle vertebral a.

Ant. spinal a.

Internal carotid a.

Ant. inf. cerebellar a.

Post. inf. cerebellar a.

CIRCLE OF WILLIS

Anterior communicating a.

Anterior cerebral a.

Basilar a.

Superior cerebellar a.

Posterior cerebral a.

Posterior communicating a.

Figure 2-26. The circle of Willis.

Blood Supply and the Watershed Area of the Brain

The anterior, middle, and posterior cerebral arteries supply blood to most of the cerebral regions. But each of these arteries end their distribution and blood supply in very small branches of arteries, resulting in a zone called the *watershed area of the brain* with somewhat inefficient blood supply. The **watershed areas of the brain** are those areas that receive blood from the small end-branches (terminal branches) of all three primary arteries that supply blood to the brain—the anterior, middle, and posterior cerebral arteries. These fine end-branches may anastomose to supply blood to the region (Bhatnagar, 2002). See Figure 2-27 for the regions of the brain that are supplied by the small end-branches of the three main cerebral arteries.

If the blood supply to the watershed region is interrupted due to vascular diseases and other potential causes, specific kinds of aphasia, especially transcortical motor aphasia and transcortical sensory aphasia, may result (Benson & Ardila, 1996).

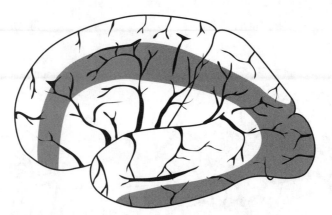

Figure 2-27. The watershed area of the brain.

For details, see Chapter 5 on transcortical motor aphasia and Chapter 6 on transcortical sensory aphasia.

The Veins and Venous Sinus System

As noted earlier, arteries carry oxygenated blood to the brain (and all other organs in the body) and a system of veins drains deoxygenated blood from organs and carries it back to the heart and eventually to the lungs where the blood is reoxygenated. In essence, the **veins** form a drainage system.

The venous system includes larger veins and many smaller, deep veins that penetrate the brain structure to collect oxygen-poor blood. Through their venules that are in contact with the capillaries, small veins throughout the brain collect the circulated oxygen-poor blood. The blood thus collected is drained into various sinuses. The venous system is complex; just one view of it is provided in Figure 2-28.

Sinuses are channels through which the blood or other fluids flow. A network of sinuses in the skull and within the cerebral structures helps collect the oxygen-poor blood from smaller veins. The sinuses in and around the brain are called *dural sinuses* because they are found within the dura. Sinuses channel the blood to the large *jugular vein,* which returns the blood to the heart.

Compared to arterial pathologies, venous pathologies cause aphasia and other communica-

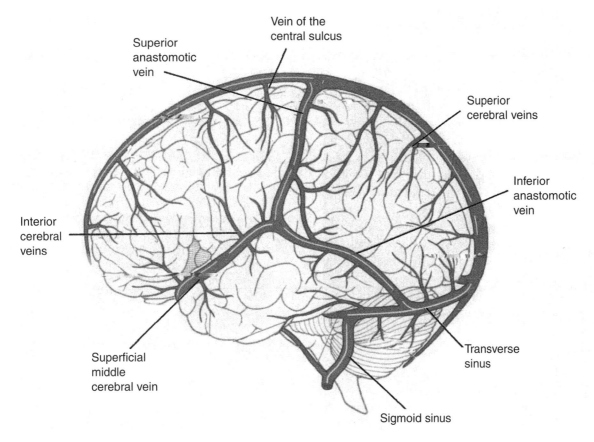

Figure 2-28. A lateral view of cerebral veins and sinuses.

tion disorders less frequently. This may be because the venous system is more interconnected and is less likely to develop occlusions and hemorrhages than the arterial system.

The Blood-Brain Barrier

The **blood-brain barrier** refers to a mechanism that prevents the cerebral penetration of harmful chemical substances and infectious microorganisms that may be present in the blood. The walls of the capillaries that help diffuse the blood nutrients to the cerebral cells are formed by endothelial cells that rest on a continuous basement membrane called *basal lamina*. Unlike the cell walls of capillaries that supply blood to the muscles and other organs, the endothelial cells of the cerebral capillary walls have continuous lining and tightly formed junctions.

Such tight junctions do not contain intercellular pores through which substances can pass.

The blood-brain barrier, while preventing harmful serum substances from reaching the neural cells, also prevents helpful medicines from needed cerebral infusion. The blood-brain barrier is weaker in babies than in adults, thus making the brains of babies more vulnerable to infections. Also, certain diseases break down the blood-brain barrier and thus allow other substances, including harmful infections, helpful medicine, and diagnostic chemicals, to penetrate the cerebral cells. Brain tumors, for example, can break down the blood-brain barrier because their cells develop intercellular pores. This disease-created vulnerability also provides an opportunity to make an accurate diagnosis of the tumor. For instance, injected radioactive amino acid will penetrate the tumor cells but not the normal brain cells. Scanning machines can then identify the tumor site.

Suggested Readings

Read the following for a more detailed and in-depth understanding of the neuroanatomy and neurophysiology relevant to speech, language, and hearing:

Bear, M. F., Connors, B. W., & Paradiso, M. A. (2001). *Neuroscience: Exploring the brain* (2nd ed.). Baltimore, MD: Lippincott Williams & Wilkins.

Bhatnagar, S. C. (2002). *Neuroscience for the study of communicative disorders* (2nd ed.). Baltimore, MD: Williams & Wilkins.

Haines, D. E. (2004). *Neuroanatomy: An atlas of structures, sections, and systems* (6th ed.). Philadelphia: Lippincott Williams & Wilkins.

Love, R. J., & Webb, W. G. (2001). *Neurology for the speech-language pathologist* (4th ed.). Boston: Butterworth.

Nolte, J. (2002). *The human brain: An introduction to its functional anatomy* (5th ed.). St. Louis, MO: Mosby Year Book.

Seikel, J. A., King, D. W., & Drumright, D. G. (2005). *Anatomy and physiology for speech, language, and hearing* (3rd ed.). Albany, NY: Thomson Delmar Learning.

Webster, D. B. (1999). *Neuroscience of communication* (2nd ed.). Albany, NY: Singular Thomson.

Zemlin, W. (1998). *Speech and hearing science: Anatomy & physiology* (4th ed.). Englewood Cliffs, NJ: Prentice Hall.

CHAPTER 3

NEURODIAGNOSTIC METHODS AND NEUROPATHOLOGY OF APHASIA

Chapter Outline

- Understanding Neuropathology of Aphasia
- Neurodiagnostic Methods
- General Neuropathology of Aphasia

Learning Objectives

After reading the chapter, the student will:

- Define neurodiagnostics.
- Define and distinguish between various brain imaging techniques.
- Describe the general neuropathology of aphasia.
- Distinguish between the different kinds of strokes and their pathologies.
- Describe the various diseases that lead to strokes.

Understanding Neuropathology of Aphasia

Both medical and communication assessments are necessary for all persons with aphasia. Soon after the stroke, when the person is a medical patient, various neurodiagnostic procedures are carried out to understand the nature of the stroke and the extent of brain damage. Of course, such diagnostic procedures are implemented in other cases of neuropathology (e.g., tumors or suspected degenerative brain diseases). How soon the communication skills will be assessed will depend on the person's physical status. While a quick bedside assessment may be made at the time of admission to the hospital, a thorough communication diagnostic assessment may have to wait until the patient's physical condition is stabilized with medical treatment.

Chapter 8 describes the speech-language assessment of persons with aphasia. This chapter describes the neurodiagnostic methods aimed at determining the type and extent of cerebral injury associated with stroke and aphasia.

Neurodiagnostic Methods

The methods of diagnosing neural pathology and its various effects are called **neurodiagnostic methods.** Most of these methods are a part of general neurological diagnostic procedures. Some methods are post hoc, some are invasive, and others are inferential. A general understanding of these methods is essential to speech-language pathologists who work with clients whose disorders of communication have a neurological basis.

Postmortem: The Post Hoc Method

Postmortem is the oldest method of relating particular areas of the brain to specific language functions. Broca and Wernicke used this method to localize certain language functions in specific brain structures. These two investigators did not have any other method available to them.

In this method:

- A patient's language problems associated with obvious neurological diseases are carefully noted.
- On the patient's death, a postmortem is performed to see pathological changes in the brain tissue.
- Observed changes then are related to the previously noted language problems.

The problem with this method is that it is post hoc and the postmortem may only be partial. Not all structures may be examined. Obviously, it is not a clinical diagnostic method that can benefit the patient. Nonetheless, the method has been valuable in gaining a scientific understanding of brain and its functions. The advantage of the method is that damaged tissue or areas can be directly observed and evaluated. Although post hoc, the evidence can be strong. The method continues to be used.

Surgical Method

Brain surgical methods, referred to as *craniotomy,* are used to remove pathological cerebral tissue that cause various neurological symptoms. The surgical method is both experimental and *in vivo* (performed on a living person in contrast to the postmortem). Many classic studies of the relation between brain and language have been conducted with this method. Two Canadian neurosurgeons, Penfield and Roberts (1959), were pioneers in this method. See Calvin and Ojemann (1980) for an excellent account of this method and its results.

The surgical method is used most often to treat severe cases of epilepsy. In these patients, the seizures are severe, frequent, and life-threatening. The only effective treatment is the surgical removal of the **epileptic focus,** the damaged or pathological area that triggers the attacks.

In this method:

- Only local anesthesia is used because the brain tissue has no pain sensors.
- The patient is fully awake during the operation, able to talk and respond in various ways.

- The neurosurgeon drills a hole or cuts open a portion of the skull and reaches the brain structures of interest.
- The surgeon maps the language cortex (brain mapping) by electrical stimulation of various areas, so that areas that control language may be spared, if that is possible.
- Sparing the mapped language areas, the surgeon then finds and destroys the epileptic focus.

Electrical stimulation of motor areas of the brain elicits motor responses. However, the same stimulation of language areas does not elicit speech but disrupts ongoing speech. The fully awake patient will be looking at a computer monitor that displays various stimulus items. The patient talks about or answers questions about the stimuli. As the surgeon stimulates different areas of the brain, the speech of the patient may be disrupted or confused. For example, while the patient is trying to name an object shown on the monitor, stimulation of a certain part of the brain may arrest the naming response or may result in interjected or repeated responses. This kind of stimulation helps localize language functions in the brain.

Electrical stimulation of language areas produces results that resemble aphasia. We have learned much about the various language areas of the brain from this kind of *in vivo* electric stimulation of the brain of a patient on an operating table. The electrical stimulation of the brain tissue is known to be safe and the disturbances it produces are temporary.

Stereotactic surgery is aimed at subcortical structures. The method is used to map and treat subcortical abnormalities. For instance, stereotactic surgery is used to treat tremor and rigidity of patients with Parkinsonism by creating lesions in the subthalamus, the ventrolateral nucleus, or the globus pallidus. The method also may be used to treat intractable pain.

Electroencephalography

Electroencephalography is a time-honored method of studying cerebral activity and pathologies by recording the electrical potential (brain waves) of the cerebral cortex. The graphic representations of the electrical activity of the brain are called *electroencephalograms* (*EEG*). The EEG is a standard clinical diagnostic method of the neurologist. Using 8 to 16 channel machines, brain waves may be simultaneously recorded from different lobes of the cortex to see differences in their pattern across and within lobes and across the corresponding areas of the two hemispheres.

In this method:

- Multiple electrodes are placed on the scalp.
- The electrical impulses the brain generates are picked up, amplified, and recorded on moving paper.
- Activity from several places on the cortex is recorded.
- Different patterns of brain waves associated with different kinds of activities (e.g., listening, talking, and thinking) are recorded.
- Any abnormal electrical activity suggesting underlying cortical pathology also is recorded.

Artifacts due to movement and unknown variables are a problem with the traditional EEG. This problem is reduced with the more recently developed signal-averaging computers that show patterns over and above the variations due to artifacts. In this method, various stimuli are presented to evoke cortical electrical responses, which are then recorded. A computer analyzes the results of stimuli presented to the patient. This method is a modification of the traditional EEG and is called the *evoked cortical response (potential) testing*. The method may involve visual-evoked response (caused by visual stimulation), somatosensory-evoked response (caused by electrical stimulation of the peripheral sensory nerves), or auditory-evoked response (caused by auditory stimulation).

The EEG is especially useful in diagnosing epilepsy as the method can detect abnormal discharges even when the patient is not experiencing seizures. Any focal lesion also is suggested by abnormal EEG patterns surrounding the site of the lesion. EEG findings, when combined with other measures and clinical evaluation, may be helpful in supporting diagnosis of herpes simplex encephalitis or such forms of dementia as the Creutzfeldt-Jakob disease (Greenberg, Aminoff, & Simon, 2002).

Electromyography

Electromyography is a method of studying muscle functions by recording the electrical potential the nerves generate when they contract (move spontaneously or voluntarily). Abnormal electrical activity in the muscles or lack of such activity may suggest neural or muscular pathology.

In this method:

- Needle electrodes are inserted into the muscle (invasive) or surface electrodes are placed on the skin just above the target muscle (noninvasive).
- Electrical activity before and during movement is recorded.
- Normal and pathological patterns of electrical activity, including their amplitude, duration, and frequency, are recorded for comparison.

Resting muscles normally do not produce electrical activity. Damaged or diseased nerves may cause abnormal electrical activity in resting muscles, referred to as *fasciculation potential*. Myographic studies help diagnose various muscles diseases, spinal motor neuron diseases, and nerve damage. It should be noted, however, that the results of myographic studies should be correlated with clinical findings to make a diagnosis. Generally, needle myography is clinically more useful than surface electrode myography.

A variation of electromyographic method is known as *nerve conduction study,* in which a peripheral nerve is stimulated to record the electrical activity in a relevant muscle. The nerve impulse generated from the stimulation also may be measured at two points on the nerve to determine the nerve conduction velocity (speed of conduction). Both sensory and motor nerves may be stimulated to study their conduction velocity. The method is useful in detecting peripheral nerve damage.

Cerebral Angiography

Cerebral angiography is a radiographic invasive procedure combined with the injection of radiopaque contrast material into selected arteries, typically the femoral artery in the groin. The X-rays do not penetrate radiopaque material; arteries that are infused with this material appear white or light on the exposed X-ray film.

In this method:

- A catheter, inserted into the femoral artery in the groin, is guided into the carotid or vertebral artery.
- A radiopaque material is then injected into the catheterized artery.
- A rapid series of X-rays is taken immediately to evaluate the health of the vascular system by examining the outline of major arteries on the film. The cerebral anterior, posterior, and middle arteries can be visualized.
- The X-rayed radiopaque material shows variations in blood circulation that might suggest vascular occlusions; arterial sections beyond a clot that blocks the blood flow will not show up, because the radiopaque material is blocked. The method also can help detect hemorrhages and aneurysm.

The use of a computer to enhance the clarity of arterial pictures is called *digital subtracting*. In this method of improved angiography, the computer subtracts image characteristics before the injection with those after. This improves the clarity of arterial images.

One limitation of cerebral angiography is that it does not outline the smaller arteries. Because it is an invasive procedure, it poses a risk of stroke.

Computed Tomography

Computed tomography, also known as *CT scan,* is a method of taking pictures of different sections of an organ without physical invasion. It is a noninvasive radiologic procedure. The term *tomos* means *sections,* and *tomography* means *imaging* the body sections. The method uses an X-ray scanning machine that rotates around structures to take images that are processed by a computer. Introduced for clinical applications in 1973, the CT scan is the early method of visualizing the brain structures in living persons.

In the CT scan method:

- A set of X-ray generators and detectors rotates 360 degrees around the head (or any other structure) of a patient and scans the structures in slices that are as thin as 1 or 2 mm.
- X-ray detectors capture the amount of radiation on the other side of the head.
- The computer constructs images of the brain (or other) scanned structures based on the amount of radiation absorbed by them.

Newer CT scanners are faster, yielding images of better resolution. Tomographic scans show internal structures, lesions, tumors, and other neuropathologies. They are especially good at detecting recent hemorrhages. CT scans are better at showing pathology caused by stroke than that caused by tumors or trauma. Therefore, tomographic scans have been used to study the location and extent of lesions in various types of aphasia (Benson & Ardila, 1996). CT scans are useful in detecting both focal and progressive pathologies. The method may fail to reveal small lesions, however. Head positioning should be carefully monitored to produce the most accurate pictures. In routine clinical practice, localization of pathology may only be approximate.

Though not invasive, CT scanning exposes patients to radiation. It is possible to introduce radiopaque material to the patient's bloodstream to improve contrast, but this increases the chances of negative side effects (e.g., pain, nausea, kidney problems). Contrast-enhanced CT scans are especially good at detecting tumors, multiple sclerosis, and hydrocephalus (Greenberg, Aminoff, & Simon, 2002).

Magnetic Resonance Imaging

Magnetic resonance imaging (MRI) is a method of generating pictures of brain structures with the help of a powerful magnetic field that alters the electrical activity of the brain. This procedure has been in clinical use since 1983. Because water is a main content of brain tissue, the behavior of atomic nuclei of hydrogen in the brain can help create images of that tissue. This method does not introduce radioactive material into the patient's body, and it does not use the X-ray. It was formerly known as *nuclear magnetic resonance imaging*. The method produces images similar to those from CT scanning.

In the MRI procedure:

- The patient's head is placed in a strong magnetic field.
- The randomly spinning hydrogen atoms of the brain produce magnetic properties that are exploited in constructing a picture of the brain structures.
- Much like iron filings lining up and pointing in the direction of a magnet, the hydrogen atoms of the brain align themselves with the magnetic field.
- When the head is placed in a strong magnetic field, the hydrogen atoms of the brain align themselves with the external magnetic field.
- When the hydrogen atoms are thus aligned with the external magnetic field, an electromagnetic pulse is introduced (the patient hears a noise similar to that produced by a washing machine).
- This pulse of energy disturbs the alignment of the hydrogen atoms of the brain for a brief moment, and then the atoms swing back to alignment as the electromagnetic pulse is withdrawn.
- While swinging back to alignment with the magnetic field, the atoms of specific areas produce particular electromagnetic signals at certain radio frequency, called *resonant frequency* (hence the name, magnetic resonance imaging); resonant frequencies are similar to faint echo.
- The computer detects, analyzes, and uses the resonant magnetic signals to construct an image of the structures.

MRI provides clearer images of body structures than the CT scan. It can detect small lesions missed by CT scans along with demyelinating and traumatic lesions. MRI is less prone to artifacts from bone tissue than are CT scans. The white and gray matter of the brain is better contrasted in MRI than in CT because the gray matter contains more water. CT scans are not especially productive during the first 48 hours of stroke, although they are still superior to MRI in detecting cerebral hemorrhage. Hematoma that is 3 to 4 days old is better revealed by MRI than CT scan, however. Although CT scans are sensitive to changes in tissue density, the MRI is sensitive to varying chemical composition of tissue.

The basic technique of magnetic resonance imaging has evolved into several newer procedures. **Functional magnetic resonance imaging (fMRI)** is one such procedure in which a contrast material is intravenously administered to the patient before MRI. The method helps detect changes in cerebral blood flow as the patient experiences different states or performs different activities (e.g., at rest versus listening to music). Functional MRI detects increased blood flow that is typically associated with cerebral activity in the regions that are activated. Currently, fMRI is a research tool and its clinical applications await further research (Greenberg, Aminoff, & Simon, 2002).

Other magnetic resonance procedures of recent origin include diffusion-weighted magnetic resonance imaging, profusion-weighted magnetic resonance imaging, MRI spectroscopy, and magnetic resonance angiography. The **diffusion-weighted MRI** procedure constructs pictures of structures based on its detection of microscopic motion of water protons in the brain tissue. The method has been found to be clinically useful because it can detect cerebral ischemia in stroke patients soon after onset and with good clarity and specificity. It also can help distinguish cerebral edema that is due to stroke from edema due to other factors.

The **profusion-weighted magnetic resonance imaging** produces images based on blood flow variations in contrast to water proton movements detected in diffusion-weighted MRI. Diffusion-weighted and profusion-weighted images may be compared to analyze ischemic damage in stroke patients.

MRI spectroscopy, often used with the traditional MRI, creates images of brain structures by detecting biochemical composition of tissue. Concentration of different brain chemicals varies in healthy and normal tissue. Therefore, this method helps detect such pathology as neuronal loss in Alzheimer's disease by measuring chemical variations across scanned tissue. The method also helps detect pathology in the absence of structural abnormality.

Magnetic resonance angiography (MRA) is a procedure in which the rate and velocity of blood supply to the selected cerebral structures are measured. Compared to the traditional cerebral angiography, MRA is noninvasive, less risky, and more economical. It is especially useful in visualizing the carotid arteries and the fast proximal intracranial blood circulation. Occlusion of vessels may be detected with this procedure although the image clarity is inferior compared to those of the traditional angiography.

Positron Emission Tomography

Positron emission tomography (PET), introduced in 1975, is mainly a research tool to study activation of brain structures associated with various activities. It studies brain activity through differences in metabolic rates of different areas of the brain.[1] Generally, differences in the rate of metabolic activity indicate differences in the health of the tissue studied.

In the PET method:

- The patient takes glucose mixed with a positron-emitting isotope[2] (carbon, nitrogen, or oxygen), which is metabolized in the cerebral cells.
- Areas of greater metabolism suggest greater neural activity and blood flow.
- The machine detects and amplifies the positrons (radiation) emitted by the isotopes.
- A computer analyzes the data to show areas of high or low metabolic activity.
- Lower glucose metabolism (hypometabolism) suggests structural and functional problems in the brain.

The PET provides information on blood flow because the greater the metabolic activity, the higher the blood flow rate. PET is useful in detecting brain

---

[1]Positron is a positively charged particle having the same mass and magnitude of charge as the electron and constituting the antiparticle of the electron.

[2]*Iso = equal; topos = place.* Any of two or more forms of an element having the same or closely related properties and the same atomic number but different atomic weights.

tumors as the tumor sites are associated with increased metabolism. However, the PET also can reveal damage to areas that have normal blood flow but reduced metabolic activity due to that damage. Furthermore, PET also can show areas that are not working, although no structural damage may be seen. In studies involving patients with aphasia, PET has shown that focal brain damage may affect functions elsewhere in the brain. This supports the view that functions in the brain are not strictly localized.

The PET is an expensive procedure. The procedure requires physicists and chemists to prepare the isotope. The PET scans may result in poor resolution of pictures (unclear boundaries of lesions). The procedure also is subject to artifacts from patient movements.

Regional Cerebral Blood Flow

Regional cerebral blood flow (rCBF) method is a technique to assess the amount of blood flow in different areas of the brain. An active cerebral region requires more blood. Thus, an estimate of the amount of blood flowing into a region indicates the presence of, or increase in, cerebral activity. Increased blood flow also is an indication of increased metabolic activity.

In the rCBF method:

- A radioactive material, often an inert gas called *xenon-133*, is prepared.
- The gas is then introduced to the patient's bloodstream, either by having the patient inhale the gas or by injecting it.
- A special camera, called a *gamma ray camera,* scans the brain for the radioactive material in the cerebral blood flow.
- The scanned information is sent to a computer that constructs the images of the regions of the brain and shows differential blood flow in different colors and hues.

Regional blood flow studies have shown that the right hemisphere is active in speech to a greater extent than previously suggested. These studies also have supported the hypothesis of localization of cerebral functions.

B-Mode Carotid Imaging

B-mode carotid imaging is a technique of constructing images of the body structures by the help of sound deflected by those structures. More specifically, B-mode carotid imaging is used to assess the health of arteries in the neck. It is similar to ultrasound imaging of the fetus used during pregnancy. This technique is also known as *echo arteriogram*.

In this procedure:

- A high-frequency sound generator is placed over the neck.
- Structures reflect this sound back to varying extent; arteries in which the blood is flowing normally do not reflect the sound.
- A computer analyzes the reflected sound to construct images of the structures, especially the arteries.

B-mode carotid imaging is noninvasive. It can help detect such arterial pathologies as stenosis and ulceration.

Carotid Phonoangiography

Carotid phonoangiography is a method of assessing the health of the carotid arteries by the characteristics of the sound generated by the blood gushing through the arteries.

In this technique, a machine:

- Picks up the sound of the blood gushing through the arteries
- Analyzes the characteristics of sounds of blood movement and thus helps assess the general health of the arteries

Arterial stenosis, or narrowing of the arteries, creates turbulence as the blood moves and this can be detected through carotid phonoangiography.

Doppler Ultrasonography

Doppler ultrasonography, also called *ultrasound*, helps assess arterial health by measuring the velocity of blood flow. Within narrowed arteries, the blood flows with increased velocity, causing an increase in the velocity of sound reflected from the arteries. The *transcranial Doppler ultrasonography* is helpful in assessing the health of cerebral arteries.

In this procedure:

- The head is exposed to high frequency sound; a computer can alter the sound characteristics and target particular arteries for study.
- Depending on the blood flow characteristics, the frequency of reflected sound changes.
- The computer analyzes the frequency changes and constructs an image of the blood flow, pressure, and velocity.

The method is clinically used to detect lesions in cranial arteries, diseases of carotid arteries, and vasospasm consequent to subarachnoid hemorrhage. Some clinicians may combine B-mode carotid imaging with the Doppler method. *Duplex* instruments in clinical use help administer the two procedures. This combination gives more complete information on the structure of the arteries and blood flow characteristics within them.

Lumbar Puncture

Lumbar puncture is a method of diagnosing infections or hemorrhages in the central nervous system by an analysis of a sample of cerebrospinal fluid. This invasive method is also known as a *spinal tap*. The method offers information that imaging techniques do not.

In this method:

- A needle is inserted, typically between the third and fourth lumbar vertebrae.
- A sample of cerebrospinal fluid is drawn.
- The pressure with which the fluid flows into the needle is measured with the help of a manometer attached to the needle.
- The fluid is analyzed for pathological conditions, including infections.

Pressure variations in the cerebrospinal fluid may suggest various pathologies, including blockage of the flow, tumors, and brain swelling. The presence of blood cells in the cerebrospinal fluid suggests cerebral hemorrhage. The method helps diagnose such conditions as meningitis and other infections, multiple sclerosis, neurosyphilis, inflammation, subarachnoid hemorrhage, meningeal malignancies, and intracranial pressure variations.

General Neuropathology of Aphasia

Aphasia has many causes, and most are chains of causes with remote and immediate elements of the chain interacting with each other. Some form of brain damage is the most immediate or even simultaneous cause of aphasia. Look at the chain of events depicted in the next section, going backward from the existing aphasia; the arrows suggest the sequence of events from the most remote (genetic predisposition) to the most recent (injury to the language structures in the brain).

An illustration of elements of a potential causal chain leading to aphasia:

APHASIA

⇧

Injury to language structures in the brain

⇧

An interrupted blood supply

⇧

Atheroscleoris

⇧

High blood cholesterol

⇧

Poor eating habits

⇧

Genetic predisposition

The causal elements are only examples, showing a potential (not certain) sequence of events. The various elements within the chain interact with each other to produce the eventual health consequence. Also, other chains of events with different causes result in damage to the language structures.

Such damage to the language structures in the brain is essential for a diagnosis of aphasia. The damage itself may have different causes; hence the site of lesion is more important in determining the kinds of aphasia symptoms than the factor that causes the lesion (Benson & Ardila, 1996).

The brains of patients who have aphasia due to various reasons (to be described shortly) show various kinds of neuropathological elements. Some of them may be seen on scanned brain images; others may be found only on autopsy. In any case, the following kinds of cerebral changes may be found in varying degrees across patients with aphasia (Greenberg, Aminoff, & Simon, 2002):

- Edema. A brain area that has recently suffered some kind of damage is typically soft and swollen. **Edema** refers to swollen tissue. The edema extends from the gray to the white matter. The edema reaches its maximum level within the first 4 to 5 days of onset. Most deaths following a stroke are due to cerebral edema.
- Cellular changes. Some cortical cells in the affected area may be dead. Others may be shrunk.
- Destruction of glial cells. The glia, the special kinds of cells that support the neural cells, may be destroyed.
- Necrosis of small blood vessels. **Necrosis** means cell damage. Damage to small blood vessels is often present.
- Ischemic penumbra. A tissue region surrounding the major locus of infarction is called **ischemic penumbra;** improving the blood supply to this region is a major medical concern following an ischemic stroke.

Transient Ischemic Attacks

Symptoms of strokes, described next, last long enough to be noticed by the patient and family members. However, *transient* (brief) "brain attacks" may be felt by the patient but may not lead to swift action because such attacks do not produce lasting effects. **Transient ischemic attacks** (TIAs) are "ministrokes" that last a few seconds, and the patient recovers without more permanent disability. However, they may be warning signs of more serious strokes that do produce lasting effects.

It is important to recognize the signs of TIAs as urgent medical attention may be needed. Prompt treatment may reduce the chance of a more serious stroke. Patients and family members should suspect a TIA when the following symptoms are experienced:

- Sudden weakness, numbness, or paralysis in facial muscles, arm, or leg (often in one side of the body)
- Sudden impairment in understanding speech
- Slurred or garbled speech
- Sudden blindness or double vision
- Dizziness, impaired balance, or disturbed consciousness

A person may have multiple TIAs and eventually a full-fledged stroke. Therefore, it is important to seek immediate medical attention by calling 911 when symptoms of the first TIA are experienced. See Appendix D for a variety of Internet resources that offer information on patient education and prompt help.

Cerebrovascular Accidents (Strokes)

Cerebrovascular accidents, popularly known as *strokes,* are a frequent and immediate cause of aphasia. A **stroke** is a syndrome with acute onset, resulting in focal brain damage, caused by disturbed cerebral blood circulation. The resulting focal brain damage leads to language problems. A neurological event that causes the most common form of disability, strokes are the third most prevalent cause of death in the United States. The annual death rate from strokes in the United States is 150,000 people; some 750,000 people experience their first stroke each year (Greenberg, Aminoff, & Simon, 2002).

To an extent, the symptom complex depends on whether the anterior or posterior brain circulation was interrupted. The internal carotid artery and its branches supply blood to the anterior portion of the brain. The vertebral and basilar arteries supply blood to the posterior portion of the brain.

Symptoms of a stroke are similar to those of TIAs, although some of the more serious symptoms associated with strokes are infrequent in TIAs (e.g., vomiting, seizures, and coma are uncommon in TIAs). A stroke is the likely problem if the patient experiences the following symptoms (Greenberg, Aminoff, & Simon, 2002):

- Severe headache combined with other symptoms (more common in anterior ischemia)
- Altered consciousness (more common in posterior ischemia)
- Impaired speech production, comprehension, or both (in anterior ischemia)
- Impaired vision, often in one eye (more common in posterior ischemia)
- Dizziness, sudden falls, inability to stand or walk (in posterior ischemia—cerebellar hemorrhage)
- Paresis (weakness) or paralysis (more common in anterior ischemia)
- Impaired sensation, especially on one side of the body (more common in anterior ischemia)
- Vomiting (in hemorrhagic stroke)
- Seizures (mostly in hemorrhagic strokes affecting subcortical white matter)
- Coma (usually in hemorrhage in pons; often fatal)

The symptoms of a stroke last at least 24 hours. In a few cases, symptoms may last more than 24 hours, and yet the patient may recover completely or nearly so. Such cases are known as **reversible ischemic neurological deficit (RIND)** or **minor strokes.** TIAs may precede strokes in many cases. It may be noted that both TIA and RIND are caused by ischemia, not hemorrhage.

Etiology of Cerebrovascular Accidents

Various vascular disorders cause strokes. Such disorders generally produce focal symptoms, the nature and extent of which depend on the site of the vascular region and that of brain tissue involvement. When such other causes as trauma or metabolic disorders produce focal symptoms, the term *stroke* is not used to describe the problem; it is reserved for a series of events triggered by vascular pathology. Based on their vascular pathology, strokes are classified as either *ischemic* or *hemorrhagic.*

Ischemic Strokes

Ischemic strokes are caused by occlusive vascular disorders that block or interrupt arterial blood flow to a region of the brain, resulting in an infarction. The word **ischemia** means interrupted blood supply to a cerebral region. When the blood supply is interrupted, the brain tissue is deprived of glucose and oxygen. If glucose and oxygen deprivation is not promptly stopped by restoring blood supply, the neural tissue will die. Such death of neural tissue is called *infarction,* or necrosis.

Blood supply may be interrupted by either cerebral thrombosis or cerebral embolism.

Thrombosis is a vascular disease involving the formation of *thrombus,* which is a collection of blood materials that get entrapped with cell material and thus block blood circulation. In general terms, a **thrombus** is a special kind of blood clot. Thrombosis may be the cause of roughly two-thirds of all ischemic strokes.

The formation of thrombi (plural of *thrombus*) are made possible by **atherosclerosis,** which is a slowly developing arterial disease process in which the arteries are hardened and narrowed from an accumulation of lipids, other fatty particles, calcium deposits, and fibrous material that result in *atherosclerotic plaque*. Atherosclerosis is associated with a variety of factors, including high blood pressure, high cholesterol (especially the low-density lipoproteins), high triglycerides, diabetes, free radicals, smoking, and use of oral contraceptives. Genetic predisposition also is suspected.

Atherosclerosis and the resulting thrombi are typically formed in large arteries (the internal carotid, middle cerebral, and basilar), small penetrating arteries, cerebral veins, and venous sinuses. Specific sites include the origins of the common carotid, middle cerebral, and vertebral carotid arteries; the basilar artery; the vertebral artery just above its entry point to the skull; and the internal carotid artery just above the common carotid bifurcation. Generally, the points at which an artery divides and bends are more vulnerable to an accumulation of material leading to atherosclerosis and consequent thrombosis.

The accumulation of materials in the arteries thickens and hardens their walls. This results in narrowed or constricted arteries through which the blood does not normally flow. Slow-flowing blood encourages the formation of thrombi (clots), which remain at the site of their formation and occlude the artery. Consequently, the tissue down the stream may die for lack of oxygen.

Thrombotic strokes tend to occur when the person is asleep or engaged only in low levels of physical activity. Transient ischemic attacks, headaches, and seizures may precede such strokes.

Embolism is another arterial disease in which a moving or traveling fragment of arterial debris blocks a small artery through which it cannot pass. Thus, an **embolus** (*emboli,* plural) is a traveling mass that may have been formed farther away from the place where it occluded a vessel. Thus, a traveling embolus contrasts with a stationary thrombus. Figure 3-1 shows plaque buildup that eventually leads to embolism

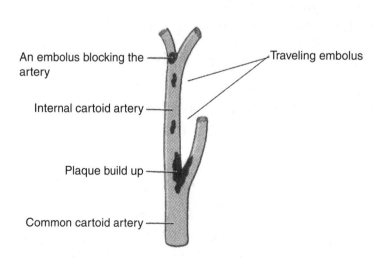

An embolus blocking the artery

Traveling embolus

Internal cartoid artery

Plaque build up

Common cartoid artery

Figure 3-1. Plaque buildup in an artery leading to anembolus that eventually blocks an artery. Brain tissue ahead of the lodged embolus will be the area of infarction.

that occludes (blocks) the blood flow in an artery, leading to cerebral cell damage in an area supplied by the blocked artery.

An embolus may be a clump of tissue from a tumor or a diseased artery, moving atherosclerotic plaque, a mass of bacteria, a blood clot or a piece of clot that has broken loose from its point of origin, or an air bubble. An embolus may have been a thrombus to begin with; when it breaks off from the site of its origin and begins to move, it is called an *embolus,* not a thrombus. Heart diseases, such as atrial fibrillation (heart palpitation), may lead to embolism because pooled blood in the heart can promote clot (embolus) formation. Emboli also may form at the site of cardiac surgery and then migrate to brain vessels to block one of them.

Emboli often occlude the middle cerebral artery and its branches, which supply 85 percent of hemispheric blood. The superior division of the middle cerebral artery supplies blood to anterior portions of the brain, including Broca's, motor, and sensory areas. The inferior division supplies Wernicke's area. Emboli also occlude blood supply to the posterior portions of the brain when they are formed in basilar and posterior cerebral arteries.

Embolic strokes tend to occur when the person is awake and active. The patient may have no warning signs, although in some cases, headaches and seizures may precede such strokes.

Hemorrhagic Strokes

Hemorrhages cause the second most common variety of strokes. **Hemorrhagic strokes** are those that result from ruptured cerebral blood vessels causing cerebral bleeding, contrasted with ischemic strokes resulting from occlusion of blood vessels (Greenberg, Aminoff, & Simon, 2002).

The common causes of blood vessel ruptures include weakened arterial walls, various malformations of the blood vessels, and high and fluctuating blood pressure. A less frequent cause is trauma to the blood vessel.

There are two main kinds of hemorrhagic strokes: intracerebral and extracerebral. The following grids show their causes and characteristics.

An **aneurysm** is a balloonlike swelling of a weak and thin portion of an artery that eventually ruptures. A common site of an extracerebral aneurysm is the base of the brain and can involve the vertebral arteries, the basilar artery, or the Circle of Willis. Anterior and middle cerebral arteries also are aneurysm sites. See Figure 3-2 for an aneurysm that might eventually rupture and produce a hemorrhagic stroke.

Intracerebral hemorrhage in basal ganglia may cause subcortical aphasia, high mortality rate, and more permanent brain damage. Hemorrhaged blood forms clots and destroys brain cells. Strokes in such cases tend to have a sudden onset. Headache, vomiting, coma, stupor, paralysis, sensory loss, confusion, memory loss, and speech-language problems are frequent symptoms.

Patients who have had ischemic or hemorrhagic strokes tend to show different patterns of recovery. These different patterns are summarized in the grid on page 89.

Intracerebral Hemorrhage	Extracerebral Hemorrhage
Hemorrhage caused by ruptures within the brain or brainstem are called *intracerebral.*	Hemorrhage caused by ruptures within the meninges are called *extracerebral.* There are three types of extracerebral hemorrhage:
Hypertension is the most common cause of blood vessel ruptures.	**Subarachnoid:** The most common of the extracerebral hemorrhages that occur on the surface of the brain, brainstem, or cerebellum; ruptures occur beneath the arachnoid; they are frequently caused by aneurysms.
Intracerebral hemorrhage is more common in small arteries deep within the brain structures, especially around the thalamus and basal ganglia.	**Subdural:** Rupture occurs beneath the dura mater; often caused by traumatic head injury.
	Epidural (Extradural): Ruptures occur above the dura, between the dura and the skull; they are often caused by traumatic head injury.

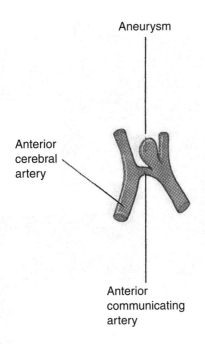

Aneurysm

Anterior
cerebral
artery

Anterior
communicating
artery

Figure 3-2. Aneurysm of an artery that might rupture and cause a hemorrhagic stroke.

Brain Trauma

Trauma to the brain is another cause of stroke. Automobile and other kinds of accidents, gunshot wounds, and blows to the head are among the frequent causes of trauma to the head and the brain. Such head injuries may cause aphasia and other disorders of communication. Generally, though, other

DIFFERENT PATTERNS OF RECOVERY FROM TYPICAL ISCHEMIC AND HEMORRHAGIC STROKES

Ischemic	Hemorrhagic
Greater and sooner recovery	Little recovery in the first 4 to 8 weeks
Noticeable recovery in the first few weeks	More rapid recovery after 4 to 8 weeks
Maximum recovery in 3 months	A slowing down of recovery, stabilizing with greater residual deficits

neurobehavioral symptoms, which are dominant in trauma patients, overshadow symptoms of aphasia.

Aphasic symptoms may be more common in patients who have open-head injury than in those who have closed-head injury (Benson & Ardila, 1996). Chapters 12 and 13 explore traumatic brain injury in greater detail.

Intracranial Neoplasms

Intracranial neoplasms (tumors) are pathological growths within the cranial structures. They are a less frequent cause of aphasia than are strokes. **Tumors** are space-occupying lesions that cause swelling in the surrounding tissue and lead to increased intracranial pressure (Greenberg, Aminoff, & Simon, 2002).

Tumors may be primary or secondary (metastatic), benign, or cancerous. Benign tumors are not cancerous and grow slowly. Malignant (cancerous) tumors grow uncontrollably because they form new blood vessels that continue to feed the tumors.

Primary intracranial tumors originate in the brain; they often are found in the cerebrum and the cerebellum. Primary intracranial tumors are common in the age group 25–50. The cause or causes of tumors are unknown, although the loss of a tumor-suppressing gene, an inappropriate expression of a cancerous gene, or a combination of both may be responsible. Heredity and former sites of injury correlate with the formation of such tumors.

Malignant primary brain tumors include several varieties, differing in their degree of malignancy and rate of growth. The term *glioma* is often used to include all forms of malignant primary brain tumors. Gliomas arise in *neuroglia* (also called glia, meaning *glue* in Greek), which are nonneural cells of the nervous system. Found between and around nerve cells, the glia support neural cells and help regulate neuronal metabolic activity and neurotransmission. Glia cells include astrocytes, oligodendrocytes, and microglia.

Astrocytomas are primary malignant tumors that arise from astrocytes. Their extent of malignancy may vary significantly, however. Astrocytomas are the most common form of glioma. The most malignant of glioma is **glioblastoma multiforme,** which is also associated with a high death rate. **Oligodendrogliomas** arise from oligodendrocytes and are typically found in the adult frontal lobes.

Intracranial tumors may cause:

- Destruction of healthy tissue
- Swelling of nearby tissue
- Headaches
- Seizures
- Focal or generalized symptoms (initially, focal; as the tumor grows, more generalized)
  - Sensory problems:
    a. Blurred vision
    b. Loss of other sensation
    c. Vertigo
  - Behavior changes:
    a. Memory problems
    b. Lethargy
    c. Personality change
  - Herniation (forcing down) of the brainstem

Most tumors are treated surgically. However, successful surgical treatment of tumors depends on their size, location, and time of diagnosis. Benign or malignant, a tumor located in an inaccessible and vital part of the brain (e.g., thalamus or brainstem) may be fatal.

Meningiomas are a variety of intracranial tumors; they form within the meninges. Benign, slow growing, and generally localized, meningiomas tend to cause focal symptoms and are most effectively removed surgically. Meningiomas are described as *extracerebral tumors* as they grow in the meninges that cover the brain to distinguish them from *intracerebral tumors* that grow within the brain structures themselves.

Secondary (metastatic) intracranial tumors are those that have grown elsewhere in the body, but have migrated into the brain. Such migration or spreading of cancer cells throughout the body is called **metastasis.** Most metastasized intracranial tumors are cancer cells that break off from their primary site elsewhere in the body and migrate into the cranial space. Most common secondary intracranial tumors come from cancer of the breast, the lungs, the pharynx, or the larynx. These cancerous cells are carried by the bloodstream. Notably, the primary intracranial tumor cells do not travel to other parts of the body.

Metastatic tumors attach themselves to brain tissue and begin to grow. They may grow in multiple brain sites. Metastatic tumors carry a high mortality rate. Death typically occurs within 2 to 3 months of diagnosis.

Tumors in the brain or elsewhere in the body are graded based on the degree of their malignancy, or the aggressiveness of their growth. By studying the tumor cells microscopically, **oncologists,** or cancer specialists, grade a tumor as either Grade I, II, III, or IV. A tumor graded I has distinct borders (circumscribed in structure) and grows slowly. A tumor graded IV grows most aggressively; it carries the worst prognosis for the patient. Glioblastoma multiforme, described previously, is typically graded IV. Tumors that fall between the least and the most aggressive are graded as II or III.

Infections

Various cerebral infections can cause aphasia. Bacterial infection, viral infection, and brain abscess are the three common forms of cerebral infections of interest. Because infections can be life-threatening and tend to produce serious physical symptoms the language disturbances they produce tend to be overlooked.

Bacterial Infections

A frequent variety of bacterial infection is bacterial meningitis. In this condition, the meninges and cerebrospinal fluid are infected. The patients experience fever, headaches, lethargy, and drowsiness; other symptoms, including coma, may follow. Treatment can be effective, but some behavioral symptoms may persist.

Bacterial meningitis has a rapid course. It may be fatal if not promptly treated with antibiotics.

Viral Infections

A variety of viral inflections can cause aphasia, along with many other kinds of symptoms. Such viral infections as rabies, AIDS, herpes simplex encephalitis, mumps, measles, and syphilis can eventually result in symptoms of aphasia. Herpes simplex encephalitis is a frequent viral infection causing aphasia.

Some experts believe that herpes simplex encephalitis is a brain infection that frequently is associated with aphasia (Benson & Ardila, 1996). The initial symptoms include headache, confusion, fever, and coma. Mortality rate is high, although the survival rate has improved with prompt treatment. As the patients recover, severe amnesia and generalized dementia may be more apparent than the naming problems they experience.

AIDS is associated with an increased incidence of transient ischemic attacks and ischemic strokes. After about 5 years of primary infection, syphilis may cause *syphilitic arteritis* (inflammation of the arteries) primarily because of meningeal inflammation (Greenberg, Aminoff, & Simon, 2002).

Brain Abscess

Bacteria, fungi, or parasites can migrate into the brain from sinuses. The course of brain abscess is slower than that of bacterial infection. Symptoms include visual problems, fever, headache, drowsiness, and lethargy.

Brain abscess is treated with surgical drainage and antibiotics. Generally, the rate of recovery is rapid, although symptoms of aphasia may persist (Benson & Ardila, 1996).

Other Factors

Several other factors that may be related to brain pathology and aphasia include cerebral toxemia, epilepsy (seizure disorders), and several progressive neurological diseases associated with aging. In the cases involving these factors, extensive neurologic and behavior disorder may be more prominent than symptoms of aphasia.

Introduction of poisonous (toxic) factors into the brain causes **cerebral toxemia.** Typical toxic factors include drug overdose, drug interactions, and heavy metal (e.g., lead and mercury) poisoning, drug abuse. Chronic use of cocaine (both the hydrochloride and alkaloidal or crack variety), amphetamines, and heroin are risk factors for stroke, especially in persons who are younger than 35 years. Use of cocaine hydrochloride most frequently causes hemorrhagic strokes, although ischemic stokes may also be observed. Crack cocaine (alkaloidal cocaine) typically leads to ischemic strokes, although hemorrhagic strokes also may occur. Amphetamines usually cause ischemic strokes (Greenberg, Aminoff, & Simon, 2002).

Epilepsy may be associated with aphasia or similar focal language impairment. Such impairments may be more often observed soon after a seizure attack. Language impairments associated with epilepsy tend to be transitory.

Among the progressive neurologic diseases associated with aging, multi-infarct dementia, dementia of the Alzheimer's type, and Pick's disease are important. Aphasia may occur in Creutzfeldt-Jakob disease. Dementia, their causes, and their language symptoms are described in Chapters 14, 15, and 16.

Suggested Readings

Read the following for a more detailed and in-depth understanding of the neurodiagnosis of and neuropathology associated with aphasia:

Bear, M. F., Connors, B. W., & Paradiso, M. A. (2001). *Neuroscience: Exploring the brain* (2nd ed.). Baltimore, MD: Lippincott Williams & Wilkins.

Benson, D. F., & Ardila, A. (1996). *Aphasia: A clinical perspective.* New York: Oxford University Press.

Bhatnagar, S. C. (2000). *Neuroscience for the study of communicative disorders* (2nd ed.). Baltimore, MD: Williams & Wilkins.

Greenberg, D. A., Aminoff, M. J., & Simon, R. P. (2002). *Clinical neurology* (5th ed.). New York: Lange Medical Books/McGraw-Hill.

Haines, D. E. (2004). *Neuroanatomy: An atlas of structures, sections, and systems* (6th ed.). Philadelphia: Lippincott Williams & Wilkins.

PREVALENCE, DEFINITION, AND CLASSIFICATION OF APHASIA

Chapter Outline

- Prevalence of Aphasia and Associated Diseases
- Definitions of Aphasia
- The Main Arguments for Classifying Aphasia into Types
- The Main Arguments Against Classifying Aphasia into Types
- An Overview of Aphasia
- General Symptoms of Aphasia
- A General Description of How Aphasic Patients Communicate
- What Aphasia IS Not

Learning Objectives

After reading the chapter, the student will:

- Summarize research on prevalence of aphasia in various populations and ethnocultural groups.
- Describe and critically evaluate the different kinds of definitions of aphasia.
- Summarize the arguments for and against classifying aphasia.
- Describe the most salient symptoms of aphasia.
- Describe the general communication patterns found in patients with aphasia.
- Distinguish the clinical conditions that may be confused with aphasia.

Prevalence of Aphasia and Associated Diseases

To understand the prevalence of aphasia, one needs to understand the prevalence of underlying diseases and pathologies. A **cerebrovascular accident (CVA),** popularly known as a *stroke,* is frequently an immediate cause of aphasia. However, heart diseases and strokes are closely related to produce a combined effect on either prevalence. Statistics on diseases are sometimes dated before they are published. An update published in a given year may have a 2 to 3 years' lag. For example, the 2005 update on stroke and heart disease summarizes data for 2002.

A comprehensive source of the most current statistics on heart disease and stroke is the American Stroke Association, a division of the American Heart Association. The association collects statistical data from various sources, including the U.S. Center for Disease Control and Prevention (and its branch, the National Center for Health Statistics). Students are encouraged to visit the various Web sites for the latest information available (see Appendix D for details). Either the key words *American Heart Association* or *American Stroke Association* will lead to the Web site that contains much valuable information. A major source for the following summary on prevalence is the 2005 update on 2002 statistics on strokes and heart diseases published on the Web by the American Heart Association (2005).

- Strokes are the third leading cause of death in the United States (coronary heart disease is #1, cancer is #2); combined, heart diseases and strokes are the number 1 cause of death; in 2002, for every 100,000 persons in the United States, about 56 deaths occurred due to stroke.
- Mortality rates differ across the types of strokes; 8 to 12 percent of ischemic (blockage of blood) strokes and 37 to 38 percent of hemorrhagic (bleeding in the brain) strokes result in death.
- About 700,000 new cases of stroke are reported each year; of these, 327,000 (47 percent) are males and 373,000 (53 percent) are females; on average, a stroke occurs every 45 seconds; 2.5 percent of total males

and 2.6 percent of total females in the country may have a stroke in a given year.

- Stroke is a leading cause of disability in the United States. More than 300,000 persons who suffer strokes are permanently disabled.

- After age 55, the incidence of strokes increases rapidly during each decade of life; about two-thirds of all strokes strike people age 65 and older; between age 45–54, 1.2 percent of men and 2.1 percent of women have a stroke; but at age 75 and older, 12 percent of men and 11.5 percent of women have a stroke.

- At comparable age levels, men have a higher risk of stroke; men's stroke incidence is 1.25 times higher than women's; however, because of increased longevity, more women than men have strokes. Each year, about 40,000 more women than men have strokes. Also, more women than men die of stroke; of every five deaths due to strokes, two are men and three are women.

- About 2 million people have survived a stroke; more than 1 million survivors will have aphasia.

- About 15 percent of the survivors of one or more strokes need institutional care; stroke patients constitute a large number of older people admitted to nursing homes.

- Strokes cause 11 to 12 percent of total mortality; 1 in every 15 deaths is due to stroke. About 163,000 people who have had a stroke die each year; this means that every 3 minutes a death due to stroke occurs. Nearly 62 percent of stroke-related deaths occur in women.

- Ischemic strokes (due to interrupted blood supply) are more common than hemorrhagic (bleeding in the brain) strokes; 88 percent of all strokes are ischemic; 9 percent are intra-cerebral hemorrhage; and 3 percent are subarachnoid hemorrhage.

- Generally, Broca's aphasia is more common in younger patients and Wernicke's aphasia in older patients.

- Generally, the prevalence of Wernicke's and global aphasia is higher in women than in men.

Strokes and aphasia are an expensive health care problem for individual families and the nation. In the past, the annual cost of treating and rehabilitating patients with aphasia exceeded $30 billion; in 2005, the cost is expected to be $57 billion (American Stroke Association, 2005). Because more than 60 percent of stroke patients who could return to work cannot because of their disability, the cost of lost wages and related expenses is enormous.

Prevalence of Aphasia and Associated Diseases in Ethnocultural Groups

The prevalence of aphasia and related diseases varies across ethnocultural groups. Because strokes and related clinical conditions that cause aphasia are associated with aging, various demographic factors of the elderly are relevant to a complete understanding of aphasia and its ethnoculturally appropriate assessment and treatment. Also, the differential prevalence of aphasia in different ethnocultural groups may partly be a function of their varying health and socioeconomic status.

Once again, for the latest statistical data on stroke and heart diseases in various ethnocultural groups, students are encouraged to visit one or more of the Web sites listed in Appendix D. A review of data reported in several sources suggests the following patterns of stroke incidence or prevalence in certain ethnocultural groups (American Heart Association, 2005; Battle, 2002; Horner, Swanson, Bosworth, & Matchar, 2003; Payne, 1997):

- Compared with whites, African Americans have nearly twice the risk of first stroke; the age-adjusted stroke incidence rates per 100,000 persons are 167 for white males, 138 for white females, 323 for African American males, and 260 for African American females (American Heart Association, 2005).

- Death rates due to stroke differ among the major ethnic groups on whom statistics are available. According to 1999–2002 statistics (American Stroke Association, 2005), stroke death rates per 100,000 were 54 for white males, 53 for white females, 82 for African

American males, 72 for African American females; 40 for Hispanics, 40 for American Indians/Alaska Natives, and 52 for Asian/Pacific Islanders. In essence, African American males have the highest death rates due to strokes, and Hispanics and American Indians/Alaska Natives have the lowest.

- In one survey in Corpus Christi, Texas, Mexican Americans had a higher incidence of strokes (168 per 100,000) compared to non-Hispanic whites (136 per 100,000) (National Heart Association, 2005).

- African American women tend to have strokes at an earlier age than white women.

- Women patients with aphasia from all ethnocultural groups combined outnumber all men with aphasia.

- Generally, ischemic attacks, transient attacks, and extracerebral strokes are more common in whites than in other groups.

- Generally, South Asians (people from the Indian subcontinent) living in the United States have a higher incidence of strokes (and heart diseases) than whites.

- Whites have a higher prevalence of ischemic strokes than Hispanics.

- Whites have a higher prevalence of heart diseases than African Americans or Hispanics.

- Native Americans tend to have more hemorrhagic strokes than whites.

- Compared to whites, Hispanics and African Americans tend to have strokes at earlier ages.

- In the age range of 44 to 55 years, more African Americans than whites die of strokes. Black and Hispanic younger adults in the 20–44 age range also have a higher incidence of strokes than whites of similar age.

- African Americans, Asians, and Hispanics are more prone to intracerebral hemorrhagic strokes than whites; these strokes are associated with higher mortality rates.

- The mortality rate from strokes in Hispanics after age 65 is lower than that in whites; this is attributed partly to Hispanic people's lower blood pressure.

- Risk factors for strokes in African Americans, from the highest to the lowest, are high blood pressure, smoking, high cholesterol levels, obesity, poor diet, and lack of exercise.

- Risk factors for Native Americans and Alaska Natives, from the highest to the lowest, are high blood pressure, smoking, lack of exercise, alcohol consumption, diabetes, and malnutrition.

- Risk factors for Hispanics, from the highest to the lowest, are lack of exercise, obesity, eating habits, alcohol, smoking, and high blood pressure.

- Risk factors for Asian and Pacific Islanders, from the highest to lowest, are lack of exercise, smoking, obesity, high-sodium diet, high cholesterol levels, alcohol, high blood pressure, and diabetes.

- The first strokes in African Americans produce more severe effects than they do in whites.

- Regardless of severity levels of their strokes, African Americans require more recovery time to return to normal activities. Eventually, African Americans tend to have lower recovery levels than whites. One reason for this is a lack of social resources, including transportation to the clinics and hospitals and supplemental in-home care, that African Americans experience.

- Increased risk of having strokes in nonwhite persons may partly be due to lack of health care; compared to white males, a higher percentage of nonwhite males report no treatment for such underlying causes as hypertension.

- Disability arising from strokes is greater for African American females and progressively lower for white females, black males, and white males.

- Disabilities due to strokes in Native Americans may often go undiagnosed or untreated.

Reliable data on prevalence of aphasia and related neurologic diseases in ethnocultural groups are limited. Different studies often report contradictory data. White men are more often over-sampled in studies, and women and ethnoculturally diverse groups are typically underrepresented. Therefore, all generalizations about prevalence of aphasia and related diseases in ethnocultural groups must be treated with caution.

Strokes and Aphasia in the Young

Strokes do occur in children although much less frequently than in adults. In a 10-year period, California hospitals admitted 2,278 children who had strokes. In a 4-year period, hospitals in Northern Manhattan treated 74 young patients with stroke (Jacobs, Boden-Albala, Lin, & Sacco, 2002). Generally:

- Boys are about 28 percent more likely than girls to have a stroke.
- As in adults, ischemic strokes are more common in children than are the hemorrhagic strokes.
- Infants (up to 1 year) are more likely to have ischemic strokes whereas teens in the 15–19 age range are more likely to have subarachnoid hemorrhage.
- Stroke risk factors in children are poorly understood although some children who have strokes have a history of head trauma, which is more common in boys than girls. Sickle cell disease is another risk factor in children.
- African American children have a higher risk of stroke than white children. While Asian and white children run the same risk, Hispanic children have the lowest risk for strokes.

Definitions of Aphasia

Definitions of aphasia vary. The varied definitions may be grouped into four categories: nontypological, typological, cognitive, and social. Nontypological definitions deny that there are different types of aphasia and suggest only one kind. Typological definitions suggest types of aphasia. Cognitive definitions define aphasia based primarily on cognitive impairments.

Each approach to defining aphasia is controversial, some more so than others. A disorder studied by different professionals, including neurologists, neuropsychologists, linguists, and speech-language pathologists, is bound to be influenced by varied perspectives.

It is neither possible nor productive to discuss all kinds of definitions of aphasia. It is useful, however, to sample a few definitions whose scope meaning or contrast in some ways and overlap in others.

Nontypological Definitions

Those who offer nontypological definitions of aphasia believe that aphasia is a unitary disorder whose somewhat varied symptoms do not justify a classification into types. In a later section, we will summarize arguments for and against classification.

Schuell, Jenkins, and Jimenez-Pabon (1964) offered an early nontypological definition of aphasia. Their definition of aphasia implies a single disorder:

> A language deficit that crosses all modalities and may be complicated by other sequelae of brain damage. (p. 113)

Darley (1982), another proponent of a nontypological approach, defined aphasia as:

> An impairment, as a result of brain damage, of the capacity for interpretation and formulation of language symbols. (p. 42)

Darley expanded his definition to include the following deficits as parts of the symptom complex:

- Reading, writing, speaking, and comprehension problems
- Deficiency in speaking and understanding language, especially morphemes and large syntactic units
- Language impairment that exceeds impairment of other intellectual functions
- Reduced access to vocabulary
- Impairment in using syntactic rules
- Impaired auditory retention span
- Disturbed input and output channel selection.

Darley's (1982) definition and description make it clear what aphasia is not. He stated that aphasia is not caused by dementia, confusion, sensory loss, or motor dysfunction.

Obviously, neither Darley nor Schuell and her colleagues believe in different types of aphasia. For them, aphasia is a single disorder. Darley and others who contend that different syndrome identification is a useless activity believe that such identification is a result of:

- The varying degrees of severity of aphasia
- Associated neuropathologies and symptoms they produce

Darley asserts that varied severity of language disturbances across patients does not mean there are different types of aphasia. This means, for instance, that although patients with Broca's aphasia may be less fluent than those with Wernicke's aphasia, there is no justification to classify them to different types because the difference is more a matter of degree than the presence or absence of a feature.

Benson and Ardila (1996), while proposing an anatomically based system of classifying aphasia, give a basic, nontypological definition:

Aphasia is the loss or impairment of language caused by brain damage. (p. 3)

Benson and Ardila (1996) believe that aphasia is an overclassified disorder and that the differences in definitions of aphasia are attributable primarily to the varying definitions of *language*. In defining language, some experts include cognition, thought, memory, and even speech; others define it more narrowly. Therefore, even though most specialists agree that the basic nature of aphasia is a disturbance in language due to recent brain injury, there still is much controversy about the scope of disturbances found in patients with aphasia.

There are thus at least two critical views on why there is classification at all. One view holds that the classification is due to paying excessive attention to differential severity levels of symptoms while failing to recognize that all modalities are affected, some to a greater degree than others (Darley, 1982). The other view holds that different ways of conceptualizing language and measuring its disturbances in people with aphasia may give an impression of apparently different types of aphasia.

Typological Definitions

As described in Chapter 1, the classification of aphasia into distinct types dates back to the time of Broca and Wernicke. Historically, types of aphasia have been based on predominant patterns of language disturbances, neuroanatomic loci of lesions, or cognitive functions. Neuroanatomically based classifications seem to have gained greater acceptance than the classifications based on other variables.

Damasio (1981, p. 51) defined aphasia as a "disturbance of one *or* more aspects" of language comprehension, formulation, or expression. The disturbance is caused by a newly acquired disease of the central nervous system.

Note that for Damasio, one *or* more language problems will define aphasia; for Darley, all should be (and actually *are*) present. Damasio's definition is typological in that aphasia could be predominantly receptive or expressive. Note, also, that Damasio's types of aphasia are based on language functions.

Goodglass and Kaplan (1983) offer another typological definition of aphasia. They stated:

> Aphasia refers to the disturbance of any or all of the skills, associations and habits of spoken or written language, produced by injury to certain brain areas that are specialized for these functions. (p. 5)

The Goodglass and Kaplan definition also gives rise to different types of aphasia based on different sets of language symptoms. The definition refers to disturbance in *any or all* skills and thus gives rise to different types, depending on the constellation of disturbances. The definition refers specifically to brain areas that specialize in language functions.

Cognitive Definitions

Some definitions may be distinguished by the importance they place on cognitive impairments in patients with aphasia. These definitions are based on the idea that cognition underlies language and that, if language is impaired, some aspects of cognition also must be impaired.

Murray and Chapey (2001) defined aphasia as:

> An acquired impairment in language production and comprehension and in other cognitive processes that underlie language.

Aphasia is secondary to brain-damage, and is most frequently caused by stroke. (p. 55)

Murray and Chapey refer to such cognitive processes as attention, memory, and thinking that may be affected in aphasia. These processes underlie and interact with language skills. In this sense, the Murray and Chapey definition places an emphasis on cognitive processes that are impaired in aphasia.

Davis (2000) defined aphasia as:

A selective impairment of the cognitive system specialized for comprehending and formulating language, leaving other cognitive capacities relatively intact. (p. 17)

Davis's definition is similar to Darley's except for its emphasis on *impairment of the cognitive system.* Darley's definition implies that intellectual functions underlie language and that these functions may be impaired to a greater extent than other intellectual skills. Nonetheless, Darley's is not a cognitively based definition. For Darley, it is sufficient to define aphasia in terms of language impairments; for cognitivists, it is necessary to make explicit reference to *impaired cognitive processes* that underlie language.

Martin (1981) offered an even more explicit cognitive definition:

Aphasia is the reduction, because of brain damage, of the efficiency of the action and interaction of the cognitive processes that support language. (p. 65)

Martin's definition of aphasia does not place the language impairment in the forefront. Reduced cognitive efficiency takes center stage. It is not clear how definitions such as those by Martin (1981) and Chapey (1981) would help distinguish aphasia from nonaphasic language or communication disorders that are also due to brain damage.

Social Definitions of Aphasia

A group of aphasiologists believe that aphasia is not limited to linguistic or cognitive deficits that figure predominantly, even exclusively, in some definitions.

The disorder has broader ramifications for the individual and his or her family members, professional caregivers, and social acquaintances. It changes the life of the individual and limits social participation. Therefore, some experts include these other, life-altering aspects in their definition of aphasia. For instance, Simmons-Mackie (2001) defines aphasia as an "impairment due to brain damage in the formulation and reception of language, often associated with diminished participation in life events and reduced fulfillment of desired social roles" (p. 248).

Such a broader view of what aphasia is probably applies to almost all serious diseases (e.g., laryngeal cancer), disorders (e.g., stuttering in children and adults or language disorders in children), and developmental disabilities (e.g., mental retardation or autism). These and many similar serious clinical conditions affect the social, personal, educational, and occupational life or goals of individuals. Nonetheless, a social approach to understanding aphasia is valuable because it broadens assessment and treatment concerns and widens the scope of treatment to include social situations, family members, and professional caregivers. The view forces clinicians to go beyond linguistic and cognitive deficits and consider goals of treatment (e.g., social integration of the person with aphasia) that may be overlooked. We will see some of the treatment implications of a more explicitly social view of aphasia in Chapter 9.

Agreement and Disagreement in Defining Aphasia

The varied definitions all suggest that aphasia (1) is a language disorder (2) found in adults (3) who have acquired a recent brain injury. Therefore, there is general consensus on some basic characteristics of aphasia. No definition implies that cerebral damage that occurred in the distant past—although a potential predisposing factor—can cause aphasia. Also, no cerebral pathological conditions with a slow and progressive course that may lead to general intellectual decline and loss of language skills—as in dementia—can lead to aphasia. To be called aphasia, the language disorder should be found in individuals who have reached the typical adult verbal skill level that abruptly declines because of a sudden or fairly sudden onset of cerebral injury. Finally, aphasia is not a motor speech disorder; it is a disorder of language formulation and expression.

Experts and their definitions disagree on mostly two dimensions. First, the need to include statements about cognition as an underlying process of language relates to unresolved theoretical issues regarding the relation between cognition and language. Some believe that it is essential to include a statement about cognition in their definitions of aphasia. Those who define aphasia as a language disorder due to cognitive impairments take a strong position on cognition as a potentially independent process that underlies language. Others who see no such need to speak to cognitive processes think that it is clinically sufficient to define the conditions of cerebral injury and the consequences it produces on verbal skills and interactions.

Second, experts disagree on the nature and extent of language impairment that may lead to a classification of aphasia. Experts generally seem to agree that patients who have aphasia tend to exhibit more or less serious impairments in almost all aspects of oral and written language. Even those who classify aphasia into types recognize that impairments overlap. Therefore, the most common reason for classifying aphasia into types seems to be the degree of severity.

Rosenbek, LaPointe, and Wertz (1989, p. 53) define aphasia as "an impairment, due to acquired and recent damage of the central nervous system, of the ability to comprehend and formulate language." They then go on to say that aphasia is a multimodality disorder, meaning that almost all aspects of communication may be affected. Their definition, in that sense, is not typological and similar to Darley's. But the authors also believe that the severity of aphasic patients' difficulties varies enough to classify them. In other words, some skills are more severely affected than others, giving different patterns of symptoms each with a predominant set of symptoms. Such patterns may be the basis to classify aphasia. It appears that Rosenbek and colleagues support a quantitatively based classification, not a categorical classification.

Each clinician will take a position on classifying or not classifying aphasia into types. To help make this decision, the arguments for and against classifying aphasia are briefly summarized.

The Main Arguments for Classifying Aphasia into Types

The following are among the most frequently cited reasons for classifying aphasia into types.

1. Different brain areas control different language functions.
2. Different types of aphasia have different cerebral sites of lesion.
3. Different lesion sites produce distinctively different syndromes (types of aphasia).
4. Some aphasic patients are more fluent than others.
5. Fluent aphasia is associated with lesions in the posterior region of the sylvian fissure; nonfluent aphasia is related to lesions in the anterior region of the sylvian fissure.
6. Comprehension of spoken language is better in some aphasic patients than in others.
7. Many other aphasic symptoms are dominant in certain patients; therefore, types may be established based on dominant symptoms.
8. Some isolated language skills—repetition, for example—are remarkably preserved in certain patients.
9. Clinical experience supports types of aphasia.
10. Different types of aphasia require different forms of treatment.

It may be noted that the justifications generally fall into two categories: different neuroanatomic sites of lesion and the differing (and dominant) patterns of symptoms.

The Main Arguments Against Classifying Aphasia into Types

The following are among the most frequently cited reasons for treating aphasia as a single entity.

1. The brain functions as an integrated unit in controlling language. Widespread anatomic connections of different parts of the brain suggest that no area functions in isolation.

2. Lesions may be localized, but not necessarily functions. Specific language functions often may be controlled by different areas of the brain in different individuals.

3. Different sites of lesion affect most, if not all, language functions or modalities.

4. A given type of aphasia may be caused by lesions in varied sites.

5. A lesion in a site associated with a particular type of aphasia in some patients may not produce the same type in other patients.

6. Variations in fluency are due to variations in severity of aphasia.

7. Comprehension of spoken language is impaired in all patients, but only to varying degrees.

8. Dominant symptoms do not create syndromes; symptoms that are dominant in one syndrome may be present, though not predominantly, in other syndromes.

9. The appearance of distinct syndromes is created by limited and biased observations that emphasize some symptoms while ignoring others.

10. Aphasia with or without associated problems (such as dysarthria) may give the impression of different types.

11. Longitudinal studies show that aphasic patients who appear different will appear similar later during the course of recovery.

12. The assertion that different syndromes of aphasia require different forms of treatment is not supported.

Some strong arguments against the classification of aphasia come from evidence showing that Broca's aphasia may not be due to damage to Broca's area. Lesions in Broca's area may produce apraxia of speech, not aphasia. However, some neurologists consider apraxic speech a part of Broca's aphasia and contend that pure apraxia is rare (Benson & Ardila, 1996).

Clinicians need to remember the entire range of symptoms found in patients with aphasia, regardless of whether they diagnose aphasia or a type of aphasia. All symptoms are not present in all cases. Symptoms that are present may be striking or subtle.

An Overview of Aphasia

Because typological approaches still dominate the aphasia literature, clinicians and researchers alike need to study them. In subsequent chapters, the major types of aphasia and several atypical varieties will be described. What follows in this section is an overview of some major types of aphasia.

Fluent and Nonfluent Aphasias

An important variable on which patients are grouped into two main types is *fluency of speech.* Some patients have relatively preserved fluency, while other patients have a marked difficulty in producing and sustaining fluent speech. Therefore, in a given patient, aphasia may be classified as either the *fluent* variety or the *nonfluent* variety. Although this classification is based on an aspect of language—fluency—it also is a classification based on anatomic consideration.

Generally, aphasia with fluent but otherwise problematic speech tends to be associated with injury in the posterior portions of the cortex. Aphasia with nonfluent speech tends to be associated with lesions in the frontal regions of the cortex. The rough anatomical division causing nonfluent and fluent aphasias is shown in Figure 4-1.

Many experts currently use this classification (Goodglass & Kaplan, 1983; Rosenbek, et al., 1989), which includes such subtypes as Broca's aphasia and transcortical motor aphasia (two non-

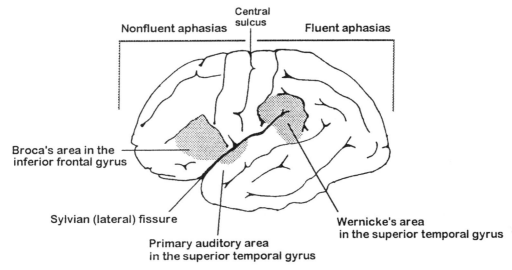

Figure 4-1. Neuroanatomical sites of fluent and nonfluent aphasias.

fluent varieties) and Wernicke's aphasia and transcortical sensory aphasia (two fluent varieties). The different varieties of nonfluent and fluent aphasias are described in Chapters 5 and 6.

Receptive and Expressive Aphasias

In a traditional classification, deficits in language comprehension versus production are the bases to categorize patients. This approach contrasts persons with more severe problems in spoken language *comprehension* against those with problems in language *expression.* Among the several experts who have proposed or used this classification, Weisenburg and McBride (1964) are notable.

This classification, too, is generally correlated with different sites of lesion. More anterior cerebral lesions tend to produce language production problems, whereas more posterior lesions tend to produce comprehension problems. Roughly, nonfluent varieties of aphasia are expressive and fluent varieties are receptive.

Perisylvian, Extrasylvian, and Subcortical Aphasias

An approach to classification based solely on anatomic site of lesion places the fluent and nonfluent aphasias into a single category. Based on this approach, Benson and Ardila (1996) propose three main syndromes of aphasia: perisylvian, extrasylvian, and subcortical aphasias. Each main syndrome has several subtypes.

The term *perisylvian* means areas *surrounding the sylvian fissure.* Recall that such language areas as Broca's and Wernicke's areas are in the vicinity of the sylvian fissure. Therefore, perisylvian aphasia is caused by lesions in the language areas surrounding the sylvian fissure. This syndrome includes Broca's aphasia and Wernicke's aphasia. Figure 4-2 shows the neuroanatomical sites of perisylvian aphasia.

The term *extrasylvian* means *areas beyond the sylvian fissure.* Therefore, extrasylvian aphasia is caused by lesions in areas other than the primary language areas that surround the sylvian fissure. This syndrome includes extrasylvian (transcortical) motor aphasia with anterior lesions and extrasylvian (transcortical) sensory aphasia with posterior lesions. In both cases, the lesion is in the arterial border zones, lying outside the sylvian fissure. Figure 4-3 shows the neuroanatomical sites of extrasylvian aphasia.

Both perisylvian and extrasylvian aphasias are traditionally recognized syndromes of cortical injury or pathological conditions. Research in recent years has shown that injury to subcortical structures, too, can cause aphasia. Subcortical aphasias are a result of injury to or pathological conditions in areas other than

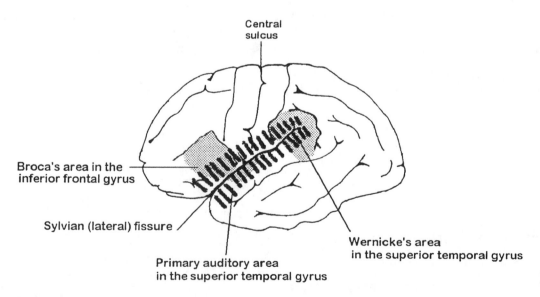

Figure 4-2. Neuroanatomical sites of perisylvian aphasia.

Arterial border zone (watershed)

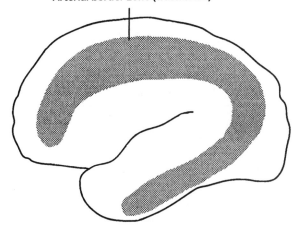

Figure 4-3. Neuroanatomical sites of extra-sylvian asphasia.

cortical structures. Subcortical aphasias are discussed in Chapter 7.

General Symptoms of Aphasia

Most patients with aphasia exhibit a set of common symptoms. A few types of aphasia are distinguished by only a few unique symptoms. Some aphasia varieties are distinguishable by a single feature. For instance, Benson and Ardila's (1996) extrasylvian syndromes are distinguished from perisylvian syndromes by a single dominant feature: patients with extrasylvian syndromes can repeat verbal stimuli whereas those with perisylvian syndromes may have difficulty with this task. Therefore, it is useful to gain an understanding of typical aphasia symptoms before considering specific types of aphasia.

Paraphasia

Paraphasias are errors in speech consisting of unintended word or sound substitutions. Many experts consider paraphasia a central sign of aphasia. There is a bewildering array of terms to classify paraphasia, and different sources give different names to the same kind of problem.

According to one classification, there are different types of paraphasia.

Verbal (Global) Paraphasia

The entire word is substituted in verbal (global) paraphasia. The substituted words may be one of two kinds, leading to two types of verbal paraphasia.

Semantic paraphasia: The substituted word is semantically related (similar in meaning) to the one intended (e.g., *son* for *daughter*).

Random (unrelated) paraphasia: Substituted and intended words are not semantically related (e.g., *window* for *banana*). As such, the paraphasia is unexplainable.

Neologistic Paraphasia

The use of a meaningless, invented word is neologistic paraphasia. Sometimes patients who cannot recall the name of an object may refer to it by their invented, nonsensical term.

Phonemic (Literal) Paraphasia

Substitution of one sound for another (*loman* for *woman*) or addition of a sound (*wolman* for *woman*) is phonemic (literal) paraphasia.

In certain patients, especially those with Wernicke's and conduction aphasia, spontaneous speech may be full of paraphasias. Paraphasias are generally absent in automatic speech (exclamations, cursing, reciting days of the week or number series, etc.).

Phonemic paraphasias are different from the articulatory errors found in patients who have Broca's aphasia and apraxia of speech. The speech errors of the latter two diagnostic categories are *phonetic,* not *phonemic.*

Paraphasia is present to a lesser or greater extent in almost all cases of aphasia. Therefore, it is not a critical factor in identifying specific types of aphasia.

Disorders of Fluency

Fluency is an aspect of language production. Fluent speech flows. It is produced with relatively less effort. It is smooth, devoid of too many interruptions, often described as dysfluencies. Traditionally, the much researched disorder of fluency is stuttering. In the study of aphasia, the terms *fluency* and *fluency disorder* have a slightly different meaning.

Aphasiologists define *fluency* as speech that approximates the normal rate, typical word output, length of sentences, and the melodic contour. Patients who produce five or more connected words may be judged fluent (Rosenbek et al., 1989). When word output is less than 50 words a minute in conversation, fluency is significantly impaired (Benson & Ardila, 1996).

Fluency or lack of it is an important consideration in assessing all patients with aphasia, although fluency is not impaired in all types of aphasia. As noted earlier, fluency is a dimension on which two major syndromes of aphasia (fluent versus nonfluent) have been identified (see Chapters 5 and 6). Patients who are nonfluent (e.g., those who have Broca's aphasia) tend to speak with a degree of muscular effort not seen in normally fluent speakers. Speech may be slow, deliberate, or limited. Their utterances may contain fewer words than normal. Their speech is generally hesitant.

Auditory Comprehension

Most aphasic patients have difficulty understanding spoken language. The degree of impairment varies across patients: Some have a mild problem, others have a profound problem.

- Among the nonfluent patients, those with global and isolation aphasia have moderate to severe impairment in comprehension.
- Among the fluent patients, those with Wernicke's and transcortical sensory aphasia also have moderate to severe problems in comprehension.
- Among the nonfluent, patients with Broca's and transcortical motor aphasia show mild-to-moderate impairment in comprehension.
- Among the fluent patients, those with conduction and anomic aphasia have mild to moderate impairment in comprehension.

TABLE 4-1 Auditory comprehension problems in the major types of aphasia. Note that patients with fluent and nonfluent aphasia may have either poor or good auditory comprehensions.

Poor Auditory Comprehension	Good Auditory Comprehension
Global aphasia (nonfluent)	Broca's aphasia (nonfluent)
Wernicke's aphasia (fluent)	Transcortical motor (nonfluent) aphasia
Transcortical sensory aphasia (fluent)	Conduction aphasia (fluent)
	Anomic aphasia (fluent)

As you can see from this summary, auditory comprehension problems do not distinguish the fluent from the nonfluent. Those problems are present in all types, although the degree varies. However, even the degree of impairment does not distinguish the fluent from the nonfluent patients. Table 4-1 summarizes auditory comprehension problems across the main types of aphasia.

Repetition

Repetition in aphasia literature is a patient's imitation of single words, phrases, and sentences a clinician models. It is an important skill to assess in aphasia, as it is impaired to varying extent in different types of aphasia. Impaired repetition is the dominant symptom of conduction aphasia, a fluent variety described in Chapter 6. And to the contrary, relatively intact repetition skills are a distinguishing feature of transcortical motor aphasia, a nonfluent variety described in Chapter 5.

Generally, repetition errors are more frequent or more severe in cases of impaired auditory comprehension (e.g., in patients with Wernicke's aphasia). Nonetheless, patients with transcortical sensory aphasia, who have relatively poor auditory comprehension, may have good repetition skills.

Similarly, some patients with good auditory comprehension may exhibit poor repetition skills. For instance, patients with Broca's aphasia cannot repeat because of impaired production, not comprehension. Hence, patients with different types of aphasia may demonstrate the same problem for different reasons. The repetition skills of major aphasia types are summarized in Table 4-2.

TABLE 4-2 Impairment of repetition skills in the major types of aphasia. Note that patients with fluent and nonfluent aphasia may have either relatively poor or better repetition skills.

Poor Repetition	Good Repetition
Broca's aphasia (nonfluent)	Broca's aphasia (nonfluent)
Wernicke's aphasia (fluent)	Transcortical motor (nonfluent) aphasia
Conduction aphasia (fluent)	Transcortical sensory aphasia (fluent)

Anomia

Anomia is difficulty in naming or finding correct words during verbal expression. Anomia typically is a symptom of aphasia, whereas anomic aphasia is a separate syndrome. Word-finding and naming problems are a common symptom of aphasia. Even those who recover from aphasia tend to retain some naming problems.

Naming problems become evident in different kinds of verbal exchanges. Naming problems may become evident in **confrontation naming,** or naming in response to a verbal demand (e.g., "What is this?"). The problem may also become evident in *word fluency* tasks, or naming as many items of a certain category as possible (e.g., "name as many California cities as you can"). Many patients may find confrontation naming easier than word fluency tasks.

Other factors that influence naming include word frequency and the semantic category to which the words to be recalled belong. Words that are of low frequency in everyday language (e.g., *perimeter*) may be more difficult to recall than words that are of high frequency. Although no particular semantic category is universally difficult for all patients, some may have pronounced difficulty with certain kinds of words. For instance, names of animals or vegetables may be especially difficult for some patients.

Because anomia is a general problem found in most patients with aphasia, it is not especially useful in distinguishing the different types. When *anomia* is the name for a special type of aphasia, persistent and severe word-finding and naming difficulty is the dominant, if not the only, problem. There is more about anomia—the type of aphasia—in Chapter 6.

Writing Problems

Writing problems associated with cerebral lesions in adults are called **agraphia.** Most, if not all, patients with aphasia have some level of impairment in their writing skills (Rosenbek et al., 1989). Hence, these problems do not distinguish different types of aphasia. The writing problems of patients with aphasia are called *aphasic agraphia.* There are several other varieties of agraphia, including pure agraphia, apraxic agraphia, and motor agraphia. These other varieties are described in Chapter 7.

Aphasic agraphia includes a variety of writing problems. Generally, the writing problems reflect the problems seen in oral communication. For instance, agrammatic, effortful, sparse speech output of Broca's aphasia is reflected in agrammatic, effortful, and sparse writing. Collectively, patients who have aphasia may write with poor letter and word formation. They may reverse, confuse, or substitute letters. There may be more errors in writing less frequently used words. Unsuccessful attempts at self-correction during writing may be common. Some words they write may be nonsensical. Errors of spelling are frequent. In the most severely impaired persons, writing may be totally unreadable.

The writing problems just described may be found in slightly different patterns, depending on the type of aphasia. Table 4-3 summarizes major writing problems associated with the main aphasia types. The table also lists the parallel language problems to show the relation between the spoken and written problems within each type of aphasia.

Reading Problems

A variety of reading problems are associated with aphasia. Some people have difficulty reading because of verbal expression problems. Others can orally or silently read printed passages but may understand little or nothing of what is read.

The terms *alexia* and *dyslexia* generally refer to reading problems. Some experts use the terms *alexia* and *dyslexia* interchangeably (Rosenbek et al., 1989; Webb, 1997). Others, especially medical specialists, define dyslexia as reading problems found in children (*Dorland's Illustrated Medical Dictio-*

TABLE 4-3 Major writing problems associated with the main aphasia types. Note that for most aphasia types, the writing problems parallel the language problems.

Type of Aphasia	Writing	Spoken Language
Broca's aphasia	Omission of grammatic elements (agrammatic writing) and letters, sparse and effortful writing, abbreviated phrases and sentences, clumsy letter formation, and poor spelling.	Agrammatic, effortful, sparse speech; poor articulation, short phrase length, and poor oral spelling.
Wernicke's aphasia	Easy and effortless writing, well-formed letters, incorrect combination or omission of letters resulting in neologistic writing, normal phrase and sentence lengths, word substitutions (paraphasic writing). Agrammatic writing of Broca's aphasia is uncommon.	Easy, effortless, fluent, normally articulated speech and language production filled with word paraphasia and neologistic, jargon-filled speech.
Transcortical motor aphasia	Clumsy and sparse writing with frequent misspellings; generally similar to the writing problems of patients with Broca's aphasia.	Sparse speech output; limited phrase and sentence length; generally nonfluent.
Transcortical sensory aphasia	Paraphasic writing with frequent misspelling; somewhat comparable to the writing problems of Wernicke's aphasia.	Paraphasic, abundant, prosodically normal speech output; generally similar to the speech and language of Wernicke's patients.
Conduction aphasia	Slow and effortful writing; letter omission, substitutions, and additions; poor spelling; generally intact grammar.	Paraphasic, fluent speech with impaired repetition skills.
Global aphasia	Severe writing problems; unintelligible writing; only a few letters and strokes may be preserved.	Severely impaired oral language skills; only a few words may be uttered.

nary, 28th ed., 1994). In this sense, dyslexia creates difficulty in acquiring reading skills. On the other hand, alexia is defined as "only the loss of ability to *comprehend* written language" (Benson & Ardila, 1996, p. 97; italics added) found in persons with good premorbid reading skills following brain injury or pathology.

Reading and writing problems often coexist in aphasia, although rare cases of *pure alexia* with only reading difficulty have been reported. Such atypical varieties of aphasia and related reading and writing problems are described in Chapter 7.

In reading, severely affected patients with aphasia exhibit a variety of difficulties. Some patients may not recognize the printed word at all. Many struggle to read and read aloud with many errors. Patients may read sentences word by word. A fairly common difficulty may be a failure to understand what is read fully or partially. Please see Chapter 7 for additional information on the classification and neuropathological factors associated with reading (and writing) deficits.

Gestures

Understanding or using gestures and pantomime in communication often is disturbed in aphasic patients. The disturbance is not entirely a function of any motor deficit (e.g., paresis or paralysis of hands) that may exist in a patient with aphasia. Impaired understanding of gestures and pantomime may reveal a difficulty in dealing with symbols used in communication, just as the difficulty shows in understanding and using verbal language.

Aphasic patients may have difficulty imitating specific gestures (such as those of the American Sign Language). Sign language users who become aphasic exhibit many difficulties in their sign expression that parallel verbal deficits found in oral language users who become aphasic. Please see Chapter 7 for a description of aphasia in sign language users.

Residual Language Performance

Across individuals, severity of aphasia varies significantly. The globally aphasic individuals have the most serious impairment in communication skills. Many patients, though, retain some communicative skills, even if they are somewhat rudimentary.

Many patients who are otherwise severely impaired may distinguish their native language from a foreign language, meaningful utterances from the nonsensical, nouns from verbs when stress is the clue (CON vict versus con VICT), and grammatical sentences from the nongrammatical. In addition, such patients may:

- Guess the first letter or the size (big, small) of the word they cannot say.
- Repeat (imitate) more words from grammatical sentences than from ungrammatical sentences.
- Produce more frequently used than the less frequently used words.
- Learn alternative modes of communication, such as gesturing, signing, or drawing.

A General Description of How Aphasic Patients Communicate

Although specific symptom complexes are associated with different types of aphasia (see Chapters 6 and 7), it is helpful to gain a general understanding of how aphasic patients talk. Due to the various symptoms described so far, the speech of most aphasic patients can be characterized as follows:

- Aphasic patients speak either little with some struggle or abundantly with ease, but without much meaning or grammar. Communication is either sparse and meaningful or abundant but full of meaningless jargon.
- When they begin to speak, most patients cannot find the words at all or the right words, resulting in a slow, halting speech. Some who cannot find words may invent meaningless "words" with better speech flow.
- In addition to invented (neologistic) words, patients may substitute sounds in words or substitute wrong or less specific words for correct or precise terms.
- Patients may omit sounds within words or whole words. However, serious articulation disorders are usually due to a coexisting dysarthria or apraxia of speech.
- Most patients may use some form of coping strategies: use a word similar in sound or

meaning, delay response so they can think of the word, try to get the word by semantic or phonemic association, or explain or describe what they are trying to say.

- With a limited range and variety of vocabulary, patients may repeat themselves or hesitate during speaking.
- Patients may have limited range and types of grammatical sentences. The utterance length may be limited, and the word order may be wrong. Some aphasic patients may produce only disjointed, brief, telegraphic utterances. They may misuse morphological elements of language or not use them at all.
- They may talk with stereotyped expressions. The patients may repeat the same utterance containing real or invented words for any type of question.
- They may not correctly repeat what they hear, especially the longer utterances, although some patients may be especially good at repetition.
- Patients may exhibit circumlocution in their speech talking in vague terms.
- Some patients may be unaware that listeners do not understand them, and they may deny that they have a communicative problem.
- Generally, the patients may have language comprehension deficits. The degree of deficit may be mild, moderate, or severe.
- Some patients may have difficulty pointing to a picture or object named.
- Some patients may give the impression that they are deaf to words ("word deafness") or say that they do not know the meaning of ordinary words. They may misunderstand words that are similar in meaning or sound.
- Patients may omit details when retelling a story. They may have difficulty with order or sequence of events in their narrations.

In spite of their communication deficits, most aphasic persons are willing to talk. Only in the first few hours of a stroke are some patients unable to make attempts at speech. Unlike patients with traumatic brain injury or dementia, patients with aphasia are generally alert and know what is going on around them. These characteristics may change, however. As the recovery slows or stops and complicating diseases or additional strokes result in physical deterioration, patients may be depressed and unwilling to talk.

What Aphasia IS Not

The age range in which aphasia is most common also is associated with several other forms of communication disorders. These other forms of communication disorders may be confused with aphasia. Therefore, it is important to distinguish them from aphasia and from each other.

Dementia

Dementia is a progressive neurological disease in which communicative and cognitive skills, along with social and personal behaviors, continue to deteriorate. The most common form of dementia is associated with Alzheimer's disease. Along with multiple brain damage, other neurological diseases, including Pick's disease and Parkinson's disease, also cause dementia.

Slow onset and general intellectual deficits and problems in abstract thinking are associated with dementia. In contrast, aphasia has a sudden onset and is not associated with general intellectual deterioration. Aphasia does not lead to behavioral deterioration (personality change) seen in dementia. The language or speech of individuals with dementia does not share many of the features of aphasia.

We will learn more about dementia in Chapters 14, 15, and 16 and about differential diagnosis of aphasia and dementia in Chapter 8.

Confused Language

Some neurological patients exhibit what is called the **language of confusion,** which is a pattern of language resulting from bilateral, traumatic brain injury. The common causes of confused language include automobile accidents, intoxication, metabolic or chemical imbalances, and central nervous system diseases.

The characteristics of confused patients include the following:

- Confused patients do not seem to be aware of their surroundings. While lying in the dull neurological ward, they may think they are walking the streets of Paris. The patients are disorientated to space and time.
- The patients tend to misidentify people and misinterpret events.
- They may have impaired memory for recent events.
- The patients often cannot follow conversation. Although unable to answer open-ended questions, the patients can answer simple questions, name objects, and read words and sentences. Their vocabulary and syntax may be normal.
- The patients tend to confabulate. For instance, when questioned "What did you do today?" a confused hospitalized patient answered: "In the morning I went on a cruise. Later I cleaned my bathroom. I talked to the president." Most patients are unaware of their bizarre, inappropriate, and confabulated responses.
- The patients have typically fluent and well-articulated speech with normal intonation. For example, when asked "What should every good citizen do?" a confused patient replied, "He should build on the right side. He should build on the left side. And he should build on the west side" (Darley, 1982, p. 25).

Irrelevant, confabulated, but syntactically correct fluent speech distinguishes the language of the confused from that of the aphasic patient. General disorientation to time, space, and person further distinguishes the confused patient from a patient with aphasia who is typically alert and aware of the surroundings. Although confused language may resemble that of Wernicke's patients, there are important differences. For instance, the confused patient shows much better auditory comprehension and better orientation to surroundings.

Confusion is often transient. When the effects of temporary metabolic disturbances and head injury clear up and the patient's physical condition improves, confusion is likely to subside.

See Chapter 8 for differential diagnosis of aphasia and confused language.

Schizophrenia

Schizophrenia is a serious psychiatric disorder characterized by disordered thought, affect, and behavior. Schizophrenic patients show irrelevant speech, but they also show a greater degree of disturbed thinking that suggests a disassociation from reality. The hallucinations, inappropriate affect, disturbed or even violent behavior, withdrawal from reality, mood changes, and regressive behaviors of schizophrenic patients clearly distinguish them from other patients. The language of the schizophrenic may be inappropriate to the question asked, appropriate in syntax, but obscured in meaning. Listening, reading, and writing skills of patients with schizophrenia may be better than those in patients with aphasia.

Schizophrenia is typically diagnosed earlier in life than most cases of aphasia. Generally, the onset of schizophrenia is more gradual than aphasia. The overall behavioral disturbances seen in schizophrenia are absent in aphasia. See Chapter 8 for differential diagnosis of schizophrenia from aphasia.

Neurogenic Speech Disorders

Neurologic diseases and trauma also may cause speech disorders, in contrast with language disorders. *Apraxia of speech* and *dysarthria* are neurogenic speech disorders, contrasted with aphasia, a neurogenic language disorder. Apraxia of speech may coexist with aphasia. In **apraxia,** the patient has difficulty in producing speech with normal articulation and prosody, but there is no muscle weakness or paralysis. Apraxia of speech is thought to be due to a speech motor planning deficit.

Dysarthria is a neurogenic speech disorder associated with weakness, slowness, or incoordination in the speech muscles and affects all basic processes of speech: respiration, phonation, articulation, and prosody. Dysarthria also may coexist with aphasia, especially with subcortical aphasia. Some patients with Broca's aphasia also may exhibit dysarthria as a separate disorder.

See Chapter 8 for differential diagnosis of aphasia from apraxia of speech and dysarthria.

Suggested Readings

Read the following (or visit the listed Web site) for additional information on the prevalence, definition, and classification of aphasia:

American Stroke Association: http://www.strokeassociation.org

Basso, A. (2003). *Aphasia and its therapy.* New York: Oxford University Press.

Benson, D. F., & Ardila, A. (1996). *Aphasia: A clinical perspective.* New York: Oxford University Press.

Davis, G. A. (2000). *Aphasiology: Disorders and clinical practice.* Needham Heights, MA: Allyn & Bacon.

Goodglass, H. (1993). *Understanding aphasia.* San Diego, CA: Academic Press.

Goodglass, H., Kaplan, E., & Barresi, B. (2001). *The assessment of aphasia and related disorders* (3rd ed.). Philadelphia: Lippincott Williams & Wilkins.

LaPointe, L. L. (Ed.) (2005). *Aphasia and related neurogenic language disorders* (3rd ed.). New York: Thieme Medical Publishers.

Murray, L. L., & Chapey, R. (2001). Assessment of language disorders in adults. In R. Chapey (Ed.), *Language intervention strategies in adult aphasia* (4th ed., pp. 55–126). Baltimore, MD: Williams & Wilkins.

Payne, J. C. (1997). *Adult neurogenic language disorders: Assessment and treatment.* San Diego, CA: Singular Publishing Group.

CHAPTER V

ETIOLOGY AND SYMPTOMATOLOGY OF NONFLUENT APHASIAS

Chapter Outline

- Four Types of Nonfluent Aphasias
- Fluency in Aphasiology
- Broca's Aphasia
- Transcortical Motor Aphasia (TMA)
- Mixed Transcortical Aphasia (MTA)
- Global Aphasia

Learning Objectives

After reading the chapter, the student will:

- Describe the concept of fluency in aphasiology.
- Describe the neuropathology of all non-fluent aphasias.
- Describe the neurological symptoms of nonfluent aphasias.

- Describe the language characteristics of nonfluent aphasias.
- Distinguish the four types of nonfluent aphasias based on neuropathology, neurological symptoms, and positive and negative language characteristics.

Four Types of Nonfluent Aphasias

As noted in Chapter 4, *fluency* of speech is a criterion for distinguishing two main syndromes of aphasia: the nonfluent and fluent aphasias. We will describe fluent aphasias in Chapter 6. In this unit, the following four types of nonfluent aphasias are described:

- Broca's aphasia
- Transcortical motor aphasia
- Mixed transcortical aphasia
- Global aphasia

Fluency in Aphasiology

That fluency is a characteristic of verbal (and nonverbal) communication is well known. In speech-language pathology, disorders of fluency are a recognized clinical entity. Historically, the most prominent and researched disorder of fluency is **stuttering,** which is characterized by excessive amounts or durations of dysfluencies (Bloodstein, 1995). **Cluttering** is another disorder of fluency that is characterized by excessively fast rate and increased number of dysfluencies. **Neurogenic stuttering** is a relatively recently researched fluency disorder found in some patients with cerebral diseases or trauma; neurogenic stuttering may or may not be associated with aphasia (Helm-Estabrooks, 1986). Added to this list is the impaired fluency of patients with aphasia.

The very concept of fluency and its impairment have somewhat different meanings in the traditional study of fluency disorders (as in stuttering) and in the study of aphasia. A main difference is that *dysfluencies* in speech are important in the study of stuttering and other fluency disorders whereas they are of little importance in the study of aphasia.

Speech fluency in aphasia is characterized by:

- Flowing speech produced with minimal or no effort. Fluent speech has a normal flow and is not associated with unusual effort.

- Normal or even increased rate of speech. Maintenance of a certain rate of speech is essential to maintain fluency.
- Normal melodic properties. Fluent speech has certain intonation patterns and melodic contour.
- Easily initiated speech. Fluent speech is easily provoked by stimulating social conditions.
- Normal amount of speech. Fluent speech should say enough (neither too little nor too much) to meet the social demands of communication.

The effect of the presence or absence of dysfluencies is not noted in the typical description of fluency in literature on aphasia. Fluency is mostly defined in terms of the degree of effort, the rate of production, the properties of intonation, the promptness of initiation, and the amount of speech production.

Nonfluency in aphasia is characterized by:

- Reduced speech rate (less than 50 wpm). An excessively slow rate of speech may give the impression of impaired fluency.
- Excessive speaking effort. Nonfluent speech is associated with struggle, facial grimaces, hand gestures, and other behaviors that suggest increased muscular effort.
- Limited phrase length. Nonfluent speech is unusually brief, limited in both length and complexity.
- Abnormal prosody. The typical patterns of intonation and rhythm may be absent in nonfluent speech. The speech may be monotonous or choppy.
- Generally depressed amount of speech. In light of the social demands of communication, the amount of speech offered may be judged too little. Answers to questions may be extremely brief.
- Speech initiated with notable difficulty. With appropriate stimulus conditions, speech is initiated with great ease. Nonfluent speech, on the other hand, requires additional or unusual stimuli to get the speech initiated. In essence, nonfluent speech is not as spontaneous as fluent speech.

• Excessive use of content words and omission of function words. Nonfluent speech contains an abundance of nouns and verbs (content words) while omitting grammatic morphemes (function words). The burden of communication is on the function words.

Generally, fluency is impaired in patients with lesions in the anterior parts of the brain. Those with lesions in the posterior parts of the brain retain fluency the best (see Figure 4-1 in Chapter 4 for this anatomical distinction).

Broca's Aphasia

Broca first described a form of nonfluent aphasia in 1861. Other names for the same syndrome include *expressive aphasia, central motor aphasia, anterior aphasia, efferent motor aphasia, agrammatic aphasia, syntactic aphasia,* and *verbal aphasia.* Benson and Ardila (1996) describe it as a variety of *perisylvian aphasic syndrome* because it is associated with damage to cerebral language areas surrounding the sylvian fissure but not extending to Wernicke's area.

Although the term **Broca's aphasia** is widely used to describe a nonfluent, effortful, and agrammatic type of language production that is generally meaningful, it is a controversial type of aphasia (Donnan, Carey, & Saling, 1999). Its symptom complex and neuroanatomical basis are both open to debate. This debate raises further questions about the localizationist or connectionist view of aphasia.

Broca's description of a language problem in a man called LeBorgne was the basis for this type of aphasia. Broca called the disorder *aphemia. Aphasia,* a term Trousseau suggested in 1864, came to be preferred over *aphemia.*

Neuroanatomical Bases of Broca's Aphasia

As noted in Chapter 2, the posterior-inferior (third) frontal gyrus of the left hemisphere is known as **Broca's area** (Brodmann's area 44, which may extend to parts of area 45). The area is also known as the *anterior language cortex*. Generally, it is the area supplied by the upper division of the middle cerebral artery. Broca's area is in the lower part of the premotor cortex that controls the movements of face, hand, and arm (Bhatnagar, 2000; Love & Web, 2001; Webster, 1999). Damage to this area may be involved in Broca's aphasia. Figure 5-1 shows the primary and the potential secondary cortical areas that may be involved in Broca's aphasia.

Broca's aphasia is controversial for several reasons. Computer axial tomography (CAT) studies, positron emission tomography (PET) studies, and a critical review of literature (e.g., see Mohr, 1980) show that involvement of Broca's area is neither sufficient nor necessary to produce what is typically described as Broca's aphasia (Damasio, 2001; Kearns, 2005). For instance:

- The lower portion of the motor strip (beyond Broca's area) may be involved.
- The areas anterior and inferior to area 44 may be affected. Again, areas other than Broca's area may be involved.
- Deep cortical damage (not a part of Broca's area) is necessary to produce Broca's aphasia. In essence, Broca's patients have more extensive cortical damage than originally thought.
- Instead of aphasia, damage limited to Broca's area is more likely to produce transient mutism and subsequent mild apraxia. Thus, damage

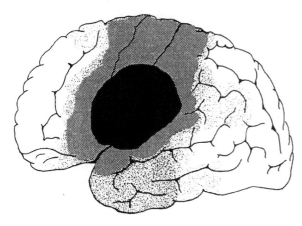

Figure 5-1. Neuroanatomical sites of Broca's aphasia. The darker area is the primary site of lesion in most cases; lighter shading shows other areas that may be involved.

limited to Broca's aphasia may not produce the syndrome with which it is associated.

- Portions of frontal, temporal, and parietal regions may be involved in producing symptoms often grouped under Broca's aphasia.

- Even Wernicke's area may be involved in Broca's aphasia.

- Patients with Broca's aphasia without damage to Broca's area may be observed. Thus, damage to Broca's area is not necessary to produce what is called Broca's aphasia.

- Some patients with injured Broca's area may have transcortical motor aphasia. Thus, in addition to producing apraxia, damage to Broca's area may produce a *different type* of aphasia.

- PET studies show that almost all aphasia patients show cerebral hypometabolism in widespread cerebral areas. Therefore, lesions alone do not explain the observed language deficits. Reduced capacity of unaffected areas also may contribute to functional deficits.

General Characteristics of Broca's Aphasia

- Neurologically, Broca's patients are more easily recognized than Wernicke's patients. Typically, Broca's patients present a contralateral (right-sided) hemiplegia[1] or hemiparesis[2] because damage to Broca's area is likely to damage the descending pyramidal tracts that run alongside that area. Weakness of muscles on the right side of the face may be evident. Patients may initially be confined to a wheelchair. In contrast, such motor problems are absent in patients with Wernicke's aphasia (Benson & Ardila, 1996; Kearns, 2005; Wertz, 1996).

- Later, patients with Broca's aphasia may use a walker or a cane. Leg and foot muscles regain functions faster than those of the hand and arm. Most motor problems improve over time.

---

[1] Paralysis of one side of the body.
[2] Muscular weakness of one side of the body. Contrasted with paralysis.

- Often depressed, Broca's patients may react emotionally when they fail on assessment tasks. Exhibiting what are called *catastrophic reactions,* patients may weep and refuse to continue or cooperate during testing and assessment.

Major Language Characteristics of Broca's Aphasia

The halting and effortful language production of patients with Broca's aphasia includes the following major characteristics (Benson & Ardila, 1996; Davis, 2000; Kearns, 2005):

- *Nonfluent and effortful speech.* The speech is filled with many pauses, interjected sounds (e.g., "*uh*"), revisions, sound and syllable prolongations, and repetitions.
- *Agrammatic speech.* Also called *telegraphic speech,* agrammatic speech is typically limited to content words (nouns and verbs) that carry the major burden of communication. The patient may omit such grammatical (function) words as articles, conjunctions, auxiliary verbs (e.g., *is, are, was, were*), copulas, prepositions, and inflections (e.g., plural and possessive forms, past tense *ed*). In essence, grammatical morphemes may be absent in speech.
- *Slow rate with uneven flow.* The frequent pauses disrupt the flow of speech and create an unnatural rhythm.
- *Limited word output and reduced length of utterances.* The speech may often be limited to just a few words and few word combinations. Phrase length may be limited and sentences tend to be short.
- *Impaired repetition of words and sentences.* When the clinician models words and sentences, the patient may be unable to imitate (repeat) them. Repetition of grammatical elements of a sentence (e.g., an article or an auxiliary verb in a sentence) may be especially missing in the patient's repetition. For instance, when asked to repeat the sentence *the boy is walking,* the patient may repeat *boy walk.*

- *Impaired confrontation naming.* This skill refers to naming an object, a picture, or a person when asked to do so. Typically, the clinician shows a stimulus and asks, "What is this?" Patients with Broca's aphasia have difficulty naming when such demands are made. Various cueing techniques (see Chapter 9 for details) often help them name the stimulus shown.

- *Some impairment in auditory comprehension.* Although patients with nonfluent aphasias have better auditory comprehension of spoken language than those with fluent aphasia, patients with Broca's aphasia rarely have completely normal comprehension of language. Although patients with Broca's aphasia comprehend language better than they produce it, their comprehension deficits are clinically significant. When asked to point to objects named in sequence, patients with Broca's aphasia may have marked difficulty. Striking difficulty also may be noted when the patients are asked to respond in such a way as to distinguish between relational words (e.g., *bigger/smaller*). Furthermore, patients may have difficulty understanding syntactic structures or meaning implied in word order. For instance, the patients may fail to distinguish the meaning of such phrases as *my sister's husband* versus *my husband's sister* even though they understand the meaning of individual words involved. The patients are especially likely to exhibit difficulty understanding grammatical morphemes they omit from their speech.

- *Generally poor oral reading.* The oral reading of patients with Broca's aphasia is effortful and nonfluent, just as their verbal expression is. Patients may have impaired comprehension of material they read. Comprehension may be limited to substantive words.

- *Writing problems.* Patients may write slowly, laboriously, and with many spelling errors and letter omissions. Letters may be poorly formed. Writing, similar to their verbal expression, may be agrammatic. They may write mostly with substantive words, omitting grammatic features. Some of the difficulty may possibly be due to their use of the nonpreferred left hand because of a paralysis of the right hand. However, their writing errors seem to exceed what might be expected from their nonpreferred hand use.

- *Monotonous speech.* Lack of intonation and other prosodic deficits may be a consequence of halting, dysfluent, arrhythmic speech that is articulated with unusual amount of effort.

See Table 5-1 for a summative overview of major language characteristics of patients with Broca's aphasia.

TABLE 5-1   The major language characteristics of patients with Broca's aphasia.

Language Parameter	In Broca's Aphasia	Positive ($+\sqrt{}$) or Negative ($-\sqrt{}$) Diagnostic Feature	Contrasted With
Speech comprehension	Better than expression; some degree of deficiency in most patients	$-\sqrt{}$	Wernicke's aphasia
Fluency	Severely impaired; agrammatic, telegraphic, dysprosodic	$+\sqrt{}$	Wernicke's aphasia
Grammar	Impaired; agrammatic	$+\sqrt{}$	Wernicke's aphasia
Paraphasia	Not a major feature	$-\sqrt{}$	
Naming	Impaired	$+\sqrt{}$	
Articulation	Impaired; possibly associated dysarthria and apraxia	$+\sqrt{}$	
Pointing	Good for single stimuli; impaired for serial tasks	$-\sqrt{}$	
Repetition	Impaired, especially for grammatic features	$+\sqrt{}$	
Reading aloud	Impaired	$+\sqrt{}$	
Reading comprehension	Impaired to some extent	$+\sqrt{}$	
Writing	Impaired	$+\sqrt{}$	
Classification	Nonfluent aphasia		
Lesion site	Broca's area (posterior-inferior frontal gyrus of the left hemisphere); other sites, including deep cortical damage, may be involved; damage limited to Broca's area may not produce Broca's aphasia.		

Associated Speech Problems

Broca's aphasia often is associated with extensive brain damage, especially in the vicinity of motor speech areas. Consequently, speech disorders that are due to central or peripheral neuropathological factors, called *motor speech disorders,* may coexist with Broca's aphasia. Therefore, Broca's aphasia may be associated with:

- *Apraxia of speech.* A neurogenic speech disorder, apraxia of speech is difficulty in motor planning of speech. It is characterized by a difficulty in initiating articulation, effortful articulation, groping articulatory movements, and articulatory inconsistency in the absence of speech musculature weakness or paralysis. Some patients may recite days of the week or month on their own without much difficulty; but the same patients may struggle with the same task when asked to perform. To some extent, the nonfluent and effortful speech of patients with Broca's aphasia may be due to their apraxia.

- *Dysarthria.* Another neurogenic speech disorder, dysarthria is caused by muscular weakness that affects respiratory, phonatory, articulatory, resonance, and prosodic features of speech. Dysarthria reduces speech intelligibility. Patients with Broca's aphasia usually have a mild form of dysarthria. Nonetheless, in combination with apraxia of speech, dysarthria may produce a notable effect on speech production and intelligibility.

It should be emphasized that apraxia and dysarthria are motor speech disorders, whereas aphasia is a language disorder associated with recently acquired cerebral damage. When they are present, apraxia and dysarthria are independent problems that coexist with aphasia. The diagnosis of aphasia does not depend on the presence of motor speech disorders.

Individual Differences in Patients with Broca's Aphasia

Because of varied neuropathology in patients diagnosed with Broca's aphasia, differences in symptom complexes across patients are especially noteworthy.

Some say just a few words; others can carry on limited conversation. Language comprehension may be good enough to carry on a basic conversation or may be impaired to a notable degree.

In some patients, even the fluency impairment—the hallmark of Broca's aphasia—may only be mild. Agrammatism may be marked or negligible. By and large, expressive skills may be more impaired than receptive skills.

Based on the severity of symptoms, extent of the underlying cerebral damage, and patterns of recovery, Benson and Ardila (1996) classify Broca's aphasia into type I and type II. In type I Broca's aphasia, the damage is limited to the cortex and immediate subcortical structures. The symptoms of type I Broca's aphasia may be limited to mild articulation and word-finding problems. Agrammatism, if present, may be mild as well. Recovery may be very good.

Broca's type II aphasia is more persistent and more severe and involves extensive cerebral damage, extending deep into the white matter. Symptoms include dysarthria and severe agrammatism, and the extent of recovery is somewhat limited by deep and extensive lesions.

Relative Strengths of Patients with Broca's Aphasia

A description of the language and speech characteristics of patients with Broca's aphasia may imply that their communication skills are seriously compromised. While that may occur in some cases, most patients with Broca's aphasia— unlike patients with Wernicke's aphasia—generally communicate well, even if they manage to communicate the most essential elements. In other words, the agrammatic and telegraphic speech of patients with Broca's aphasia can still express the basic meaning, as does an agrammatic telegram.

Patients who are confused may exhibit irrelevant speech, but those with Broca's aphasia are generally relevant in their responses. Their speech, no matter how limited or agrammatic, is meaningful, relevant to the question asked, and socially appropriate. Unlike patients with Wernicke's aphasia, those with Broca's are aware of their speech difficulty. They try to self-correct, even if their efforts are not successful. They exhibit the normal reactions of frustration at their failure to communicate.

Patients with Broca's aphasia are usually cooperative during assessment and treatment. Most patients are task-oriented.

Transcortical Motor Aphasia (TMA)

Transcortical motor aphasia is another variety of nonfluent aphasia in which repetition skills are well preserved. Its other names include *dynamic aphasia* and *isolation syndrome.* Both Wernicke and German physician Ludwig Lichtheim (1845–1928) suggested the term *transcortical motor aphasia,* which has gained acceptance.

Benson and Ardila (1996) describe transcortical motor aphasia as a form of *extrasylvian aphasic syndromes* because the neuropathological factors lie outside the perisylvian language zones. There is nothing truly *transcortical* about transcortical aphasia, but it is an established term to describe a type of nonfluent aphasia with good repetition (Benson & Ardila, 1996; Cimino-Knight, Hollingsworth, & Gonzalez Rothi, 2005; Helm-Estabrooks & Albert, 2004).

Neuroanatomical Bases of TMA

The lesions causing TMA are usually outside Broca's area. Most often, the anterior superior frontal lobe is involved. The lesions often are found in deep portions of the left frontal lobe or below or above Broca's area. The most common sites of TMA are shown in Figure 5-2.

Other observations about the neuroanatomical basis of TMA include the following:

- Lesions often affect *association pathways.* Such pathways connect perisylvian regions with other cerebral regions. Generally, damage to anterior superior frontal lobe is associated with TMA.
- Supplemental motor areas may be involved. To highlight the importance of this involvement, the term *supplemental motor area apha-*

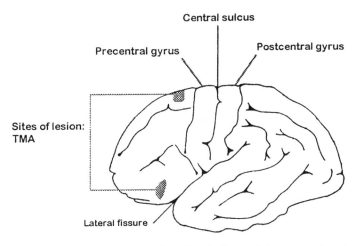

Figure 5-2. Neuroanatomical sites of transcortical motor aphasia. The two common sites of lesions are identified.

sia has been suggested. It is thought that lesions may separate the supplemental motor cortex[3] from Broca's area.

- The areas supplied by the anterior cerebral artery and the anterior branch of the middle cerebral artery are affected. The watershed region between the middle cerebral and anterior arteries often is involved.

- Head trauma with frontal lobe damage, tumors, herpetic encephalitis, and progressive neurological diseases affecting the frontal lobe also may cause TMA.

General Characteristics of TMA

In most respects, TMA is similar to Broca's aphasia. The neurological deficits may vary across patients. General characteristics of patients with TMA include (Benson & Ardila, 1996; Cimino-Knight, Hollingsworth, & Gonzalez Rothi, 2005):

- *Motor disorders.* Rigidity of upper extremity, akinesia (absence or poverty of movement), and bradykinesia (slowness of movement) may be seen to varying extents in patients, especially soon after the onset of aphasia. Hemiparesis (leg more involved

---

[3] The supplemental motor cortex is in the premotor area, which is in front of the motor cortex.

than the arms) may characterize some patients. Buccofacial apraxia may be seen in a few cases.

- *Apathy or behavioral withdrawal.* Most patients show little or no interest in using language.

Major Language Characteristics of TMA

The patients with TMA exhibit the following language characteristics (Benson & Ardila, 1996; Cimino-Knight, Hollingsworth, & Gonzalez Rothi, 2005):

- *Muteness.* Soon after the onset, patients may be speechless (mute), possibly due to akinesia.
- *Echolalia and perseverative speech.* As the patient recovers from speechlessness, the patient may exhibit echolalia (repetition of heard speech), and perseveration (multiple repetitions of one's own utterances) often may be evident.
- *Reduced spontaneous speech.* Lack of interest in verbal communication and a disinterest in spontaneous speech are common.
- *Nonfluent, paraphasic, agrammatic, and telegraphic speech.* As speech is recovered, the patient may begin to offer limited spontaneous speech that is similar to that found in Broca's aphasia. Single words that need to be coaxed and unfinished sentences characterize the speech. Failure to use complex and precise syntactic structures may persist even as speech generally improves.
- *Naming problems.* Patients may have difficulty naming when asked to (confrontation naming). Naming may improve with various cues.
- *Intact repetition skill.* The unique and diagnostic feature of TMA is a remarkably preserved repetition skill. The patient who typically gives a single word response after much coaxing may repeat long and complex sentences the clinician models for imitation. This is in contrast to patients with Broca's aphasia whose repetition skills are impaired.

- *Relatively intact serial speech.* The patient, although needing assistance to initiate it, may produce serial speech with little or no errors. For instance, the patient, once initiated, may count numbers and recite days and months.

- *Intact knowledge of grammar and meaningfulness.* Patients may correct a grammatically incorrect model the clinician provides and repeat it in its correct form (e.g., *These is books* may be corrected and repeated as *These are books*). Patients may refuse to repeat nonsense syllables.

- *Limited word fluency.* The patient may have difficulty generating word lists (e.g., production of as many *names of flowers* as possible). Some patients who attempt a list generation may mix words from different categories.

- *Use of motor prompts to initiate speech.* Patients may try to facilitate the initiation of speech by such motor activities as clapping, vigorous head nodding, or hand waving.

- *Better comprehension than production.* Auditory comprehension is generally good for simple conversation. Comprehension may be impaired for complex speech, however.

- *Reading problems.* Reading aloud and reading comprehension both are better preserved than either speaking skills or writing skills. Nonetheless, reading aloud may be slow and difficult to maintain. Reading comprehension may be intact for simple printed material and impaired for syntactically complex material.

- *Writing problems.* Disinterested in writing, the patient who is coaxed to write may write little and with poor spelling and large and ill-formed letters.

In essence, a discrepancy between language production problems (impaired) and repetition skills (spared) characterizes TMA. Of these, spared repetition skills most clearly distinguish TMA from Broca's aphasia.

See Table 5-2 for a summative overview of language characteristics of patients with TMA.

TABLE 5-2 The major language characteristics of patients with transcortical motor aphasia (TMA).

Language Parameter	In Transcortical Motor Aphasia	Positive (+√) or Negative (−√) Diagnostic Feature	Contrasted With
Speech comprehension	Good; some subtle problems, especially for complex material	−√	
Fluency	Impaired; initially mute; later, paraphasic, agrammatic, telegraphic; limited word fluency; similar to Broca's	+√	
Grammar	Impaired	+√	
Paraphasia	Some paraphasia		
Naming	Mildly impaired		
Articulation	Good	−√	Broca's aphasia
Pointing	Good		
Repetition	Good; echolalia and perseverative speech	+√	
Reading aloud	Impaired	+√	
Reading comprehension	Good, except for syntactically complex material	+√	
Writing	Impaired	+√	
Neuromotor skills	Right hemiparesis or hemiplegia; difficulty initiating motor tasks	+√	
Classification	Nonfluent aphasia		
Lesion site	Deep portions of the left frontal lobe below or above Broca's area; association pathways; supplemental motor area; lesions in areas served by the anterior branch of the middle cerebral artery		

Individual Differences in Patients with TMA

Apraxic difficulty in producing speech sounds may be evident in some individuals. Across individuals, the similarity between TMA and Broca's aphasia can vary; the closer the lesion to the Broca's area, the greater the resemblance between the two syndromes.

Depending on the site and extent of lesions, a few patients may show sensory loss or visual-field loss. Some patients may ignore the use of their right limb.

Benson and Ardila (1996) suggest that there may be two types of transcortical motor aphasia. They believe that marked lower extremity paresis, lower extremity sensory loss, and mild dysarthria distinguish the two types; they are absent in type I and present in type II. Language characteristics are common.

Relative Strengths of Patients with TMA

- *Good repetition skills.* TMA's distinguishing feature is the patients' most important strength: intact verbal repetition skill. When echolalia is dominant, repetition skills may be nonfunctional, however. This may result in parrotlike imitative responses.
- *Preserved overlearned speech.* As noted, the patients can recite number series or nursery rhymes once such speech is somehow initiated. Perseveration, however, may adversely affect this skill.

Mixed Transcortical Aphasia (MTA)

A rare variety of nonfluent aphasia, mixed transcortical aphasia also is known as *isolation aphasia* or *isolation of the speech area.* Most experts (e.g., Benson & Ardila, 1996; Cimino-Knight, Hollingsworth, & Gonzalez Rothi, 2005) describe MTA, although it is not a part of the Boston classification of Goodglass and Kaplan (1983).

Mixed transcortical aphasia combines symptoms of TMA and transcortical sensory aphasia, a fluent form of aphasia, described in Chapter 6. Both production and comprehension of language are impaired. MTA is similar to global aphasia in that the language impairment is extensive and often severe. Patients with MTA retain their speech repetition skills, a feature that distinguishes them from patients with global aphasia. This isolated preservation of the repetition skill in the presence of impaired language skills is the reason for suggesting the name *isolation aphasia* for this syndrome.

Neuroanatomical Bases of MTA

Various conditions that reduce blood flow through the cerebral arteries can cause MTA (Benson & Ardila, 1996; Cimino-Knight, Hollingsworth, & Gonzalez Rothi, 2005). These conditions include:

- *Hypoxia of various origin.* Carbon monoxide poisoning, reduced oxygen supply to tissue in spite of normal blood supply, anoxia (total lack of oxygen supply), chronic hypo-perfusion (reduced blood flow), and acute carotid occlusion or stenosis have all been suggested or documented in individual cases.
- *Cardiac arrest.* Sudden cardiac arrest also may deprive the cerebral structures of oxygen.
- *Cerebral edema.* Cerebral shock resulting in severe cerebral swelling may be associated with MTA.
- *Multiple embolic strokes.* Such strokes involving especially the peripheral branches of the middle cerebral artery can cause TMA.

The damage most often is found in the cerebral border zone or the watershed area (see Figure 4-3 in Chapter 4 for a graphic representation of this area). This area lies between the areas supplied by the middle cerebral artery on the one hand and the anterior and posterior cerebral arteries on the other. Typically, Broca's area is spared as is Wernicke's area and the arcuate fasciculus. However, both these spared areas may be isolated from the rest of the brain.

General Characteristics of MTA

Patients with MTA may have a varied clinical picture because of different and often extensive neuropathology (Benson & Ardila, 1996; Cimino-Knight, Hollingsworth, & Gonzalez Rothi, 2005). Depending on the individual case, these patients are likely to show:

- *Bilateral upper motor neuron paralysis.* This spastic paralysis affects volitional muscle movements.
- *Severe spastic quadriparesis.* This is weakness in all four limbs, suggesting bilateral brain damage.
- *Visual field defects.* The typical problem is a right hemianopia.

- *Weakness in hip and shoulder muscles.* Except for such weakness, a few patients may not have any other marked neurologic deficit.
- *Severe brain damage.* This may result in a variety of sensory and motor problems.

Major Language Characteristics of MTA

MTA resembles global aphasia, with profoundly impaired communication skills except for repetition skills. Language production and comprehension are both impaired, often severely (Benson & Ardila, 1996; Cimino-Knight, Hollingsworth, & Gonzalez Rothi, 2005). Patients with MTA are characterized by:

- *Extremely limited spontaneous verbal expressions.* Some patients may have no spontaneous speech.
- *Echolalia.* Parrotlike repetition of what is heard may be notable. Patients may repeat what others say. The patients' speech often may be limited entirely to this type of echolalia. The length of phrases repeated, however, may be limited to three or four words only. The patients also may repeat nonsense syllables or words from foreign languages.
- *Repetition combined with sentence completion.* If an examiner says the initial part of a familiar statement or song, the patient may immediately repeat it and then go on to complete it.
- *Severely impaired fluency.* This is understandable because of the extremely limited spontaneous speech of patients with MTA.
- *Severely impaired auditory comprehension.* The patient may not comprehend even simple conversation.
- *Marked naming difficulty.* The patient may respond with neologism but often does not respond when asked to name stimuli (confrontation naming). A rare case of MTA with good confrontation naming has been reported, however.
- *Mostly unimpaired automatic speech.* Once initiated and left to continue without interruption, the patient may recite the months in a

year or a number series. Once interrupted, the patient cannot reinitiate, however.

- *Normal articulation.* While many aspects of language are impaired, patients with MTA have relatively normal articulation skills.
- *Severe reading deficits.* Oral reading and comprehension of read material both may be severely impaired. The impairment is often total.
- *Severe writing impairments.* The writing impairment, too, may often be total.

Patients with MTA are reported to show little recovery of language skills. Because of the limited number of cases studied, prognostic statements are difficult to make.

See Table 5-3 for a summative overview of language characteristics of patients with MTA.

TABLE 5-3   The major language characteristics of patients with mixed transcortical aphasia.

Language Parameter	In Mixed Trancortical Aphasia	Positive (+√) or Negative (−√) Diagnostic Feature	Contrasted With
Speech comprehension	Impaired, often severely	+√	
Fluency	Impaired, often severely	+√	
Grammar	Impaired	+√	
Paraphasia	Not a significant feature	−√	
Naming	Impaired	+√	
Articulation	Good	+√	
Pointing	Impaired	+√	
Repetition	Good; but parrotlike, nonfunctional repetition	+√	Global aphasia, because of other similarities
Reading aloud	Impaired, often severely	+√	
Reading comprehension	Impaired, often severely	+√	
Writing	Impaired	+√	
Classification	Nonfluent aphasia		
Lesion site	The watershed area (border zone); spared but isolated Wernicke's and Broca's areas		

Relative Strengths of Patients With MTA

Except for preserved repetition skills, which may not serve them well, the patients with MTA have limited assets. MTA affects all modes of communication, language production, comprehension, reading, and writing. Nonetheless, the patients may sing along and repeat some sentences.

Global Aphasia

Various studies report that global aphasia may account for 30 percent to 55 percent of aphasic patients. The higher percentage may especially be documented if the patients are assessed in their acute stage (Peach, 2001). **Global aphasia** is the most severe form of aphasia and has a generalized (global) effect on communication skills (Collins, 2005). The disorder affects all modes of communication, including nonverbal communication, and spares no particular skill.

Neuroanatomical Bases of Global Aphasia

The lesions that produce global aphasia are likely to involve the entire perisylvian region. Both Broca's area and Wernicke's area are affected. Therefore, all speech and language centers in the dominant hemisphere tend to be affected. The damage may extend into deeper white matter of the brain. In some cases, basal ganglia, the internal capsule, and the thalamus may be damaged (Collins, 1991, 2005; Peach, 2001).

Exceptional cases of global aphasia with limited damage have been reported. In some patients the lesion was restricted to the anterior region, the posterior region, or subcortical structures (Peach, 2001).

Typically, the more common lesion sites are supplied by the middle cerebral artery, the largest branch of the internal carotid artery. Occlusions of the middle cerebral artery, especially if they occur before it branches out to supply the various areas of the brain, can produce devastating effects. Most severe deficits are found in patients who have lesions

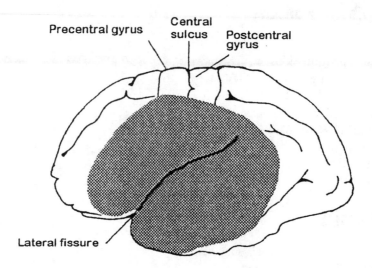

Figure 5-3. Neuroanatomical basis of global aphasia. The entire language zone surrounding the sylvian fissure (the shaded area) is involved in global aphasia.

in the frontal, temporal (especially the posterior temporal gyrus), and parietal lobes. Figure 5-3 shows the areas that are commonly affected in global aphasia.

In essence, widespread destruction of the left fronto-temporo-parietal regions involved in speech and language is common in globally aphasic patients. However, atypical global aphasia cases with other damage sites have been reported.

General Characteristics of Global Aphasia

Patients with global aphasia, generally with their severe impairments, show the following general characteristics (Collins, 1991, 2005; Peach, 2001):

- *Presence of strong neurological symptoms.* Because of large lesions, patients with global aphasia have significant neurological impairment. Right hemiparesis (muscular weakness or partial paralysis on one side) or hemiplegia (paralysis on one side) is present. Right-sided sensory loss is commonly observed.

- *Apraxia.* Both verbal and nonverbal apraxia may be present.

- *Hemineglect.* The patient may exhibit a tendency to neglect one side of his or her body. Hemineglect, especially left neglect, is more common in right hemisphere damage, described in Chapter 10.

Major Language Characteristics of Global Aphasia

Generally extremely limited language skills distinguish global aphasia from other forms (Collins, 1991, 2005; Peach, 2001):

- *Globally impaired communication skills.* In most cases, all verbal and nonverbal language skills are profoundly impaired. Consequently, there may be no significant profile of differential communicative performance on assessment tasks or during social communication.
- *Severely reduced fluency.* Extremely limited speech in most cases results in equally restricted fluency.
- *Extremely limited verbal expressions.* The patient's language may be limited to a few recognizable or unrecognizable words, exclamations, and serial utterances. Some patients may repeat such consonant-vowel combinations as do-do-do or ma-ma-ma (Peach, 2001). Patients may keep repeating short utterances (perseveration).
- *Impaired repetition.* The patient may be unable to repeat even simple words.
- *Impaired naming.* Lack of meaningful verbal expression obviously extends to problems in naming.
- *Impaired auditory comprehension.* Comprehension may be limited to single words, although some evidence suggests that patients understand more than they can express. A few patients who could comprehend a certain category of words (e.g., famous personal names) have been described, however.
- *Impaired reading and writing skills.* These problems generally parallel their severe language deficits.

See Table 5-4 for a summative overview of language characteristics of patients with global aphasia.

TABLE 5-4 The major characteristics of patients with global aphasia.

Language Parameter	In Global Aphasia	Positive (+√) or Negative (−√) Diagnostic Feature	Contrasted With
Speech comprehension	Impaired	+√	
Fluency	Severely impaired	+√	
Grammar	Impaired; agrammatic	+√	
Paraphasia	Not a significant feature	−√	
Naming	Impaired	+√	
Articulation	Impaired	+√	All other types in severity of deficits
Pointing	Impaired	+√	
Repetition	Impaired	+√	
Reading aloud	Impaired	+√	
Reading comprehension	Impaired to some extent		
Writing	Impaired	+√	
Classification	Nonfluent aphasia		
Lesion site	Widespread damage, surrounding the entire perisylvian region		

Individual Differences in Patients with Global Aphasia

As in all types of aphasia, there may be significant individual differences in the extent of impairment. These differences may be mostly explained by the extent of lesions. Some individuals may retain restricted auditory comprehension.

Some patients with global aphasia may not have obvious neurological symptoms. More limited lesions that spare the motor areas may leave patients with intact motor skills. Some data suggest a better prognosis for patients without hemiplegia or hemiparesis (Peach, 2001).

Prognosis for recovery from global aphasia is limited and worse than what is seen in other types of aphasia. Some may show a slightly better recovery of their comprehension skills than expressive skills.

Nonetheless, several studies report that global aphasia at the onset may eventually evolve into another type of aphasia in some patients (Peach, 2001). Global aphasia may evolve into Broca's, Wernicke's, anomic, or conduction aphasia. Global aphasia in younger patients is more likely to evolve into a less severe type. Presumably, patients who evolve into other types of aphasia show significant improvement. Furthermore, compared to those who do not receive treatment, those who do improve in their communication skills.

It is important not to offer unduly pessimistic prognosis at the time of onset as many patients are acute at that time. Classification of aphasia is tenuous at the time of onset. Global aphasia that remains stable even after one year post-stroke, especially without treatment, may indeed have a poor prognosis.

Relative Strengths of Patients with Global Aphasia

Although they are thought of as the most severely impaired of patients with aphasia, globally aphasic patients may retain some strengths that might be useful in treatment sessions. For instance, some patients follow whole body commands (e.g., "sit down" or "stand up").

Globally aphasic patients may distinguish between meaningful and meaningless speech and correctly identify environmental sounds. They may recognize familiar places, persons, melodies, humor, absurdities, and metaphor.

Some patients may grasp the meaning of spoken speech by interpreting gestures and facial expressions. Compared to questions related to impersonal or objective information, they may respond better to personally relevant questions. Globally aphasic patients are generally alert, task-oriented, and responsive during assessment and treatment. They are socially appropriate (Brookshire, 2003).

Globally aphasic patients' alertness, social appropriateness, and task orientation help distinguish them from patients with confused language or dementia.

Suggested Readings

Read the following for additional information on nonfluent aphasias and their differential diagnosis:

Basso, A. (2003). *Aphasia and its therapy.* New York: Oxford University Press.

Cimino-Knight, A. M., Hollingsworth, A. L., & Gonzalez Rothi, L. J. (2005). The transcortical aphasias. In L. L. LaPointe (Ed.), *Aphasia and related neurogenic language disorders* (3rd ed., pp. 169–185). New York: Thieme Medical Publishers.

Collins, M. J. (2005). Global aphasia. In L. L. LaPointe (Ed.), *Aphasia and related neurogenic language disorders* (3rd ed., pp. 186–198). New York: Thieme Medical Publishers.

Damasio, A. (2001). Neural basis of language disorders. In R. Chapey (Ed.), *Language intervention strategies in aphasia and related neurogenic communication disorders* (4th ed., pp. 18–36). Philadelphia: Lippincott Williams & Wilkins.

Kearns, K. P. (2005). Broca's aphasia. In L. L. LaPointe (Ed.), *Aphasia and related neurogenic language disorders* (3rd ed., pp. 117–141). New York: Thieme Medical Publishers.

CHAPTER 6

ETIOLOGY AND SYMPTOMATOLOGY OF FLUENT APHASIAS

Chapter Outline

- Fluency in Aphasia
- Wernicke's Aphasia
- Transcortical Sensory Aphasia
- Conduction Aphasia
- Anomic Aphasia

Learning Objectives

After reading the chapter, the student will:

- Describe the neuropathology of all fluent aphasias.
- Describe the neurological symptoms of fluent aphasias.
- Describe the language characteristics of fluent aphasias.

- Distinguish the four types of fluent aphasias based on neuropathology, neurological symptoms, and positive and negative language characteristics.

Fluency in Aphasia

As noted in the previous chapter, fluency is a dimension on which aphasic syndromes are distinguished. Previously, we considered four varieties of aphasia in which fluency is significantly impaired. In contrast, we will now consider four varieties of aphasia in which fluency is relatively unimpaired. Although there are differences (and similarities) between the varieties of fluent aphasia, a common dominant element is relatively well preserved fluency.

Patients who are fluent are described as those whose speech is abundant. Their verbal output may consist of 100 to 200 words per minute. In contrast, the speech of the patients with nonfluent aphasia is often described as sparse and limited. In addition, aphasic patients who are fluent produce their speech with ease, good articulation, and normal prosody. The phrase length is normal (5 to 8 words per phrase).

Fluent speech in fluent aphasia does not imply normal language, however. Fluent patients tend to omit meaningful and semantically significant words. Their verbal expression may be full of paraphasias. In spite of their flowing and copious speech, the patients are less effective in their communication than those with nonfluent aphasia.

We will consider four varieties of fluent aphasia: Wernicke's aphasia, transcortical sensory aphasia, conduction aphasia, and anomic aphasia.

Wernicke's Aphasia

As noted in Chapter 1, the German neuropsychiatrist Carl Wernicke first described a form of aphasia in 1874. He called it *sensory aphasia.* Other names include *receptive aphasia, acoustic-amnestic aphasia, verbal agnosia, word deafness, syntactic aphasia, posterior aphasia,* and *central aphasia.* The name *Wernicke's aphasia* has come to prevail over the others.

Wernicke's aphasia is clinically well established as it is one of the early aphasia syndromes to be described. Some experts believe that it is the least controversial aphasia syndrome, certainly less controversial than Broca's aphasia.

Wernicke's aphasia is characterized by fluent and sometimes excessive verbal expressions that are grammatically intact but are full of paraphasias and neologisms that can render the speech unintelligible. Such verbal expressions are combined with significant auditory comprehension deficits. The combination of fluent and jargon-filled speech and poor auditory comprehension characterizes Wernicke's aphasia.

Neuroanatomical Bases of Wernicke's Aphasia

Wernicke himself localized the damage associated with what he called *sensory aphasia* to the superior temporal gyrus in the dominant hemisphere. Many subsequent studies and more recent brain imaging techniques have confirmed that in most patients the lesion that causes Wernicke's aphasia is often in Wernicke's areas (posterior portion of the superior temporal gyrus in the left hemisphere). The area also is known as the *posterior language cortex.*

Accumulated evidence now suggests that the lesion may extend to the second temporal gyrus, the surrounding parietal region, the angular gyrus, and the supramarginal gyrus (Benson & Ardila, 1996; Caspari, 2005; Damasio, 2001; Helm-Estabrooks & Albert, 2004). In addition, subcortical damage that impairs connections to the temporal cortex also may produce Wernicke's aphasia (Benson & Ardila, 1996). Figure 6-1 shows the primary and secondary areas of lesion often found in patients with Wernicke's aphasia.

Embolic or thrombolic cerebrovascular accidents and intracranial hemorrhage in the posterior temporal lobe and trauma or tumor in the same area are among the more common causes of damage to Wernicke's and surrounding areas. The sites of lesion associated with Wernicke's area are supplied by the posterior branches of the left middle cerebral artery. Untreated ear infections also may cause damage to Wernicke's area.

A curious finding is that damage to Wernicke's area may not always produce symptoms consistent with Wernicke's aphasia. However, those with such symptoms almost always have lesions in the dominant superior temporal gyrus, whether extended to

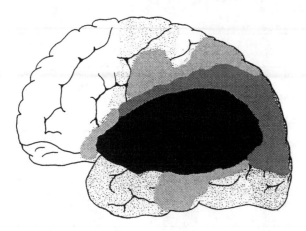

Figure 6-1. Neuroanatomical bases of Wernicke's aphasia. The darker area shows the primary site of lesion found in many cases; lighter shades show other areas that may be involved.

other areas or not. Therefore, although the lesion may not necessarily predict the symptoms, the symptoms seem to predict the lesion.

General Characteristics of Wernicke's Aphasia

Unlike patients with Broca's aphasia, those with Wernicke's aphasia may appear physically normal. Often, neurological examination of these patients is negative (Benson & Ardila, 1996; Caspari, 2005; Damasio, 2001; Helm-Estabrooks & Albert, 2004). Patients with Wernicke's aphasia:

- *Do not have paresis or paralysis.* Most patients do not have muscle weakness or paralysis. Such motor symptoms are absent because the typical site of lesion is away from motor centers of the brain.
- *May sound confused.* Jargon-filled, irrelevant sounding but somewhat incessant speech may give the impression of confusion.
- *Lack insight into their disability.* Patients with Wernicke's aphasia do not seem to appreciate their communicative disorder and its effects on the listener.
- *Lack frustration in failed communication.* Most patients with Wernicke's aphasia are

not as frustrated as Broca's patients, possibly because they do not understand the nature of their disability.

- *Exhibit psychiatric symptoms.* The patients may be paranoid, homicidal, suicidal, or depressed. They may accuse others of speaking in a code they cannot decipher. Such paranoia may partly be due to their severe auditory comprehension problems. Their depression may partly be due to social isolation they experience in spite of their verbosity. People who do not understand their meaningless speech may ignore them. It should be noted, however, that depression is a common reaction to stroke, and patients with Wernicke's aphasia do not seem to be more susceptible to it than patients with other types of aphasia (Graham-Keegan & Caspari, 1997).

Because of their confused and irrelevant speech, paranoia, and depression, combined with normal or near-normal neurological findings, patients with Wernicke's aphasia may be mistakenly diagnosed as psychiatric patients and treated, for instance, as schizophrenic patients. A mild form of Wernicke's aphasia may be especially difficult to diagnose (Benson & Ardila, 1996).

Major Language Characteristics of Wernicke's Aphasia

Fluent but jargon-filled speech and defective auditory comprehension are the hallmarks of this syndrome (Benson & Ardila, 1996; Caspari, 2005; Damasio, 2001; Helm-Estabrooks & Albert, 2004). A careful examination of the symptom complex of patients with Wernicke's aphasia reveals:

- *Normal or even abnormal speech fluency (logorrhea or press of speech).* Unlike patients with Broca's aphasia, those with Wernicke's aphasia are generally prolific and excessive in their word output. The patients may add extra syllables to some of the words they produce. Their speech is incessant and produced effortlessly. Some patients with Wernicke's aphasia speak so incessantly that they may need frequent and strong signals to stop talking.

- *Rapid rate of speech.* Most patients, as they have a lot to say in response to even simple questions, speak rapidly.

- *Normal prosodic features.* Patients with Wernicke's aphasia speak with normal rhythm, intonation, and linguistic stress. Even when they produce meaningless utterances, the patients' speech may sound normal.

- *Good articulation.* Patients with Wernicke's aphasia may not exhibit symptoms of apraxia and dysarthria.

- *Normal phrase lengths* (5 to 8 words). Unlike patients with Broca's aphasia, those with Wernicke's aphasia produce phrases and sentences that are either normal or excessively long.

- *Generally intact grammatical forms.* The language productions of patients with Wernicke's aphasia have apparently normal grammatical forms. Nonetheless, their morphological and syntactic use is not entirely normal. For instance, the patients may exhibit *paragrammatism,* which is an excessive use of grammatical morphemes. Goodglass (1993) characterized the language production of Wernicke's patients as "pseudogrammatical sentences" (p. 211).

- *Severe word-finding problems.* The patients may completely fail to name objects shown or may produce a semantic substitution or an incomprehensible neologistic response. They may begin to describe the object instead of naming it (circumlocution). The patients may do slightly better when asked to point to objects, especially when only a few choices are displayed.

- *Empty speech.* Wernicke's patients produce much but convey little because their speech is filled with semantic and literal paraphasia, extraneous syllables, and meaningless word creations (neologism). Unlike patients with Broca's aphasia who retain meaningful content words in their speech (and thus communicate more effectively), those with Wernicke's retain grammatical words and omit content words or substitute them with neologistic words. In response to a question "How are you today?" a patient replied: "Well for the umpig and it is leedwa in the geebud." (Note the preserved *grammatical words* but essentially empty speech.) The patients' speech also may be filled with such general words as *this, that, stuff,* and *thing.*

- *Poor auditory comprehension.* This is a dominant and distinguishing feature of Wernicke's aphasia. This deficit may be highly variable across patients. Some may have difficulty in comprehending only certain elements of spoken speech, while others may have extreme difficulty in understanding most, if not all, spoken speech. Most have difficulty in comprehending the names of common objects and even greater difficulty in comprehending sentences. Patients have difficulty distinguishing spoken words that contain minimally different phonemes (e.g., the /p/ and /b/ in *pat* and *bat*).

- *Impaired conversational skills.* This impairment may be due to poor auditory comprehension. Those who seem to understand conversation on a topic may cease to understand when a new topic is introduced. Most may need extended time to establish new conversational topics. Comprehension of conversation is most seriously impaired in the presence of background noise, movements, and background speech. Comprehension, when good, usually is short-lived in a given conversational context. Conversational turn taking may be minimally acceptable in mildly involved patients but grossly impaired in cases of severe involvement; patients may fail to yield to their conversational partners.

- *Impaired repetition skill.* The degree of impairment may correspond to the degree of auditory comprehension deficit. Patients who cannot understand anything will not repeat anything and those who understand certain words and phrases may repeat them.

- *Impaired reading comprehension.* Most patients may not recognize sounds associated with written words. They may fail to understand the meanings of printed words. They may not match alphabets or recognize the names of the alphabets.

- *Impaired writing skills.* Patients with Wernicke's aphasia may write a lot, write freely, and write meaninglessly; their writing parallels their speech. Unlike patients with Broca's aphasia, they write with their dominant hand and in cursive style. Their writing, as copious as their speech, may be full of misspelling of words and nonexistent words. The patients may be unaware of their writing problems.

See Table 6-1 for a summative overview of major language characteristics that are diagnostic of Wernicke's aphasia.

Most of the communication problems associated with Wernicke's aphasia are explained on the basis of lack of sensory monitoring of speech and writing. The patients do not get sensory feedback to regulate and correct their speech errors. The inference is that they may not understand that they are not making sense.

The extent and the nature of auditory comprehension deficits are not well understood. These

TABLE 6-1   The major language characteristics of patients with Wernicke's aphasia.

Language Parameter	In Wernicke's Aphasia	Positive (+√) or Negative (−√) Diagnostic Feature
Speech comprehension	Severely impaired	+√
Fluency	Good; even excessive; paraphasic empty speech	−√
Grammar	Good; paragrammatism; pseudogrammatical sentences	−√
Paraphasia	Semantic and neologistic	+√
Naming	Severely impaired, frequent word substitutions	+√
Articulation	Good	−√
Pointing	Impaired	+√
Repetition	Impaired, comparable to speech comprehension deficit	+√
Reading aloud	Impaired	+√
Reading comprehension	Impaired	+√
Writing	Impaired; paraphasic, neologistic	+√

deficits are difficult to measure. Better auditory comprehension is related to greater and earlier recovery of language functions, which is true in all aphasic patients.

Individual Differences in Patients with Wernicke's Aphasia

As noted previously, damage to Wernicke's area in some patients may not produce Wernicke's aphasia. Although auditory comprehension deficits are a hallmark of the syndrome, some patients have better auditory comprehension than others. Varying size and location of the lesion cause individual differences in the symptoms.

Based on individual differences in Wernicke's aphasia symptom complex, Benson and Ardila (1996) describe a type I and a type II variety. Wernicke's aphasia type I is characterized by a poor comprehension of spoken language but better comprehension of written language. Marked difficulty in understanding spoken words is described as *word deafness,* and a similar difficulty in understanding printed material is called *word blindness.* Type I patients have greater word deafness than word blindness. Patients with Wernicke's aphasia type II, on the other hand, exhibit greater word blindness than word deafness. That is, type II patients comprehend spoken speech better than printed word.

Relative Strengths of Patients with Wernicke's Aphasia

Some patients retain better comprehension for redundant or personally meaningful material. Clinicians may exploit this in treatment by starting with personally meaningful material. Most patients maintain correct syntactic arrangement, articulation, and prosody.

Although they may not understand many commands, most patients may correctly follow *whole-body commands.* For instance, a patient who cannot *clap hands* on command may promptly *stand up* when commanded.

Transcortical Sensory Aphasia

Wernicke first described **transcortical sensory aphasia (TSA)** in 1881. Four years later, in 1885, Lichtheim described the same syndrome. TSA also is known as *posterior isolation syndrome.* Benson and Ardila (1996) call it *extrasylvian (transcortical) sensory aphasia.*

Most early descriptions of patients with TSA highlight their tendency to echo and imitate what is heard. Because in some respects TSA is similar to Wernicke's aphasia, some have called it *Wernicke's aphasia type II* (which should not be confused with Benson and Ardila's Wernicke's aphasia type II). Because of their similarities, TSA and Wernicke's aphasia may be confused with each other. However, the distinguishing feature is that repetition is intact in TSA and impaired in Wernicke's aphasia.

In Chapter 5, we discussed transcortical motor aphasia (TMA), a nonfluent form of aphasia with lesions in the extrasylvian cortical regions. TMA also is characterized by intact repetition skills; thus, TSA is a *fluent counterpart* of the nonfluent TMA.

Neuroanatomical Bases of TSA

The most frequent cause of TSA is a lesion in the temporoparietal region. In some cases, the lateral aspects of the occipital lobe also may be involved. Damage to the posterior portion of the middle temporal gyrus is typical. In some cases, the angular gyrus and visual and auditory association cortex also may be involved. Wernicke's area, Broca's area, and the arcuate fasciculus are typically intact (Benson & Ardila, 1996; Cimino-Knight, Hollingsworth, & Gonzalez Rothi, 2005; Damasio, 2001; Helm-Estabrooks & Albert, 2004).

The cortical regions of the dominant hemisphere that are typically damaged in TSA are in the watershed areas of the middle cerebral artery. In addition to ischemic lesions, head trauma also can cause TSA, but the symptoms are transient. The most common site of TSA is identified in Figure 6-2.

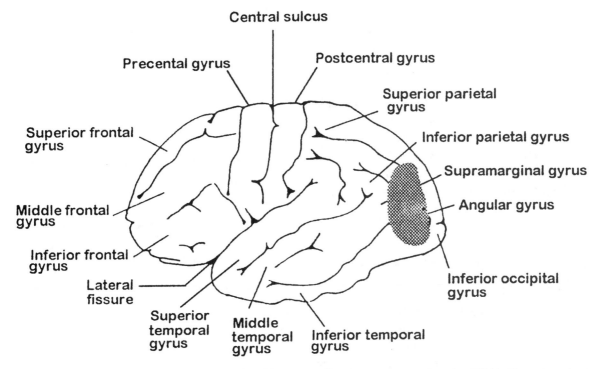

Figure 6-2. Neuroanatomical basis of transcortical sensory aphasia (TSA). The shaded area is the most common site of lesion.

General Characteristics of TSA

The general and neurological characteristics of patients with TSA may change over time. Because of the site of lesion, patients with TSA exhibit a number of related deficits (Benson & Ardila, 1996; Cimino-Knight, Hollingsworth, & Gonzalez Rothi, 2005; Damasio, 2001; Helm-Estabrooks & Albert, 2004):

- Onset of TSA is associated with hemiparesis. Soon, the patient recovers from hemiparesis. Therefore, in the later stages, there may be no significant physical symptoms.

- Patients in the initial stages of Alzheimer's disease[1] exhibit symptoms that are similar to those of TSA, but the problem evolves into an irreversible dementia. Dementia of the Alzheimer type and other forms of dementia are described in Chapters 14, 15, and 16.

_____

[1] Patients with Alzheimer's disease have lesions in bilateral, posterior association cortex.

- TSA also is associated with the Gertsmann syndrome, a neurological syndrome with finger agnosia, agraphia, confusion of laterality, and acalculia. Occipital and angular gyrus lesions are present.

- Unilateral inattention (neglect of one side of the body) is common. Left neglect is a diagnostic feature of right hemisphere syndrome; see Chapters 10 and 11 for details.

- Sensory loss may or may not be present. Some patients are reported to have visual problems.

Major Language Characteristics of TSA

TSA is characterized by fluent, well-articulated, paraphasic, somewhat echolalic, empty speech in the context of poor auditory comprehension (Benson & Ardila, 1996; Cimino-Knight, Hollingsworth, & Gonzalez Rothi, 2005; Damasio, 2001; Helm-Estabrooks & Albert, 2004). Specifically, patients with TSA exhibit:

- *Fluent speech.* Fluency of patients with TSA is similar to those with Wernicke's aphasia. With good articulation and normal phrase length, the patients speak with acceptable intonation and stress patterns. In essence, the phonemic, phonetic, and prosodic features of patients with TSA are intact.

- *Generally good syntactic skills.* Comparable to the language production of patients with Wernicke's aphasia, language of the patients with TSA do not exhibit agrammatic speech found in Broca's aphasia.

- *Paraphasias.* The speech of patients with TSA is full of semantic and neologistic paraphasia.

- *Empty speech.* The fluent speech of patients with TSA fails to communicate because of their paraphasia and neologism. Although they are fluent speakers, patients with TSA do not exhibit logorrhea or press of speech that characterizes patients with Wernicke's aphasia.

- *Impaired naming.* This problem may be severe in patients. Consequently, there may be many pauses in speech although their tendency is to find neologistic and nonspecific words instead of specific names during conversation. In confrontation naming tasks, the patients may fail to name the object shown. The patients also may fail to point to the object when the examiner names it. Any attempt to describe the object (instead of naming it) may result in paraphasic neologistic expressions.

- *Good repetition skills.* Unlike fluent patients with Wernicke's aphasia, those with TSA can repeat words and phrases modeled for them. The patients may not comprehend the meaning of the words they repeat, however.

- *Echolalic behavior.* This feature, also absent in Wernicke's patients, is a significant aspect of TSA. Patients may repeat words and phrases they hear. More significantly, they may incorporate the clinician's words and phrases into their own expressions, with no regard for meaning. This echolalia extends to grammatically incorrect forms, nonsense syllables, and words from foreign languages, a feature not found in patients with transcortical motor aphasia.

- *Impaired auditory comprehension of spoken language.* The comprehension deficits may be severe in some cases. Many patients fail to understand a simple request to point to objects shown, motor commands, and simple yes/no questions. Therefore, their repetition and echolalia of heard speech are puzzling.

- *Once initiated, normal automatic speech.* The patients may need help in getting initiated on a serial task, but once initiated, they may complete it. For example, they may count numbers or recite the days of the week when they get started with the clinician's help.

- *Completion of poems and sentences.* When a clinician starts a sentence or a poem, the patient may promptly complete it, another puzzling aspect of the patient's otherwise poor comprehension of spoken language.

- *Poor reading comprehension.* Many patients can read aloud normally, albeit with word substitutions. The comprehension of what is read, however, may be extremely limited or totally absent.

- *Relatively preserved oral reading skills.* Compared to other language skills, patients with TSA read better, although they may not understand what is read.
- *Writing problems.* The writing of patients with TSA resembles that of patients with Wernicke's aphasia. In general, the writing problems parallel expressive language problems.

In essence, a puzzling echolalic and repetition behavior in the presence of defective auditory comprehension distinguishes TSA from Wernicke's aphasia. In most other respects, the two types of aphasia are more similar than different.

See Table 6-2 for a summative overview of major language characteristics that are diagnostic of TSA.

TABLE 6-2   The major language characteristics of patients with transcortical sensory aphasia.

Language Parameter	In Transcortical Sensory Aphasia	Positive (+√) or Negative (−√) Diagnostic Feature
Speech comprehension	Impaired	+√
Fluency	Good, but paraphasic, echolalic, empty speech	−√
Grammar	Good	−√
Paraphasia	Neologistic and semantic	+√
Naming	Impaired	+√
Articulation	Good	−√
Pointing	Impaired	+√
Repetition	Good; echolalic repetition	+√
Reading aloud	Good	−√
Reading comprehension	Impaired	+√
Writing	Impaired	+√
Awareness, self-correction	Not noted	+√

Individual Differences in Patients with TSA

As with all syndromes of aphasia, the symptom complex of patients with TSA may vary, depending not only on the extent of the lesion but also on the presence of associated syndromes. For instance, a form of TSA in which language problems show progressive deterioration has been reported. In some patients, an initial Wernicke's aphasia may evolve into a chronic form of TSA. An initial TSA in some patients may evolve into anomia; some of these patients may recover fully. In some patients, TSA may persist with little or no change over time. Such persistent TSA is associated with parietal damage.

Relative Strengths of Patients with TSA

Patients with TSA have the same strengths as those found in Wernicke's patients: good fluency, prosody, phrase length, and so forth. An additional positive feature of TSA is the intact repetition skills, although this may or may not serve them well in their everyday communication or during language treatment.

Conduction Aphasia

Another form of fluent aphasia, conduction aphasia also has been called *central aphasia, efferent conduction aphasia,* and *repetition aphasia.* Benson and Ardila (1996) consider it a form of perisylvian aphasia syndrome. Wernicke first postulated the existence of conduction aphasia. It is among the more controversial of aphasia syndromes. **Conduction aphasia** is characterized by paraphasic fluency, good comprehension, and impaired repetition. Patients with conduction aphasia are mostly similar to those with Wernicke's aphasia. A notable exception is the good to normal auditory comprehension of patients with conduction aphasia.

Conduction aphasia is a rare syndrome. Only about 5 to 10 percent of aphasic patients are diagnosed with it.

Neuroanatomical Bases of Conduction Aphasia

The neuroanatomical bases of conduction aphasia is more controversial than it is for most other types. A left parietal lobe damage is often mentioned in the literature (Benson & Ardila, 1996). The supramarginal gyrus, inferior parietal gyrus, and lower part of the postcentral sulcus may be damaged. Some experts have suggested that the arcuate fasciculus that connects Broca's area with Wernicke's also may be damaged. The other possible site of lesion is the left temporal lobe, the auditory association area (Benson & Ardila, 1996; Damasio, 2001; Helm-Estabrooks & Albert, 2004; Simmons-Mackie, 2005).

Wernicke hypothesized that in conduction aphasia, the damage disconnects the motor language area (Broca's area) from the sensory language area (what came to be known as Wernicke's area).

Others have suggested that conduction aphasia may result from a lesion or lesions anywhere between Broca's and Wernicke's area. Both the site of lesion and the resulting symptoms vary.

Goldstein (1948) disagreed with Wernicke's interpretation of conduction aphasia. Instead, he proposed that conduction aphasia is due to a damage to a central region that integrates form and meaning of language. Hence, he called it *central aphasia*.

A more frequently shown site of lesion in conduction aphasia is depicted in Figure 6-3.

More anteriorly located lesions produce less fluent aphasia with better auditory comprehension, and the more posterior lesions may produce more fluent aphasia with poorer auditory comprehension. This is known as the bimodal distribution model.

General Characteristics of Conduction Aphasia

Patients with conduction aphasia present varied neurological and other symptoms, perhaps an indication of varied sites of brain damage. Some patients may present no neurological symptoms while others may present paresis of the right side of the face and right upper extremity. In its severity, this paresis may range

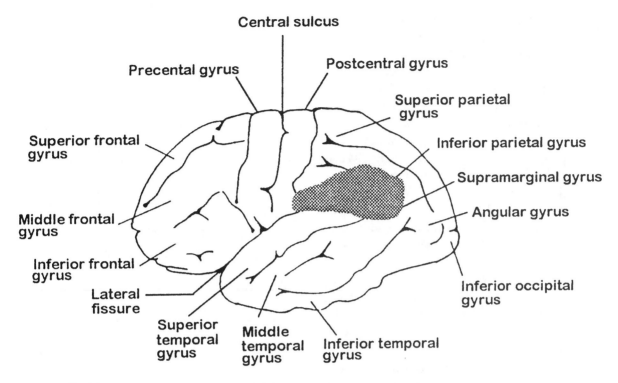

Figure 6-3. Neuroanatomical basis of conduction aphasia. The shaded area is the most common site of lesion.

from a mild to a severe degree. Most patients may recover well from their motor problems. On the other hand, some patients may possibly have oral and limb apraxia. Some patients may possibly have right sensory impairment (Benson & Ardila, 1996; Damasio, 2001; Helm-Estabrooks & Albert, 2004; Simmons-Mackie, 2005).

Major Language Characteristics of Conduction Aphasia

Impaired repetition and fluent and paraphasic speech with naming difficulties characterize patients with conduction aphasia (Benson & Ardila, 1996; Damasio, 2001; Helm-Estabrooks & Albert, 2004; Simmons-Mackie, 2005).

Patients with conduction aphasia tend to exhibit:

- *Impaired repetition.* The distinguishing feature of conduction aphasia is the marked difficulty in repeating modeled productions, even though the patients comprehension of spoken language is good. Disproportionately impaired repetition with good auditory comprehension is a key diagnostic feature of conduction aphasia. In Broca's and Wernicke's aphasia, impairments in repetition and other language skills are proportionate; in conduction aphasia, repetition impairment is disproportionate to other impairments. When asked to repeat modeled productions, the patient's repetition may consist of added or deleted phonemes (phonemic paraphasia). The patients with conduction aphasia may find repetition of longer words, phrases, sentences, and unfamiliar phrases the most difficult. They also may find function words to be more difficult to repeat than content words. Nonetheless, the patients may use words in spontaneous speech that they cannot repeat.

- *Varied speech fluency.* The patients with conduction aphasia may be variable in their speech fluency. Some are more fluent than others, but generally even the more fluent patients are less fluent than those with Wernicke's aphasia. Hesitations and self-corrections interrupt the fluency of patients with conduction aphasia. Therefore, conduction aphasia is a fluent aphasia but not as fluent an aphasia as Wernicke's.

- *Paraphasic speech.* Although patients with conduction aphasia exhibit paraphasias, semantic paraphasias and neologisms are less frequent than in other fluent aphasias.

- *Marked word-finding problems.* There may be more word-finding problems on content words than on function words. Consequently, their speech may be devoid of content words, leading to empty speech.

- *Recognition of errors.* Patients with conduction aphasia seem to be aware of their errors as they tend to make efforts to correct them. Unfortunately, their efforts at self-correction are no more successful than those with Broca's aphasia.

- *Typically good syntactic and prosodic features.* Patients with conduction aphasia use normally varied syntactic structures, a feature that distinguishes them from those with Broca's aphasia.

- *Typically normal speech articulation.* However, literal paraphasia (sound substitutions) are frequent in the speech of patients with conduction aphasia and are actually more prominent in repetition tasks. Patients tend to substitute difficult phonemes with simpler ones. Phoneme deletions are also common, but phoneme additions are rare. Generally, articulation may be better in singing than in speech.

- *Naming problems.* Patients with conduction aphasia may exhibit mild to severe naming deficits. When asked to name objects, an occasional patient may simply fail to name, but most patients produce a plethora of literal paraphasia. Interestingly, the patients who cannot name objects may easily point to the objects named for them.

- *Normal or near-normal auditory comprehension.* In most patients, comprehension may be adequate for typical conversation. Those who show comprehension deficits may find it difficult to understand only the grammatically more complex structures.

- *Variable reading problems.* Most patients have difficulty reading aloud. Their oral reading may be filled with paraphasias, and they may simply fail to read short printed material. Nonetheless, the patients can silently read *and* comprehend such long and complex material as a novel or a scientific book.

- *Writing problems.* Most patients have some level of difficulty writing. The patients can write a few words with well-formed letters; spelling errors, letter omissions, reversals, and substitutions may be common in these and extended writing.

- *Buccofacial apraxia.* Difficulty in performing buccofacial movements when requested may be present in most patients. Some patients may fail to perform limb movements upon request.

In essence, a disproportionate impairment in repetition, fluent speech that is not as fluent as the speech of Wernicke's patients, phonemic paraphasias, and good comprehension are among the more important distinguishing features of conduction aphasia (Simmons-Mackie, 1997).

See Table 6-3 for a summative overview of major language characteristics that are diagnostic of conduction aphasia.

Individual Differences in Patients with Conduction Aphasia

Patients with conduction aphasia may vary more widely than patients with other types of aphasia because of varied lesion sites. The degree of fluency varies across patients.

Depending on the site of lesion, some patients may have visual problems. Others may have limb apraxia.

Relative Strengths of Patients with Conduction Aphasia

Patients with conduction aphasia have an excellent chance for significant to near-complete recovery from motor and language problems. Most patients

TABLE 6-3   The major language characteristics of patients with conduction aphasia.

Language Parameter	In Conduction Aphasia	Positive (+√) or Negative (−√) Diagnostic Feature
Speech comprehension	Good; mild impairment	−√
Fluency	Good, but some pauses and paraphasia	−√
Grammar	Good	−√
Paraphasia	Literal paraphasia	+√
Naming	Impaired	+√
Articulation	Good	−√
Pointing	Good	−√
Repetition	Severely impaired	+√
Reading aloud	Impaired	+√
Reading comprehension	Good	−√
Writing	Impaired	+√
Awareness, self-correction	Aware; unsuccessful self-correction attempts	−√

with residual problems can supplement their verbal expressions with appropriate gestures and intonation. The periodic phonemic paraphasia these patients exhibit (e.g., "pepperoni bitza") may not erect communication barriers.

Anomic Aphasia

Anomic aphasia also is known as *amnesic aphasia, amnestic aphasia,* and *nominal aphasia.* Many investigators have described a predominant naming problem as anomic aphasia, when most other language functions, including repetition, are within the normal range. Benson and Ardila (1996) classify anomic aphasia as an extrasylvian aphasia, a classification that includes transcortical aphasias. In fact, Benson (1979a) considered anomic aphasia and transcortical sensory aphasia as two points on a continuum.

There is much doubt about its existence as a reliable syndrome of aphasia (Benson & Ardila, 1996). The undetermined or highly variable lesion sites is one reason for doubting the validity of this diagnostic category.

Anomia is naming difficulty; it is a symptom of almost all types of aphasia. **Anomic aphasia** is a syndrome whose overriding feature is a persistent and severe naming problem in the context of relatively intact language skills. Therefore, it is necessary to distinguish *anomia* as a symptom from *anomia* as a *syndrome.*

As a symptom, anomia is found not only in aphasia but also in several forms of dementia (see Chapters 14, 15, and 16), encephalitis, increased intracranial pressure, subarachnoid hemorrhage, concussion, right-hemisphere injury (see Chapters 10 and 11), and all cases with generalized (diffuse, nonfocal) brain damage. Furthermore, anomia is the most commonly found residual symptom in persons who have recovered from all types of aphasia.

Neuroanatomical Bases of Anomic Aphasia

Lesions that cause anomic aphasia are controversial or generally varied; in some cases, the loci may not be identified with any degree of certainty. Damage in multiple sites may be associated with anomic aphasia. Some frequently cited sites of lesions include the angular gyrus and the second temporal gyrus (Davis, 2000; Helm-Estabrooks & Albert, 1991; Raymer, 2005). The juncture of temporoparietal lobes also maybe involved. These sites that may cause anomic aphasia are shown in Figure 6-4.

Major Language Characteristics of Anomic Aphasia

Although the lesion site is not definite and multiple sites may be involved, the syndrome of anomic aphasia may be identified with a cluster of positive and negative signs. The most significant positive sign is the persistent naming problem. Fluent if somewhat empty speech may be another positive sign. Other signs are either negative or somewhat variable (Davis, 2000; Helm-Estabrooks & Albert, 2004; Raymer, 2005).

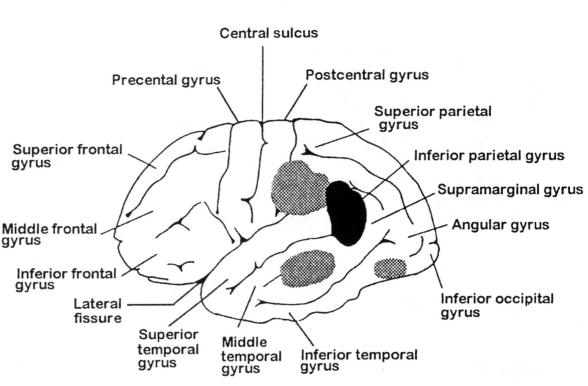

Figure 6-4. Neuroanatomical bases of anomic aphasia. The dark and the lighter shaded areas are among the multiple sites of lesion.

Patients with anomic aphasia tend to exhibit:

- *Debilitating and pervasive word-finding difficulty.* This is the hallmark of anomic aphasia. To diagnose anomic aphasia, the extent of this problem should exceed all other communication problems of a patient.

- *Unimpaired pointing.* The patient who cannot name may easily point to the named objects, suggesting good comprehension of spoken names.

- *Fluent speech.* The speech of patients with anomic aphasia is often described as fluent, but this is not fully accurate. Their serious and pervasive naming problems force them to pause and repeat excessively. Their speech may be full of nonspecific words and circumlocution. Their substitution of words such as *this, that,* and *thing* for specific words results in empty speech.

- *Normal syntax.* Generally, the syntactic structures of patients with anomic aphasia are within nominal limits.

- *Verbal paraphasia.* A common problem found in patients with anomic aphasia is word substitutions. As noted before, nonspecific words replace specific words, resulting in both empty speech and circumlocution (beating around the bush).

- *Good auditory comprehension.* Most patients can follow normal conversation although in some a subtle problem may be found.

- *Intact repetition.* Patients have no difficulty imitating a clinician's modeled words, phrases, and sentences.

- *Good articulation.* Anomic aphasia generally is not associated with articulation problems.

- *Normal or near-normal oral reading and writing.* The patients can comprehend what they read or write.

See Table 6-4 for a summative overview of major language characteristics that are diagnostic of anomic aphasia.

TABLE 6-4   The major language characteristics of patients with anomic aphasia.

Language Parameter	In Anomic Aphasia	Positive ($+\sqrt{}$) or Negative ($-\sqrt{}$) Diagnostic Feature
Speech comprehension	Good; mild impairment	$-\sqrt{}$
Fluency	Good, but frequent pauses and some paraphasias	$-\sqrt{}$
Grammar	Good; normal syntactic and morphologic features	$-\sqrt{}$
Paraphasia	Occasional paraphasic errors	$+\sqrt{}$
Naming	Severely impaired	$+\sqrt{}$
Articulation	Good	$-\sqrt{}$
Pointing	Good	$-\sqrt{}$
Repetition	Good	$-\sqrt{}$
Reading aloud	Good	$-\sqrt{}$
Reading comprehension	Good	$-\sqrt{}$
Writing	Good	$-\sqrt{}$

Individual Differences in Patients with Anomic Aphasia

Except for the naming problem, most other symptoms may vary across patients. Such variability is not surprising in view of the varied sites of lesion that can produce anomic aphasia. For instance, patients who have more frontal lesions may be able to name objects if a phonemic cue (the first sound of the word) is provided.

When the lesion is in the angular gyrus, the patients who cannot name an object may also fail to recognize it when the examiner says the name. They may repeat a word endlessly with no comprehension of its meaning.

Relative Strengths of Patients with Anomic Aphasia

Generally, most language functions, except for naming, are relatively unimpaired. As noted, the consequence of this serious naming problem is paraphasic speech. Clinically, treatment is concerned with the single debilitating problem of word finding (naming).

Suggested Readings

Read the following for additional information on fluent aphasias and their differential diagnosis:

Benson, D. F., & Ardila, A. (1996). *Aphasia: A clinical perspective.* New York: Oxford University Press.

Cimino-Knight, A. M., Hollingsworth, A. L., & Gonzalez Rothi, L. J. (2005). The transcortical aphasias. In L. L. LaPointe (Ed.), *Aphasia and related neurogenic language disorders* (3rd ed., pp. 169–185). New York: Thieme Medical Publishers.

Collins, M. J. (2005). Global aphasia. In L. L. LaPointe (Ed.), *Aphasia and related neurogenic language disorders* (3rd ed., pp. 186–198). New York: Thieme Medical Publishers.

Kearns, K. P. (2005). Broca's aphasia. In L. L. LaPointe (Ed.), *Aphasia and related neurogenic language disorders* (3rd ed., pp. 117–141). New York: Thieme Medical Publishers.

Raymer, A. (2005). Naming and word retrieval problems. In L. L. LaPointe (Ed.), *Aphasia and related neurogenic language disorders* (3rd ed., pp. 68–82). New York: Thieme Medical Publishers.

Simmons-Mackie, N. (1997). Conduction aphasia. In L. L. LaPointe (Ed.), *Aphasia and related neurogenic language disorders* (2nd ed., pp. 63–90). New York: Thieme Medical Publishers.

ATYPICAL APHASIAS AND APHASIA IN SPECIAL POPULATIONS

Chapter Outline

- Atypical Syndromes
- Alexia
- Agraphia
- Agnosia
- Aphasia in Special Populations

Learning Objectives

After reading the chapter, the student will:

- Describe the distinction between cortical and subcortical aphasias.

- Specify the neuropathology of subcortical aphasias.

- Describe the speech and language characteristics of patients with subcortical aphasias.

- Define and describe alexia, agraphia, and agnosia.

- Describe and distinguish aphasia in bilingual, left-handed, and sign language users.

- Define and describe crossed aphasia, its neuroanatomic bases, and language characteristics.

Atypical Syndromes

As the literature on aphasia has expanded over the years, two factors have become apparent. First, in spite of proliferating syndromes, up to 50 percent or more patients with aphasia do not fit the description of standard syndromes (fluent and nonfluent and their varieties). Several unusual or rare syndromes of aphasia and related disorders do not fit the traditional classification. These forms of aphasia are described as *atypical syndromes* (Coppens, Lebrun, & Basso, 1998).

Additional atypical syndromes include reading and writing problems that are disproportionately greater than other language and cognitive problems. Finally, sensory disorders in the absence of peripheral sensory problems, which are called *agnosias,* also are included in a discussion of atypical language disorders based on cerebral pathology. The list of such atypical forms of aphasia gets periodically expanded with the addition of new forms, as described in this chapter.

Second, aphasia in certain specific populations has been of both research and clinical interest. Aphasia in such populations may not be entirely atypical, but their special study may be worthwhile. For instance, a study of aphasia in people who are illiterate, bilingual, or left-handed and those who use tonal or signed languages may illuminate aspects of aphasia in all speakers.

This chapter provides brief descriptions of atypical aphasias and various manifestations of alexia, agraphia, and agnosia. The chapter also includes aphasia in selected specific populations. Atypical syndromes include subcortical aphasias, alexia and its different forms, agraphia, and agnosia.

Subcortical Aphasias

That aphasia is a language disorder associated with cortical pathology is the classic view. In recent years, however, language and speech disorders associated with subcortical pathology have been reported. **Subcortical aphasias** are those that are often associated with damage to basal ganglia and the thalamus. Recently developed brain imaging techniques have been useful in understanding the role of sub-cortical structures in language. Nonetheless, many unresolved issues surround the concept of subcortical aphasia:

- It is doubtful whether lesions in subcortical structures alone produce aphasia; it is believed that in addition to subcortical pathology, damage to other left hemisphere gray matter is necessary to produce aphasia. In many cases of subcortical aphasia, CT scans may have failed to detect existing cortical damage.

- Language disorders associated with subcortical structures do not necessarily mean that the structures have language functions; the disorders may be due to general swelling and reduction in cerebral blood flow following subcortical damage. In essence, reduced metabolic rate in the structurally intact left cerebral cortex may be responsible for the symptoms.

- Nonetheless, evidence for linking certain subcortical structures to aphasia has been reported and likely more such evidence will be forthcoming.

- Some structures (e.g., the insula, which is suspected to have an unspecified language function) are deep within the brain, but they still are cortical, not subcortical.

- To produce aphasia, subcortical damage must be extensive.

Neuroanatomical Bases of Subcortical Aphasia

Two major structural regions have been associated with subcortical aphasias: basal ganglia, along with their surrounding structures, and the thalamus. Lesions in or surrounding the left basal ganglia are reported to have been involved in several cases of subcortical aphasia. Aphasia resulting from such areas are often described as nonthalamic and classified into three varieties. The first variety of nonthalamic aphasia is associated with anterior damage in the internal capsule and the putamen. The second variety is associated with a posterior damage to the capsular-putamenal regions. The third variety is caused by anterior-posterior damage to the internal capsule and the putamen. However, this damage may extend to the thalamus.

Lesions in the left thalamus also are reported to be the cause of subcortical aphasias in several cases. Hemorrhage in the thalamus region has been the most frequently reported cause of subcortical aphasia. A few case studies have supported the diagnosis of thalamic aphasia by demonstrating CT or MRI findings that suggest hemorrhagic damage to the thalamus (Benson & Ardila, 1996). To the contrary, there is evidence that damage to the thalamus may not necessarily produce aphasia. For instance, surgical destruction of the thalamus (performed to relieve symptoms of Parkinson's disease) has not produced aphasia in many patients.

Major Language Characteristics of Subcortical Aphasia

Patients who have lesions in the basal ganglia and surrounding structures in the left hemisphere tend to exhibit a variety of language disorders. The specific pattern of deficits depends on the site of lesion. For instance, patients with *anterior damage in the internal capsule and the putamen* tend to exhibit:

- A severe form of dysarthric articulation
- Phrases of four to six words, indicating adequate phrase length
- Mild repetition problems
- Moderate naming or word-finding problems
- Some auditory comprehension problems
- Moderate reading problems
- Severe writing difficulties

Patients with *posterior capsular-putamen lesions* may exhibit:

- Fluent speech
- Severe auditory comprehension deficits
- Significant naming and word-finding problems
- Mild repetition problems
- Moderate reading difficulties
- Moderate writing problems

Patients who have both *anterior and posterior damage* that extends to the thalamus may exhibit:

- Global aphasia
- Nonfluent and extremely limited spontaneous speech
- Speech limited to stereotyped monosyllabic utterances or single-word productions
- Severely dysarthric articulation
- Severely impaired auditory comprehension
- Significant naming and repetition problems
- Serious reading and writing problems

Patients who have lesions or hemorrhages in the *thalamus* tend to exhibit:

- A serious clinical condition with hemiplegia, hemisensory loss, right-visual field problems, and, in some cases, coma
- Mutism as the patient begins to recover from the initial condition
- Fluent, but paraphasic speech, as the patient recovers from mutism
- Severe naming problems
- Good auditory comprehension for conversational speech, which may be poor for complex material
- Relatively intact repetition
- Significant decrease in paraphasia while repeating modeled phrases
- Impaired reading and writing skills
- Significant improvement in language skills as aphasia due to thalamic hemorrhage tends to be transient if the patient recovers from the subcortical pathology (many patients, however, do not recover from the brain pathology)

Alexia

Alexia is loss of reading proficiency or impaired reading proficiency due to recent brain damage. **Dyslexia** is difficulty in learning to read, even though the instruction was adequate. Some experts use the term *dyslexia* to mean all kinds of reading problems, including those found in patients with recent cerebral pathology. They then use the term *developmental dyslexia* to refer to reading problems in children with no demonstrated cerebral pathology and *acquired dyslexia* to refer to reading problems found in patients with cerebral pathology. To avoid any reference to reading problems in children, the term *alexia* is preferred in this book (Benson & Ardila, 1996).

Several varieties of alexia are found in persons who have acquired normal reading skills and who then have lost them to varying degrees due to cerebral pathology. The three more common varieties include alexia without agraphia, alexia with agraphia, and frontal alexia.

Alexia Without Agraphia (Pure Alexia)

Alexia without agraphia refers to reading problems due to recent brain injury with intact writing skills. Reading problems associated with brain injury were known for centuries. However, it was Joseph Jules Dejerine (1849–1917), a French neurologist, who gave the first systematic and clinical description of alexia in adult patients with cerebral pathology.

In 1892, Dejerine described the case of a patient who could not read but had all other language functions intact, including writing. He could copy printed material, although he could neither read nor understand what he copied.

A postmortem of Dejerine's patient showed lesions in the medial and inferior regions of the occipital lobe and the splenium of the corpus callosum. Later, this syndrome came to be known as *pure alexia, alexia without agraphia, occipital alexia, pure word blindness, agnosic alexia, optic aphasia,* and *posterior alexia* (Benson & Ardila, 1996). Although alexia without agraphia is a rare syndrome, it is easily recognized because of its unique and dramatic effect.

Neuroanatomical Bases of Alexia Without Agraphia

Serious damage to the left visual cortex and to the posterior corpus callosum fibers that connect the left hemisphere with the right visual cortex is the main cause of alexia without agraphia. Medial and inferior regions of the occipital lobe and splenium of the corpus callosum are often involved. The left hemisphere is rendered visually incompetent and the right hemisphere, which is still visually competent, cannot communicate with the left. Two causes of this type of damage have been identified:

- Occlusion of the posterior cerebral artery is the frequent cause of damage to the left visual cortex in the parietal lobe.
- Tumors and malformation of arteries also may cause parietal lobe damage.

Reading and Related Problems of Patients with Alexia Without Agraphia

Pure alexia is characterized by the following symptoms:

- An inability to read normally. Except for a few commonly used words (e.g., patients may read and understand their name and the name of their city), the patients cannot read in the typical manner. However, the patient can read "letter-by-letter" in a laborious manner, because printed letter or number recognition, if lost at the onset, may soon be regained. Printed word recognition may continue to be seriously impaired.
- Normal recognition of words spelled out orally. The patient will have lost only the meaning of the written word.
- Normal recognition of letters and words an examiner traces on the patient's palm. Thus the patient can recognize words and letters in nonvisual sensory experiences.
- Near-normal writing skills, although the patient cannot read what he or she writes. Letter omissions and substitutions may be seen, however.
- Slowly deteriorating writing skills. This difficulty may be due to lack of visual monitoring of writing.
- Difficulty copying written words and sentences. The patient may write the same material to dictation.
- Good recognition of words spelled out by the examiner. The patient also can spell words the examiner says.

- Right hemianopia (visual defects or blindness in half the visual field) in some right-handed individuals. In left-handed individuals, left hemianopia may be observed.
- Generally near-normal oral language skills. Some patients may have naming difficulties, however.
- Especially impaired color naming in many but not all patients. This difficulty extends to pointing to a named color. Nonetheless, the patients may have no difficulty using color names in conversation or answering a question about color (e.g., "What is the color of spinach?").
- No neurological symptoms of significance. Hemianopia may be the only exception.

Most patients show slow but significant recovery of reading skills, especially with reading therapy. However, the recovery rarely reaches the premorbid level.

Alexia with Agraphia

Alexia with agraphia refers to writing and reading problems due to recent neurological impairment. In 1891, Dejerine was the first neurologist to give a clinical description of a patient who had both reading and writing problems (alexia with agraphia). Generally, the severity of reading and writing problems is roughly equal. Reading of any kind of symbols, including musical notations and mathematical formulae may be affected. This syndrome also is known as *angular alexia, parietal-temporal alexia, central alexia, semantic alexia,* and *letter blindness.*

Neuroanatomical Bases of Alexia with Agraphia

Patients who have alexia with agraphia may or may not present serious and obvious neurological symptoms. At the onset, the patients may experience a temporary paresis of their upper extremities. A more permanent effect might be a right-sided sensory loss or right visual field defect. Investigations with CT, MRI, isotope brain scan, surgical exploration, and autopsy have confirmed the following neuroanatomical factors associated with alexia with agraphia:

- The lesion is in the angular gyrus, toward the back end of the sylvian fissure at the parietal-temporal lobe junction (hence the name, parietal-temporal alexia).
- The most common cause of the lesion is cerebrovascular pathology involving the angular branch of the middle cerebral artery.
- Tumors, metastatic tumors, trauma, and gunshot wounds are among the other causes of a lesion.

The lesion isolates the visual cortex from Wernicke's area and Broca's area. Furthermore, the lesion disconnects Wernicke's area from the anterior motor planning area. Therefore, what the patient reads is not communicated to Wernicke's area, leading to an inability to read. The motor area, not receiving any information from Wernicke's area or visual cortex, cannot execute motor actions involved in writing.

Reading and Writing Problems of Patients with Alexia and Agraphia

Alexia with agraphia is characterized by dominant reading and writing problems and some symptoms of aphasia. As noted previously, an initial paresis of the upper extremities and right-sided sensory deficits complete the clinical picture:

- Loss or serious impairment in reading and writing skills. The loss often is partial; the two skills often are impaired to about the same extent.
- Difficulty in reading aloud. The difficulty extends to letters and words; this is unlike patients with pure alexia who can recognize letters of the alphabet.
- Difficulty in comprehending what has been read. This difficulty extends to a comprehension of musical notations, mathematical formulae, and other symbolic notations.
- Difficulty in comprehending words spelled out loud. This problem also is unlike that found in patients with pure alexia who can recognize words spelled out loud.
- Writing problems that parallel reading problems. Patients can write letters and letter

combinations that appear like words; however, the letter combinations they produce are nonsensical.

- Letter and word copying skills that are better than spontaneous writing skills. Patients cannot transpose printed writing to cursive writing and vice versa.
- Difficulty in solving arithmetic problems (acalculia). This difficulty may be compounded by the patient's inability to understand abstract number systems.
- Certain symptoms of aphasia. These may include deficient auditory comprehension of spoken language, paraphasia, impaired repetition, and anomia; only in rare cases are these aphasia symptoms absent.

Many patients recover their reading and writing skills to some extent. Residual problems probably are common, limiting reading comprehension and writing skills. A patient's premorbid literacy skills and the need and motivation to maintain those skills may influence the rate of recovery.

Frontal Alexia

Frontal alexia refers to poor reading skills in patients who have suffered damage to areas in the frontal cortex. In addition to other kinds of reading problems, frontal alexia is characterized by refusal to read or inability to read when requested. Of all the types of alexia, frontal alexia has generated the most controversy. Frontal alexia most often is associated with Broca's aphasia. Early investigators thought that poor reading skills of patients with Broca's aphasia were due to their limited literacy. Also, not all patients with Broca's aphasia have frontal alexia, leading to the controversy. Founding psychoanalyst Sigmund Freud, who practiced neurology early in his career, was one of the first to draw attention to the coexistence of frontal alexia and Broca's aphasia, which has now been confirmed (Benson & Ardila, 1996).

Neuroanatomical Bases of Frontal Alexia

Patients who have frontal alexia may present right hemiplegia. In addition, visual problems may be seen in a few patients. Neuroimaging techniques and autopsies have confirmed the neuroanatomical bases of frontal alexia.

- The most frequent site of lesion is the posterior portion of the inferior frontal gyrus.
- The lesion may extend into the anterior insula, an oval region buried in the depths of the lateral fissure.
- The most frequent cause of lesion, as in Broca's aphasia, is a cerebrovascular accident (CVA); tumors and trauma also may be involved.

When present, the reading difficulties of patients with Broca's aphasia may be described as alexia. However, it should be noted that alexia is not a diagnostic feature of Broca's aphasia.

Reading and Related Problems of Patients with Frontal Alexia

Patients with frontal alexia exhibit a pattern of symptoms that distinguish them from those with other forms of alexia and agraphia. The disorder is characterized by the following symptoms:

- Significant reading problems. Most patients can read only individual words, especially nouns and verbs that have individual meanings (substantive words).
- Limited comprehension. Patients may comprehend only the individual words they can read aloud.
- Difficulty comprehending relational words. Patients may not understand the meaning conveyed by such relational words as adjectives, conjunctions, and prepositions. Negatives and qualifiers also may give problems. They may interpret pairs of positive and negative statements as the same.
- Refusal to read. Patients may insist they have lost the capacity to read and thus avoid reading.
- Failure to read on command. Even though patients can read the words spontaneously, they may be unable to comply when asked to read.
- Morphological errors in reading. Patients may omit printed morphological elements or fail to understand them.

- Significant writing problems. These problems may partly be due to writing with the nonpreferred left hand because of right paresis. Writing may include grammatic and syntactic mistakes, spelling errors, and poor letter formation. Omission of letters while copying may be common.
- Differential impairment in comprehending spoken versus written language. Patients can better comprehend spoken language than written language.
- Limited verbal output. Patients' conversational speech output may be greatly reduced.

Although both reading and writing are affected in frontal alexia, it is different from alexia with agraphia. Compared to those who have frontal alexia, patients who have alexia and agraphia have much more serious reading and writing problems, approaching near illiteracy. In those patients who have had both frontal alexia and Broca's aphasia but recover from their aphasia, reading problems may remain the most serious residual symptoms (Benson & Ardila, 1996).

Agraphia

Agraphia is writing disorders associated with recent cerebral pathology. The term implies a loss or impairment of previously acquired writing skill. Hence, it does not refer to writing problems in children who still are learning to write. The term also does not refer to writing problems seen in psychiatric conditions, including confusional states.

The 19th century British neurologist John Ogle introduced the term *agraphia* in 1867 to describe writing problems seen in neurologically involved patients. In 1881, the Austrian physiologist Sigmund Exner proposed that the foot of the second frontal gyrus (portion of the premotor cortex close to the hand region of the motor cortex lying above Broca's area) is the cerebral writing center. This area is sometimes referred to as *Exner's area* (Benson & Ardila, 1996; Tseng & McNeil, 1997). Exner's area has not been accepted by later researchers, and many have suggested that writing involves the participation of several brain centers.

Lesions in the left hemisphere tend to produce more pronounced structural and syntactic writing problems than those in the right hemisphere. Writing of patients with left hemisphere damage may contain agrammatic, syntactic, and neologistic errors. Anterior lesions may produce structurally poor writing (misspellings, poor letter formation). Posterior lesions may cause problems in word order and word omissions, but the letters may be well formed.

Right hemisphere lesions may affect certain spatial aspects of writing. For example, giving adequate margins and spaces in writing may be more severely impaired in patients who have right hemisphere damage. Left neglect in reading and drawing also may be evident.

As noted in the previous units on aphasia, most aphasic patients have writing problems of varying severity. In this sense, agraphia is associated with such major aphasia types as Broca's, Wernicke's, and conduction. Major writing problems associated with these and other types of aphasia have been described in the previous units.

In this section, a few additional forms of agraphia are briefly described. Benson and Ardila (1996) and Tseng and McNeil (1997) provide additional information on varieties of agraphia.

Pure Agraphia

Pure agraphia refers to an isolated writing disorder with all other language functions, including auditory comprehension, being normal or nearly so. Patients who exhibit pure agraphia do not have aphasia, apraxia, or alexia, although a case or two described as pure agraphia have included alexia (Benson & Ardila, 1996). The existence of this syndrome is debated, although a few cases of writing problems with no other language difficulties have been noted.

The patient may be unable to write anything, although there is no aphasia and no motor involvement. Some patients with pure agraphia may make errors in spontaneous writing but their automatic writing, copying, and letter formation may be well preserved. The damage is reported to be in the premotor cortex (Exner's area). Lesions in the left superior parietal lobe also have been linked to pure agraphia. Both auditory comprehension and expressive language are normal or near-normal.

Apraxic Agraphia

Apraxic agraphia refers to writing problems associated with apraxia. The disorder involves serious problems in letter formation. Some patients may only produce a scribble for each letter. Others may write with numerous spelling errors and repeated words. Still other patients may write only in capital letters. Spontaneous writing, copying, and writing to dictation all may be equally affected. Patients with apraxic alexia may spell words correctly and write words with block letters. The patients could say the letters of the words they were asked to write but produce only a scribble.

Descriptions of symptoms of apraxic agraphia are sometimes contradictory. While some patients so described could not copy, others could. While some could not print block letters, others could. Focal brain lesions, often in the parietal lobe, cause apraxic agraphia.

Motor Agraphia

Motor agraphia is a group of writing disorders that are due to neuromotor problems. Several varieties have been described. For example, in paretic agraphia, peripheral nerve problems create writing difficulties; both lower and upper motor neuron pathology can affect the muscles of hands (paresis, weakness, spasticity) and in turn affect writing.

Hypokinetic agraphia (micrographia) is a motor disorder of writing with unusually small letters or letters that get progressively smaller in a piece of writing. This disorder often is associated with Parkinson's disease.

Hyperkinetic agraphia is a disorder of writing associated with tremors, tics, chorea, and dystonia. When upper limbs have involuntary hyperkinetic movements, writing is extremely disturbed or even impossible.

Research on normal and disordered writing is extremely limited. Treatment of spoken language deficits in patients with cerebral lesions has been a priority. Generally, treatment directed at improving writing skills ends with improved oral communication skills. We need more research on treating writing skills in patients who have aphasia and specific forms of agraphia.

Agnosia

A group of disorders involving cerebral pathology and affecting recognition of sensory stimuli is called agnosia. **Agnosia** is difficulty grasping the meaning of certain stimuli, even though there is no sensory impairment. Patients with agnosia can see, hear, or feel stimuli, but do not recognize them for what they are, although the inability typically is limited to one modality. This kind of pure agnosia is rare. An impression of agnosia may be sometimes gained by difficulty in sensory discrimination, intellectual deterioration, or difficulty in simple comprehension.

Agnosia is not due to intellectual impairment or deficiency. It is not due to dementia. Once recognized, the person can name the object or the stimulus. A stimulus whose meaning is not grasped in one sensory modality (e.g., visual) is easily grasped in another modality (e.g., tactile). For instance, a patient who fails to name an object on sight may readily name it when the same object is placed in his or her hand. Here are a few major types of agnosic disorders.

- *Auditory agnosia* is an inability to recognize or understand the meaning of auditory stimuli in persons whose peripheral hearing is within normal limits. Bilateral damage to the auditory association area is the typical neuropathology causing auditory agnosia. Patients with auditory agnosia can respond to sound but cannot grasp its meaning. Although they can visually recognize objects, patients cannot match objects with sounds with which they are associated.

- *Auditory verbal agnosia* or *pure word deafness* is a disorder in which the patients cannot understand the meaning of spoken words though they can hear them. Recognition of nonverbal sounds and that of printed or written words is unimpaired. Spontaneous speech, reading, and writing are normal or only minimally affected. Bilateral temporal lobe lesions that isolate Wernicke's area cause this rare disorder.

- *Visual agnosia* is a rare disorder in which the meaning of objects seen normally is not understood. The patients can recognize the stimuli by hearing the sounds they make or by touching and feeling (tactile sensation). This intermittent and inconsistent disorder is typically caused by bilateral occipital lobe damage, posterior parietal lobe damage, or damage to fiber tracts that connect the visual cortex to other brain areas.

- *Tactile agnosia* is a disorder in which the patients cannot recognize objects they touch and feel when blindfolded (they do not see the objects) or hear the sounds the objects make. The patients can feel the objects and report touch and other tactile stimuli but cannot name them or describe them. When they see or hear the characteristic sound, the patients readily recognize the objects or stimuli. The typical lesion site is in the parietal lobe; the lesion isolates the somatosensory cortex from other parts of the brain.

Aphasia in Special Populations

Aphasia in certain special populations has been a subject of research and writing (Coppens, Lebrun, & Basso, 1998). In this section, we will take a brief look at selected populations in which aphasia has been of special interest to clinicians and researchers.

Aphasia in Bilingual Individuals

Bilingual individuals who have aphasia present a special opportunity to study the potentially differential decline in their two languages. A varied symptom complex in the two languages, if present, may shed some light on how the brain processes two or more languages.

Unfortunately, careful studies of aphasia in bilingual persons, with equally competent analysis of deficits in both the languages, are few and fraught with methodological problems. Clinicians generally tend to ignore the bilingual status of the patient. Bilingual patients with aphasia are common in almost all societies, as 80 percent of the people worldwide may be bilingual. In the United States, it is estimated that more than 150,000 patients are bilingual and 45,000 new bilingual cases may be reported each year. Nonetheless, bilingual patients are typically assessed and treated in the dominant language of the society, the region, or the hospital (Paradis, 1998).

Most people who are bilingual do not have a perfect knowledge of both the languages just as very few monolingual individuals have a perfect knowledge of their language. Bilingual individuals may be equally proficient in the two languages, somewhat deficient in both, and more proficient in one and less in the other. See Table 7-1 for definitions of terms that suggest different degrees of bilingualism.

There has been a suggestion that in a bilingual person, the right hemisphere is dominant for language (perhaps the second language). An overwhelming body of research evidence has contradicted this suggestion, however. As in unilingual speakers, the left hemisphere is dominant for language in bilingual speakers. The right hemisphere participation may be limited to some aspects of pragmatic use of language (see Chapters 10 and 11 on right hemisphere syndrome for details). As in unilingual speakers, aphasia in bilingual speakers is associated with left hemisphere damage. Types of aphasia and the way they evolve are similar across unilingual and bilingual speakers (Paradis, 1998).

TABLE 7-1 Bilingualism is a matter of degree.

Term	Definition
Unilingual	A person who speaks only one language.
Ambilingual (perfect bilingual)	A person who speaks each of the two languages in the same, native manner.
Equilingual (balanced)	A person who speaks two languages with equal proficiency, regardless of the mastery level.
Semilingual	A person who speaks two languages, but neither is native-like; the person needs both to express himself or herself.
Dominant bilingual	A person who speaks two languages, but one with a greater proficiency than the other.

The research on aphasia in bilingual speakers and its course of change with or without treatment consists mostly of uncontrolled observations and individual and unreplicated case histories. Reliability of such observations is difficult to establish. All generalizations about patterns of recovery summarized here are subject to change as new and systematic observations are reported. Available observations have revealed that performance and patterns of recovery in the two languages of a bilingual speaker may vary in all possible way (Benson & Ardila, 1996; Paradis, 1998):

- The recovered language may or may not be native, preferred, dominant, or that of the surrounding environment.
- Recovery of one or the other language of a patient with aphasia bears no systematic relationship to the site or severity of lesion.
- Some patients recover their dual language skills to roughly the same premorbid level (parallel recovery).
- Some patients may recover one language better than the other, even though they spoke both the languages equally proficiently before the onset of aphasia.
- Some patients who spoke one of the two languages better before the onset of aphasia may recover both equally, to the pleasant surprise of family members.
- Generally, the premorbidly better-spoken language may be recovered sooner or to a greater extent than the one spoken not as well; however, certain patients may recover better the premorbidly poorly spoken language than the one spoken more efficiently.
- Some patients may never recover one of the two languages (selective recovery).
- Some patients may recover a language only months after they recovered the other language (successive recovery).
- Some patients may begin to lose the language they first regained just when they begin to regain the skills in the other, hitherto unregained, language (antagonistic recovery). Other patients may alternately lose and gain the two languages in a seesaw pattern of recovery.

- Some bilingual patients may intermingle phrases and sentences (not just individual words) between languages.

- A few patients may automatically translate their own or other person's utterances in one language into another. Strangely, some patients may translate into a language they cannot spontaneously speak now (but they did before) but not to a language they do speak now.

- Some patients may begin to recover a language that they now speak with the accent of the other language, even though they did not use that accent premorbidly.

- In some rare cases, the little-used and long-forgotten native language may be better retained to the dismay of younger family members who have not heard that language.

- The known patterns of recovery may mix over time or across languages in the same patients.

- Generally, individual differences are more important than known patterns; a patient may not fit any known pattern.

The clinician should collect detailed information on the premorbid skill levels in the two (or more) languages an individual patient spoke. The clinician then should carefully evaluate the current skills and the emerging patterns of recovery of the languages throughout the treatment period. Because most clinicians cannot do this efficiently, the help of an expert translator is typically necessary.

Aphasia in Left-Handed Individuals

Roughly 4 percent of the population are left handed, 30 percent are mixed handed, and 66 percent are right handed (Basso & Rusconi, 1998). Of the small number of left-handed people, only 50 percent may have a right hemisphere dominance for language. In essence, no more than 2 percent of the general population (who also are left-handed) may have language represented in their right hemisphere. Therefore, it is now well established that handedness is no indication of cerebral language dominance.

Methodologically sound research on aphasia in left-handed individuals is limited. Available evidence seems to support the following statements:

- The incidence of aphasia due to left hemisphere lesions in left-handed speakers may be roughly the same as that in right-handed individuals with left hemisphere lesions.
- The incidence of aphasia due to right hemisphere lesions in left-handed individuals is greater than the incidence of aphasia due to similar lesions in right-handed individuals.
- Aphasia that results from right or left hemisphere lesions does not seem to differ substantially.
- Recovery from aphasia produced by left hemisphere lesions does not seem to be related to handedness.

In general, research on aphasia in left-handed individuals has not produced data that make significant differences in assessment or treatment. By and large, differences between right- and left-handed aphasia patients have been overestimated in the past (Basso & Rusconi, 1998).

Aphasia in Sign Language Users

Whether sign language users, including the deaf, have a different cerebral language representation than those who use oral language has been researched and debated. Available evidence shows that for deaf signers, as in hearing speakers of oral (spoken) language, left hemisphere lesions cause aphasia. Right hemisphere lesions in sign language users do not severely disrupt signing skills but lead to effects that are similar to those produced in oral language speakers with normal hearing. In essence, cerebral language dominance is independent of the type of language used (oral or signed); it is typically the left hemisphere that dominates language functions.

A more fascinating line of research is the nature of aphasia in sign language users, rather than the cerebral dominance of signed versus spoken languages. Several case studies of aphasia in deaf individuals who use sign language have been reported. Many early studies analyzed impairments in only finger spelling, not the use of full-fledged sign language (Corina, 1998). More recent studies done with better methods have suggested the following:

- Deaf sign language users who suffer posterior temporal lobe damage may have difficulty understanding the signs (sign language comprehension deficit).

- Generally, impaired comprehension deficits may be associated with impaired sign production skills. Nonetheless, impaired comprehension but intact production of signs has been reported in individual cases whose occipital areas were involved.

- Deaf sign language users may have difficult producing signs when they sustain left and anterior frontal lobe damage. These production deficits resemble those of oral speakers with similar damage. Signing may be effortful and dysfluent (not smooth flowing) and restricted mostly to single sign productions.

- Similar to verbal paraphasia, aphasic sign language users may exhibit hand shape paraphasias in which correct movements are substituted with incorrect ones.

- Aphasic sign language users may omit movements that are suggestive of morphologic features of their language.

- Nonfluent signing in premorbidly fluent sign language users is typically associated with a lesion in Broca's area and further involvement of cortical regions controlling hand and arm movements.

- Fluent but somewhat meaningless signing in deaf individuals is associated with a more posterior cerebral damage, although Wernicke's area may not necessarily be involved. Such patients' comprehension of sign language may be severely impaired.

- Right hemisphere lesions in deaf sign language users may produce discourse deficits, including excessive attention to detail or omitting essential features in describing events or stimuli.

In essence, the left and right hemisphere damage in hearing and deaf individuals produces similar effects. Although brain imaging studies have shown bilateral activation in sign language users, its clinical significance is not clear (Corina, 1998).

Crossed Aphasia

Crossed aphasia is a rare form of aphasia in right-handed individuals who sustain a single right hemisphere lesion. In a majority of cases, vascular pathology in the right hemisphere causes crossed aphasia. Tumor in the right hemisphere is a distant second cause.

Aphasia in right-handed individuals is *uncrossed* if the language dominance is clearly established in the right hemisphere. Because the left hemisphere dominance of language is demonstrated in right-handed and even many left-handed individuals, crossed aphasia has been a puzzle and a fertile ground for speculation. Several hypotheses have been proposed to account for crossed aphasia:

- Crossed aphasia may be the result of either right-hemisphere, bilateral, or diffuse language representation in the brain. Evidence of language representation in patients who exhibit crossed aphasia is inconclusive and contradictory.

- Crossed aphasia may be due to a concomitant and undiscovered lesion in the left hemisphere. This hypothesis has been difficult to sustain in the absence of demonstrated left hemisphere lesions.

- Crossed aphasia may be due to subcortical lesions in the right hemisphere, thus denying the existence of a rare or unique *crossed* aphasia. Although some patients with crossed aphasia had subcortical lesions, many did not. Therefore, most experts reject this view (Coppens & Hungerford, 1998).

- Crossed aphasia may be due to the effects of a right hemisphere lesion that spreads to the left hemisphere. For instance, the lesion could reduce the metabolic rate in the unaffected regions of the brain. Evidence on this hypothesis has been contradictory.

Currently, there is no satisfactory explanation of crossed aphasia that is unequivocally supported by data and agreed upon by experts. It is possible that the syndrome has multiple causes, supporting somewhat contradictory claims (Coppens & Hungerford, 1998).

Beyond its etiology, there is disagreement on most all aspects of crossed aphasia. The incidence of crossed aphasia in right-handed aphasic persons is reported to be as low as zero and as high as 18 percent. Many studies report incidence in the range of 1 to 3 percent. Although some studies report a younger mean age of onset, others have reported no such trend. While some have claimed more women than men may exhibit crossed aphasia, others have disputed this.

The symptoms of crossed aphasia, too, are not without controversy. The following characteristics, each with a dose of contradictory evidence, have been reported:

- Crossed aphasia is typically nonfluent and agrammatic, with initial mutism. But nonfluent aphasia is more common in uncrossed aphasia as well.
- Naming skills are preserved in most patients.
- Language comprehension skills may be varied across patients.
- Repetitions skills also may be varied.
- Although the nonfluent variety is more common among patients with crossed aphasia, all other forms, including global, Wernicke's, transcortical, and conduction aphasia, roughly in that order of frequency, have been reported.
- Generally, the symptoms of crossed aphasia are similar to uncrossed aphasia. However, some differences have been noted, although all varieties of uncrossed aphasia also show certain unexpected features:
  - Some patients with crossed Broca's aphasia may have intact reading skills.
  - Some patients with crossed Wernicke's aphasia may only have a mild auditory comprehension deficit.
  - Some patients with crossed and mixed transcortical aphasia may have intact naming skills.
  - Some patients with crossed aphasia may have better oral language skills than written language skills, although the opposite tendency also has been reported.

- Symptoms typical of right hemisphere syndrome (e.g., visual neglect, visuospatial problems, and emotional indifference; see Chapters 10 and 11) may be found in patients with crossed aphasia. The severity of those symptoms may vary significantly.

- There is a suggestion that patients with crossed aphasia recover faster than patients with uncrossed aphasia; however, data do not seem to support this claim. Most experts now believe that pattern of recovery and response to treatment are similar for crossed and uncrossed aphasia.

Little treatment research involves crossed aphasia. Until treatment research begins to guide professional practice, making a careful analysis of deficits to be treated and applying treatment procedures that have been effective with other aphasia syndromes may be the clinician's best approach.

Suggested Readings

Read the following for additional information on atypical aphasias and related syndromes:

Basso, A., & Rusconi, M. L. (1998). Aphasia in left-handers. In P. Coppens, Y. Lebrun, & A. Basso (Eds.), *Aphasia in atypical populations* (pp. 1–34). Mahwah, NJ: Lawrence Erlbaum Associates.

Coppens, P., & Hungerford, S. (1998). Crossed aphasia. In P. Coppens, Y. Lebrun, & A. Basso (Eds.), *Aphasia in atypical populations* (pp. 203–260). Mahwah, NJ: Lawrence Erlbaum Associates.

Corina, D. (1998). Aphasia in users of signed languages. In P. Coppens, Y. Lebrun, & A. Basso (Eds.), *Aphasia in atypical populations* (pp. 261–309). Mahwah, NJ: Lawrence Erlbaum Associates.

Paradis, M. (1987). *The assessment of bilingual aphasia.* Hillsdale, NJ: Lawrence Erlbaum Associates.

Tseng, C., & McNeil, M. (1997). Nature and management of acquired neurogenic dysgraphias. In L. L. LaPointe (Ed.), *Aphasia and related neurogenic language disorders* (2nd ed., pp. 172–200). New York: Thieme.

Webb, W. G. (2005). Acquired dyslexias: Reading disorders associated with aphasias. In L. L. LaPointe (Ed.), *Aphasia and related neurogenic language disorders* (3rd ed., pp. 83–96). New York: Thieme.

ASSESSMENT OF APHASIA

Chapter Outline

- Assessment of Aphasia: Some Practical and Professional Considerations

- The Most Frequently Assessed Behaviors

- Activities Used in Assessment

- Direct and Repeated Observation of the Patient

- Standardized Tests in Assessing Aphasia

- Assessment of Functional Communication

- Independent Tests of Specific Skills

- An Outline of Aphasia Assessment

- Assessment of Clients from Varied Ethnocultural Backgrounds

- Differential Diagnosis

Learning Objectives

After reading the chapter, the student will:

- Describe target communication skills that need to be assessed in patients with aphasia.

- Specify a variety of methods of assessing communication skills.

- Describe and evaluate the most commonly used aphasia assessment tools.

- Write assessment plans for patients with different forms of aphasia.

- Describe the guidelines one might use in evaluating patients of varied ethnocultural backgrounds.

- Summarize the differential diagnostic guidelines that help distinguish aphasia from other, potentially confusing conditions.

Assessment of Aphasia: Some Practical and Professional Considerations

In a general sense, the goal of assessment is to understand the patient's past, present, and future. The emphasis will be on the client's communication skills, but those skills must be understood in the context of the client's health problems, prospects for improvement or stabilization of the physical condition, overall quality of life, and family and social support systems. A crucial consideration is what the client can or cannot do now but may be able to (or wishes to do) with the help of treatment and rehabilitation. The patient's family and occupational (if relevant) structure, the social dynamics he or she faces, and the cultural background of the person are a part of this understanding. What the client and family members expect from treatment and rehabilitation and the client's future plans also are important to understand. Furthermore, what the medical and communication prognosis might be for the client needs to be understood as well. As described in Chapter 9, the treatment realm is expanding into social and family structures and support systems of clients. Therefore, it is no longer sufficient to evaluate just a client's neurological or communication problems. Such a view of assessment and treatment also is supported by the World Health Organization's International Classification of Function, Disability and Health (IFC) (WHO, 2001). See Appendix C for a brief review of the revised WHO classification.

An adequate aphasia assessment is time-consuming. Although student clinicians in university speech-language and hearing clinics can extend assessment into a second session, clinicians in most medical and rehabilitation settings do not have the luxury of time. Clinicians are typically expected to complete an assessment in an hour or less. Even with the most efficient use of time, clinicians cannot collect all the kinds of information needed during this time. Some comprehensive standardized test batteries may take more than an hour to administer (e.g., the Boston Aphasia Diagnostic Examination alone can take up to 4 hours!). Therefore, clinicians need to use creative strategies to maximize their assessment time and adopt other methods to collect needed information. For instance, the clinician may:

1. Assess the problems that are functional for the patient, the family, or the immediate caregivers; ask the patient what troubles him or her the most (e.g., "I can't think of the words"). Ask family members and institutional caregivers about the most troublesome skill deficits; this will help limit the parameter of assessment and complete the task in time.

2. Assess the most prominent features of aphasia and probe for less prominent features later, or make an evaluation based on an interview. For instance, use a brief test of naming, and evaluate auditory comprehension problems in Broca's aphasia during the interview, thus avoiding the administration of a time-consuming auditory comprehension test. If warranted, such tests may be administered later.

3. Interview the client and family over the phone and go over the case history to clarify the information before the assessment session.

4. Consider assessment an ongoing activity; keep an eye on behaviors not assessed and be ready to make a quick assessment as the treatment moves from one set of skills to another. Also, some skills may be assessed during the initial treatment sessions, taking only a few minutes each time.

5. Select tests that are relatively brief yet as reliable and valid as some of the longer ones.

6. Use client-specific assessment procedures if they save time compared to the administration of lengthy standardized tests.

7. Obtain a previous but recently conducted assessment report and judge whether the information on the report is credible and still applicable; if so, omit or postpone the administration of certain procedures.

In medical and rehabilitation settings, experienced clinicians can quickly review the patient's medical charts, assess the most critical problems, and suggest an initial treatment plan in about an hour. The student clinician, however, needs to learn all aspects of assessment done in sufficient detail. Only the clinician who has mastered the details of a comprehensive assessment can truncate it and do it efficiently without compromising reliability and validity of assessment data. Therefore, the assessment plan presented in this chapter is more detailed than what is often implemented by expert clinicians. But this may be the way to achieve that expertise.

Technically and clinically, a thorough assessment and understanding of the client help make an accurate diagnosis of aphasia and possibly a differential diagnosis of aphasia type. This differential diagnosis may further help rule out other types of communication disorders. In addition, such an understanding helps the clinician devise a flexible treatment plan for the patient and possibly suggest a prognosis under specified conditions.

Extended, systematic, reliable, valid, flexible, and client-specific measurement of a patient's behavior and skills of interest is the key to fully understanding the patient and to making a comprehensive and reliable assessment of communicative disorders. Aphasia presents no exception to this general rule.

Measurement of the patient's behavior and skills must be *extended.* Superficial observations done over short periods of time may give a wrong picture of the client's communicative skills, although increased clinical expertise will decrease the amount of time needed. Symptoms of aphasia change over time; one type of aphasia may evolve into another. Therefore, assessment-oriented observation is necessary even after treatment has started. Due to practical restraints of time, the traditional assessment is done in a relatively short time, perhaps an hour or so. Extended base rates of communicative behaviors, established before starting treatment, will counter this limitation. Base rates extend the pretreatment observations of the client and his or her communication skills. Periodic assessment as changes seem to occur in the patient will help make continuous assessment.

Measurement must be *systematic.* Systematic measurement involves clearly defined target skills and relatively constant measurement procedures. For instance, if the patient with aphasia shows variability in naming skills, the conditions under which the naming skills are measured, the stimuli used to measure them, and the conditions under which they are measured must be held constant across measurement periods.

Results of measurement must be *reliable*. **Reliability** of measures is assured when repeated measures of the same skill result in consistent scores. Repeated measures, especially baselines established before starting treatment, will help ensure reliability. Results of measurement must be *valid*. **Validity** of measures is assured when the clinician measures only the targeted skills. Measurement of naming skills, for example, should only measure naming skills, and not something else.

Measurement must be *client specific*. **Client-specific measures** are those designed specifically for an individual person. Because individual differences are significant even within a diagnostic type (e.g., Broca's aphasia or Wernicke's aphasia), the assessment methods must suit the individual. Individual differences within and across ethnocultural groups also require flexible and client-specific procedures. The methods should not depend exclusively on standardized tests that make it easier to collect assessment information but may not always assure the reliability, validity, and clinical usefulness of information obtained.

Measurement and analysis should include *adequate sampling of behaviors*. Behaviors are adequately sampled when sufficient numbers of opportunities are given to produce each target skill. Each communicative skill of a patient should be sampled in sufficient numbers. The patient should be offered multiple opportunities to produce a skill being measured. Whether it is naming or conversational turn taking, the clinician should create multiple conditions under which the skills may be exhibited. For instance, instead of asking a patient to name just a few pictures, the clinician should show several, personally relevant pictures for naming. Inadequate behavior sampling is a major cause of unreliable measures. This problem is often aggravated when the clinician exclusively relies on standardized tests to assess communicative and related behaviors. Adequate sampling of behaviors without the use of standardized tests is possible and may even be preferred. To do this, the clinician must know what kinds of behaviors should be sampled and how.

Many symptoms are common to different types of aphasia. Therefore, many common behaviors are frequently assessed across types of aphasia. An understanding of most commonly observed and assessed skills will help clinicians design client-specific and flexible procedures.

The Most Frequently Assessed Behaviors

In assessing aphasia, all forms of communication, including nonverbal and written forms of communication, must be adequately sampled (Davis, 2000; Golper, 1996; Holland, 1996; Murray & Chapey, 2001; Spreen & Risser, 1998). With the help of standardized and nonstandardized methods, the clinician should sample the following aspects of communication:

- *Fluency of speech.* Fluency is one of the dimensions of speech on which two broad categories of aphasia are distinguished. Therefore, the clinician needs to assess the fluency of a patient's speech.

- *Syntactic and morphologic features.* This aspect of communication also is a basis for distinguishing certain types of aphasia. Therefore, an assessment of syntactic and morphologic aspects of speech will help make a differential diagnosis.

- *Conversational speech samples.* An adequate sample of a patient's discourse will help assess various aspects of verbal as well as nonverbal communication. Beyond fluency and syntactic and morphologic aspects, conversational speech samples help assess such conversational language skills as turn taking and topic maintenance.

- *Auditory comprehension skills.* Greater or lesser degree of impairment in auditory comprehension of spoken language is also of diagnostic value in assessing aphasia and in diagnosing certain types of aphasia.

- *Repetition skills.* Repeating modeled speech productions is variously impaired in aphasia. As noted, some patients may have intact repetition skills. Therefore, an assessment of repetition skills is a standard procedure in aphasia diagnosis.

- *Naming skills.* Naming problems of greater or lesser magnitude characterize most patients with aphasia. As they are a more pervasive and common problem across patients with aphasia, naming skills are routinely sampled in assessing aphasia.

- *Speech production.* Although speech problems are technically not a part of aphasia, many patients may have a concomitant dysarthria. Therefore, speech production is typically sampled.

- *Writing.* Depending on the premorbid literacy skills, writing skills of patients will help make a specific diagnosis in some cases. In all cases, this mode of communication needs to be explored with a focus on rehabilitation.

- *Reading aloud and reading comprehension.* These two skills may be differentially impaired in some cases. As with writing skills, an assessment of reading skills with a view to exploit and strengthen them will be useful in most cases.

- *Automatic speech and singing.* Automatic speech, echolalic speech, and singing may offer diagnostic clues in some patients. They also may have to be dealt with in treatment. Therefore, these skills need to be addressed during assessment.

- *Nonverbal communication.* The use of gestures and other forms of nonverbal communication may be important for certain patients and may be a means of communication that needs to be taught to others. Therefore, a patient's current nonverbal communication skills and the need for teaching such skills should be assessed.

The skills selected for assessing a client depend on the kinds of impairment that are dominant and the expected kinds of impairments that may be subtle. Skills that are obviously unimpaired may be sampled more briefly than those that are expected to be impaired. Also, because assessment is a continuous process, treatment sessions may reveal the need to assess skills that have not been previously assessed.

Activities Used in Assessment

A variety of activities may be used to assess the behaviors of interest. Most clinicians use a combination of standardized and nonstandardized procedures to sample behaviors that will help diagnose aphasia and plan for treatment (Davis, 2000; Golper, 1996; Holland, 1996; Murray & Chapey, 2001; Spreen & Risser, 1998). Many nonstandardized and client-specific procedures may be designed to suit an individual patient. The following kinds of activities are used in a comprehensive assessment procedure:

- *Conversation.* An extended conversational sample will help assess various aspects of speech and language, including fluency, articulation, syntactic and grammatic structures, naming difficulties, comprehension of speech, such automatic speech as echolalia, and such nonverbal communication skills as the use of gestures.

- *Answering questions.* Beyond normal conversation in which questions may be asked, the clinician may use formal, structured, and prepared questions to assess the speed and accuracy of responses, relevant and irrelevant information that may be offered, confabulation, and auditory comprehension of speech.

- *Describing pictures.* Some standardized tests of aphasia offer opportunities to show pictures that patients are asked to describe. Clinicians also can select pictures from various sources (e.g., magazines and cartoons) and present them to evoke descriptions. While some pictures help evoke descriptions of events specific to what is depicted, others may help evoke sequential events that help weave a story. Picture descriptions, especially the kind that involves sequential elements, help assess adequacy and comprehensiveness of language functions, including temporal and logical sequences of narration, to meet social communication demands.

- *Producing rapidly alternating movements.* This specialized task is designed to assess the speed and accuracy of speech-related movements.

- *Reciting days of the week and months of the year.* This task helps assess whether automatic speech is either intact or impaired.

- *Naming objects or pictures.* As naming is impaired to varying degrees in most patients with aphasia, the clinician needs to assess this skill routinely.

- *Naming friends, colleagues, and family members.* This may be called the *functional* naming task. In this task, the patient is asked to name individuals who are significant in his or her life. For example, the patient may be asked to name photographs of family members. The results of this assessment will be useful in planning treatment.

- *Naming with various cues.* The patient may be asked to name objects and pictures and then be immediately provided with a cue. The cue may consist of the first phoneme (or letter) of the target word or the use of the object shown. The results of this task will help plan for a treatment strategy to improve naming skills.

- *Pointing to named objects or pictures.* This task will help assess the patient who may not verbally respond to commands and requests but can respond appropriately in nonverbal ways. The task also is helpful in assessing auditory comprehension in a restricted context.

- *Matching printed words to pictures.* Asking patients to match printed words to pictures helps assess reading comprehension at its simplest level.

- *Repeating clinician-modeled words, phrases, and sentences.* The clinician models selected productions the patient repeats. This task is especially designed to assess repetition skills that are differentially impaired in different types of aphasia.

- *Saying as many words as possible that belong to a specified category.* This is a standard task to assess an aspect of speech fluency and potential naming difficulties. Some patients may have a marked difficulty in producing words that belong to specific categories (e.g., plants or animals).

- *Saying as many words as possible that start with a specified letter.* This task helps assess phonemically triggered speech fluency and potential naming difficulties. The results will be valuable in treatment planning.

- *Telling the meaning of proverbs and metaphors.* This task will help assess the understanding and use of the abstract language.

- *Defining word meanings.* This task is essential to assess an understanding of literal or multiple and abstract meaning of words.

- *Telling and estimating time.* This task helps assess temporal aspects of experience and general orientation to time.

- *Detecting absurdity in oral or written statements.* A failure to detect absurdity in written or oral statements may suggest impaired abstract reasoning and inference. This problem may need to be addressed in treatment.

- *Naming environmental sounds.* This task will help assess whether the patient still understands the various auditory stimuli commonly found in his or her environment. A difficulty found in this task may suggest auditory comprehension problems.

- *Completing incomplete sentences.* Sentence completion tasks are useful in assessing a variety of skills, including naming, grammatical connection between words, semantic associations, and generally intact verbal behavioral chains.

- *Carrying out spoken commands.* This task is generally useful in assessing auditory comprehension of language. Simpler and complex commands help assess breakdown in comprehension at different levels of complexity.

- *Carrying out written instructions.* Failure to follow written instructions may suggest problems in reading comprehension.

- *Reading aloud printed numbers, letters, words, phrases, or paragraphs.* These are the various levels at which a patient's reading skills are assessed. The results will be helpful in planning reading remediation.

- *Silently reading printed sentences or passages and answering questions about what is read.* This task helps evaluate reading comprehension, a skill often impaired in patients with aphasia.

- *Writing dictated numbers, letters, words, phrases, and sentences.* Problems in writing accuracy, letter and number formation, and general organization of writing may be assessed through this task.

- *Copying printed numbers, letters, words, phrases, and sentences.* Impaired copying skills suggest serious writing problems and help identify the need for writing remediation programs.

- *Giving written description of pictures.* Another test of writing skills, this task also will help evaluate written expression of sequential events, understanding of story themes, implied meanings, and sentence construction.

- *Drawing.* Patients' drawing of human figures and common objects may reveal such associated problems as spatial perception and organization, constructional impairment, left neglect, and general drawing skills.

- *Performing math operations.* Addition, division, and multiplication tasks may reveal problems that need to be addressed in treatment to promote functional recovery for everyday living.

- *Gesturing, signing, and pantomiming.* These skills are especially helpful in assessing the rehabilitation potential of patients with severe impairments in oral expression. Treatment in such cases may target functional nonverbal communication modes.

- *Responding to gestures, signs, and pantomime.* This task will help evaluate a patient's understanding of nonverbal communication modes.

- *Demonstrating the use of objects.* Patients who cannot name objects may be asked to demonstrate their use. The results may help design cues that might be useful in teaching naming.

- *Making block designs.* Several tests of intelligence include block design tasks (subtests). Impaired block designing suggests problems with abstract and geometric perceptual skills.

- *Performing selected actions (praxis).* Patients may be asked to show how they would brush their teeth, drink from a glass, cut a piece of paper with a pair of scissors, or hold a pencil to write. Such tasks help evaluate various kinds of (nonverbal) apraxia that may be associated with aphasia.

The activities selected for assessing a patient depend largely on the dominant and subtle symptoms. Most activities are common across patients, and some may receive a special emphasis (e.g., activities designed to assess nonverbal apraxia) because of a patient's unique condition. Many standardized tests include some of those activities. In most cases, the clinician may design particular and client-specific activities to assess a given patient.

Direct and Repeated Observation of the Patient

Before administering standardized diagnostic tests to a patient, a clinician should repeatedly and directly observe the patient. Brief and informal conversations with the patient at an earliest opportunity will be a good starting point. Observing the patient's interaction with the family or health care professionals will be useful. These observations may help select standardized tests and design client-specific procedures of assessment. These observations will help formulate initial impressions of the patient. For instance, the results of a set of observations might suggest that the patient's fluency is or is not intact, the use of syntactic and morphologic features are intact or impaired, auditory comprehension is good or bad, and nonverbal gestures seem to help or hinder communication.

The observations need to be repeated, often even beyond the point of standardized test administration. The clinical picture of patients who have had cerebral injury due to CVA and other causes changes over time. These changes may be observed in informal situations. To document changes over time, the clinician should continue to make systematic observations of the patient during all phases of rehabilitation. The speech-language pathologist also should encourage other health care workers and family members to report changes in the patient's general behavior, including communication skills.

Standardized Tests in Assessing Aphasia

Both screening and diagnostic aphasia tests are available. Some standardized diagnostic tests are designed to assess and classify aphasias into specific types (e.g., conduction aphasia or transcortical sensory aphasia). Other tests assess various behaviors of interest and do not attempt a typological classification.

An initial screening test, a more detailed diagnostic test, and client-specific assessment procedures (including direct observations and conversational speech samples) will help assess both the needs and strengths of the patient. What follows is a review of a few commonly used screening and diagnostic tools.

Selected Screening Tests of Aphasia

Most screening tests are brief instruments that help make a quick, initial, and bedside assessment of patients who have had a CVA or exhibit other signs of cerebral injury. Screening tests sample only a few language and related functions. They are typically followed by the administration of a diagnostic test and other client-specific procedures.

Most clinical facilities that serve a large number of patients with aphasia have their own structured procedures to screen patients. Some experienced clinicians may have their own informal but uniform means of screening patients for aphasia. A few minutes of conversation; some common objects to name or point to; questions that evoke brief descriptions; a request to recite numbers and days of the week; and repetition of words, phrases, and sentences may give an expert clinician sufficient information to screen a patient (Davis, 2000). Therefore, not all clinicians use standardized screening instruments. Those who wish to use one may select one or more of the screening tests listed in Table 8-1.

Most screening tests take 10 to 20 minutes to administer. Although there is some variability, most tests include items to assess verbal expression, auditory comprehension, repetition, naming, automatic speech, and limited reading and writing. Because the screening tests will not sample all behaviors of

TABLE 8-1 Selected screening tests of aphasia.

Screening Test	Author and Reference
Aphasia Language Performance Scales (ALPS)	Keenan and Brassell (1975)
The Boston Diagnostic Aphasia Examination (BDAE) (3rd ed.)—the short form	Goodglass, Kaplan, and Barresi (2001)
Sklar Aphasia Scale (SAS)	Sklar (1983)
Acute Aphasia Screening Protocol (AASP)	Crary, Haak, and Malinsky (1989)
Aphasia Screening Test (2nd ed.)	Reitan (1991)
Aphasia Screening Test (2nd ed.)	Whurr (1996)
Bedside Evaluation Screening Test (BEST) (2nd ed.)	Fitch-West and Sands (1998)
Quick Assessment for Aphasia	Tanner and Culbertson (1999)

interest and not sample screened behaviors in depth, they should never replace diagnostic tests and extended client-specific observations. Furthermore, screening tests are not designed to provide sufficiently reliable and valid information to plan treatment. Used according to their design and intent, screening tests are useful.

Selected Standardized Diagnostic Tests

Standardized tests give a format to assess various skills of interest. They provide standard procedures for scoring and interpreting the patient's responses.

THE MINNESOTA TEST FOR DIFFERENTIAL DIAGNOSIS OF APHASIA (MTDDA) (SCHUELL, 1973)

One of the earliest standardized tests of aphasia that was frequently used in earlier decades, MTDDA contains 47 subtests with the number of test items ranging from 5 to 32. MTDDA evaluates five areas of performance: auditory disturbances, visual and reading disturbances, speech and language disturbances, visuomotor and writing disturbances, and numerical and arithmetic disturbances.

Although MTDDA does not classify aphasia into the traditional types, it does classify the disorder into five groups:

- Group 1. Simple aphasia
- Group 2. Aphasia with visual involvement
- Group 3. Aphasia with sensorimotor involvement
- Group 4. Aphasia with scattered findings (generalized brain damage)
- Group 5. Irreversible aphasic syndrome

The test results also help group patients into two minor aphasia syndromes as follows:

- Minor syndrome A: Aphasia with partial auditory perception
- Minor syndrome B: Aphasia with persisting dysarthria

MTDDA is a comprehensive test. It takes from 4 to 6 hours to administer; consequently, some clinicians might administer only selected subtests that are especially relevant for a given client. Acceptable validity has been reported, but its reliability is unknown.

THE BOSTON DIAGNOSTIC APHASIA EXAMINATION (BDAE) (GOODGLASS, KAPLAN, & BARRESI, 2001)

A widely used test, the BDAE aims to classify aphasia into types. The results suggest the site of brain lesion in given patients. The test evaluates articulation, fluency, word-finding difficulty (naming), repetition, serial speech, grammar, paraphasias, auditory comprehension, oral reading, reading comprehension, writing, and musical skills (e.g., singing). The test allows for conversational speech sampling.

The test contains 27 subtests. It takes from 1 to 4 hours to administer. A 5-point severity rating scale and a profile of speech characteristics help determine the severity and type of aphasia.

The Boston Naming Test is a part of the BDAE, although it can be obtained and administered independently to assess naming skills in-depth. The test contains 60 naming items. The third edition of the test also contains a short form that takes 30 to 45 minutes to administer.

BDAE is a comprehensive test, although its reliability measures are not reported. Acceptable validity data are reported. However, it fails to classify many patients into particular types of aphasia.

The Boston Assessment of Severe Aphasia (BASA) (Helm-Estabrooks, Ramsberger, Nicholas, & Morgan, 1989)

This relatively comprehensive test may be administered soon after the stroke, even at the bedside. It contains 15 subtests and 61 items that help assess a variety of skills, including auditory comprehension, repetition, social greetings and simple conversation, yes/no questions, orientation to time, signing one's name, buccofacial or limb apraxia, gestural recognition, oral and gestural recognition, reading comprehension, writing, and visuospatial skills.

The BASA may be administered in less than 40 minutes. Responses may be scored as fully or partially correct.

The Western Aphasia Battery (WAB) (Kertesz, 1982)

This test also seeks to classify aphasia into types. The test evaluates speech content, fluency, auditory comprehension, repetition, naming, reading, writing, calculation, drawing, nonverbal thinking, and performance on block designs.

The WAB takes 1 to 2 hours to administer. It is relatively easy to score and comprehensive in its coverage. Adequate validity and reliability have been demonstrated. Nonetheless, the test has been criticized for being unable to classify many patients into an aphasia type.

The BDAE and the WAB correlate well, but they classify only about 27 percent of patients into the same types. One test may indicate anomic aphasia and the other Wernicke's. This problem may be due to unreliable classification of aphasia or insensitivity of the tests to different patterns of deficits. Furthermore, the WAB does not correlate well with clinician judgments. That is, the clinician and the test may disagree about the differential diagnosis of a patient. Another limitation of WAB is that it does not allow for patients who cannot be classified into a particular type of aphasia; it forces all into one or the other type.

The Porch Index of Communicative Ability (PICA) (Porch, 2001)

This test does not classify aphasia into types. Eighteen subtests and 181 test items help assess auditory comprehension by pointing to objects; reading printed words; oral expressive language mainly through object descriptions, naming, sentence completion, and repetition; pantomime to demonstrate functions of objects; visual matching of pictures to objects or objects to pictures; writing names and functions of objects, writing words when spelled, and writing to dictation; and copying names and geometric forms. The test uses pen, pencil, matches, scissors, key, quarter, toothbrush, comb, fork, and knife as the same 10 test stimulus objects in all of its subtests. The test items are arranged in a decreasing order of difficulty.

Acceptable levels of validity and reliability have been reported, although the measures may not reflect communication skills in daily living conditions (Davis, 2000). The Porch helps assess skills that other tests do not. However, the Porch gives only a limited measure of speech and language. The test can be administered in 1 hour or less. It requires intensive training to administer and score; new users need about 40 hours of training. The patient response scoring system is complex, involves 1 through 16 scores, and requires examiner judgment. The Porch Index has been used extensively to assess aphasic patients' improvement with and without treatment.

THE NEUROSENSORY CENTER COMPREHENSIVE EXAMINATION FOR APHASIA (NCCEA) (SPREEN & BENTON, 1977)

This extensive test contains 20 language subtests. It has additional tests for visual and tactile functions. The test evaluates such functions as language comprehension and production, reading, writing, copying, word fluency, digit and sentence repetition, visual object naming, sentence construction, and articulation. Scores may be adjusted for age and education of the patient. Percentile scores may be derived from the adjusted scores. The NCCEA yields profiles of patients' strengths and weaknesses. The test does not use difficult or infrequently used items or objects; therefore, its ceiling is low. Consequently, the test may be good at assessing patients who are severely impaired but may miss those with mild difficulties.

See Table 8-2 for a list of standardized diagnostic tests and other kinds of assessment tools for aphasia.

TABLE 8-2 Standardized aphasia diagnostic test batteries.

General Diagnostic Tests	
Test Name	**Author and Reference**
The Minnesota Test for Differential Diagnosis of Aphasia (MTDDA)	Schuell (1973)
The Boston Diagnostic Aphasia Examination (BDAE)	Goodglass, Kaplan, and Barresi (2001)
The Boston Assessment of Severe Aphasia and (BASA)	Helm-Estabrooks, Ramsberger, Nicholas, Morgan (1989)
The Western Aphasia Battery (WAB)	Kertesz (1982)
The Porch Index of Communicative Ability (PICA) (4th ed.)	Porch (2001)
The Neurosensory Center Comprehensive Examination for Aphasia (NCCEA)	Spreen and Benton (1977)
Functional Communication Assessment	
Functional Communication Profile	Sarno (1969)
Communication Abilities of Daily Living (2nd ed.)	Holland, Frattali, and Fromm (1998)
The Communicative Effectiveness Index (CETI)	Lomas et al. (1989)
Communication Profile: A Functional Skills Survey	Payne (1994)
Functional Assessment of Communication Skills for Adults (ASHA FACS)	Frattali, Thompson, Holland, Wohl, & Ferketi (1995)
Amsterdam-Nijmegan Everyday Language Test (ANELT)	Blomert, Kean, Koster, and Schokker (1994)
Bilingual Aphasia Tests	
Multilingual Aphasia Examination (Rev. ed.)	Benton and Hamsher (1978)
Bilingual Aphasia Test (BAT)	Paradis (1987)

Assessment of Functional Communication

One limitation of certain standardized tests is that the behaviors sampled may not reflect a patient's everyday communication skills. Formal stimulus presentation under structured situations to evoke limited responses may not resemble everyday communication situations in which the environment is less structured, highly variable, and rich in contextual cues. In addition, the responses a patient easily gives in a structured situation may not be forthcoming in a social communication situation. To at least partially overcome such problems of traditional, standardized tests, clinicians have developed functional assessment tools.

Functional assessment tools target communication in relatively natural settings. These tools require systematic observation of a patient's social interactions in everyday situations, including health care settings. Functional assessment instruments tend to be less standardized than the traditional tests and allow for more informal and spontaneous measures of communication. Furthermore, in functional communication assessment, social (pragmatic) use of language and effective communication are more important than phonologic, morphologic, and syntactic accuracy of productions.

Functional assessment of communication is especially useful in documenting treatment outcome (Frattali, 1998). The patients who regain their functional communication skills in treatment will have achieved personally and socially meaningful results.

It should be noted that in a comprehensive assessment of aphasia all varieties of procedures—including the traditional, standardized diagnostic tests, client-specific procedures, and functional communication evaluation—play an important role. Each kind of assessment helps evaluate a dimension of communication that the other might miss or underevaluate. Table 8-2 lists aphasia diagnostic tests, including the functional communication assessment tools.

FUNCTIONAL COMMUNICATION PROFILE (SARNO, 1969)

One of the earliest attempts to assess functional communication skills of patients with aphasia, Sarno's (1969) *Functional Communication Profile* seeks to assess 45 behaviors in five categories: movement, speaking, understanding, reading, calculation, and writing. An examiner needs to observe patients and make judgments about the adequacy of behaviors exhibited.

To fully interpret the results of assessment, the clinician needs to gather extensive information on the premorbid language skills of the patient through interviews of family members and case history. A 9-point rating scale helps evaluate such communicative skills as indicating *yes* or *no,* reading newspaper headlines, and making change.

COMMUNICATION ABILITIES OF DAILY LIVING (2ND ED.) (HOLLAND, FRATTALI, & FROMM, 1998)

This is another leading assessment procedure that emphasizes daily communication in everyday situations; Holland published the first edition in 1980. The test contains 50 items and seeks to evaluate reading, writing, and using numbers; social interaction; divergent communication; contextual communication; nonverbal communication; sequential relationships; and humor/metaphor absurdity. For the most part, simulated situations that involve interaction with others (e.g., a receptionist or a physician) and daily activities such as driving, shopping, and making phone calls are used to assess communicative behaviors.

An interview and simulated situation (e.g., shopping or visiting a doctor's office) help assess various targeted skills. During the interview, the patient may be addressed with a wrong name to evaluate an understanding of one's own name. The patient may be asked to read a map and tell how he or she might get from point A (e.g., a bank) to point B (e.g., post office). The patient may be asked to list three items from a grocery store. As test items emphasize communication effectiveness as against grammatic accuracy, it provides useful information on social and pragmatic communication skills. This test also has Italian and Japanese versions.

THE COMMUNICATIVE EFFECTIVENESS INDEX (CETI) (LOMAS ET AL., 1989)

This instrument helps assess four domains of functional communication skills: basic needs (e.g., toileting, eating, grooming); life skills (e.g., shopping, understanding traffic signals, using the telephone); social needs (e.g., playing cards, writing to a friend); and health threats (e.g., calling for help, letting someone know about one's own medical condition). The authors selected these four domains for assessment after interviewing stroke survivors and their spouses who suggested them as essential communication skills. The 16 test items evaluate such specific skills as giving yes/no answers, expressing physical pain or discomfort, and starting a conversation. The skills may be rated as "not at all able" to "as able as before the stroke."

A spouse, another family member, a friend, or a neighbor may rate the skills, which helps evaluate communication skills in natural settings.

COMMUNICATION PROFILE: A FUNCTIONAL SKILLS SURVEY (PAYNE, 1994)

Most aphasia assessment instruments, including those that evaluate functional communication skills in natural settings, have not adequately sampled ethnic minorities in their patient selection process for standardization. A notable exception is the *Communication Profile* by Payne (1994). The sample included patients from African American, American Indian/Alaska Native, Asian American/Pacific Islander, and Asian American ethnic groups.

The *Communication Profile* uses a 5-point scale to rate the importance of selected skills in daily living. Either the client or the caregivers may evaluate the importance of everyday understanding, reading, speaking, and writing skills.

FUNCTIONAL ASSESSMENT OF COMMUNICATION SKILLS FOR ADULTS (ASHA FACS) (FRATTALI, THOMPSON, HOLLAND, WOHL, & FERKETI, 1995)

This tool, developed for the American Speech-Language-Hearing Association, requires direct observations of clients to rate behaviors in four domains: social communication (e.g., use of familiar names; understanding of TV/radio; explanation of how to do something); communication of basic needs (e.g., expression of likes and dislikes, request for help); reading, writing, and number concepts (e.g., following written instructions, completion of forms; making money transactions); and daily planning (e.g., telling time, following a map). Speech-language pathologists or significant others may make the observations and complete the rating form.

The domains are rated on a 7-point scale of independence. A rating of 7 on a skill means the patient performs it with no assistance, and a rating of 1 means he or she failed to perform even with assistance. The rated dimensions take into consideration adequacy, appropriateness, promptness, and communication sharing. The results of assessment can be summarized into mean scores for domains and dimensions, overall scores, and profiles of both communication independence and qualitative dimensions. The tool has been found to be valid and reliable when used with adults with left-hemisphere stroke with aphasia. The tool, however, is more appropriate to evaluate a rehabilitation program's effectiveness rather than making a detailed analysis of a patient's strengths and weaknesses.

AMSTERDAM-NIJMEGAN EVERYDAY LANGUAGE TEST (ANELT) (BLOMERT, KEAN, KOSTER, & SCHOKKER, 1994)

This test has two parallel forms, each containing 10 items. The test helps assess pragmatic language skills described in terms of scenarios of familiar daily living activities. For instance, one of the items describes a situation in which the patient has to change a doctor's appointment. The examiner then asks the patient to indicate what he or she might say to the physician. The validity of the measure depends on the accurate comprehension of the scenarios presented.

The communication skills are rated in two 5-point scales. One scale evaluates the understandability of messages and the other evaluates the intelligibility of utterances.

Assessment of Bilingual/ Multilingual Patients

Assessment of patients who speak English as a second language or do not speak English at all would pose special problems for a unilingual English-speaking speech-language pathologist. Even when an aphasia diagnostic test is available in the patient's first language, the clinician who does not speak that language will be unable to administer it. In such cases, the clinician may have to use interpreters of test items. When no tests are available, nonstandardized assessment in the patient's first language may need to be attempted with the help of an interpreter.

Assessment of bilingual patients who speak English as a second language may be accomplished with an English test, but a test in the patient's first language, if available, may be more or equally appropriate. See Table 8-2 for a list of aphasia diagnostic tests, including tests for bilingual individuals.

Several tests are now available to assess multilingual or bilingual patients. One such test is the *Multilingual Aphasia Examination* by Benton and Hamsher (1978). Similar to NCCEA in its contents, this test evaluates such language functions as naming, repetition, fluency, auditory comprehension, spelling, and writing. The test has English, French, German, Italian, and Spanish versions. Repeated testing of the same patient may be accomplished by alternate forms.

Another useful test is the *Bilingual Aphasia Test (BAT)* by Paradis (1987). A unique test that allows evaluation in 40 languages with parallel forms, the BAT is one of the most comprehensive tests available (Benson & Ardila, 1996). The test can evaluate a patient's relative performance in a primary and a secondary language. BAT helps assess phonologic, morphologic, syntactic, lexical, and semantic aspects of the languages. It also helps assess language use in auditory, visual, oral, and digitomanual modalities. The bilingual section of the test evaluates skills in pairs of languages.

Several well-established English tests have been translated to other languages. For instance, the Boston Diagnostic Aphasia Examination, the Boston Naming Test, and Communication Abilities in Daily Living are available in various languages, including Spanish, Italian, and Chinese. A potential problem with translated tests is that culturally inappropriate test items may evoke invalid responses. A test should select items from the linguistic milieu and should be standardized with a sample from the relevant population.

Independent Tests of Specific Skills

Comprehensive test batteries of aphasia provide subtests for most skills that need to be assessed. Subtests of large tests may not sample a given skill adequately, however. When a given skill (e.g., naming or auditory comprehension) needs to be evaluated more extensively and in-depth, specific tests designed for that purpose may be more useful than subtests. The following are just a few examples of independent tests of specific skills.

Tests of Auditory Comprehension

Several tests of auditory comprehension are available, but the original *Token Test* (DeRenzi & Vignolo, 1962) and its variations (DeRenzi & Faglioni, 1978) are well known and widely used. Placing small tokens that vary in size, color, and shape, the clinician asks the client to touch one or multiple tokens in a specified sequence. The client may also be asked to manipulate the tokens. Correct responses indicate auditory comprehension of sentences. A limitation of the test is that it samples auditory comprehension in a highly restricted context. The functional significance of the results may be limited as well. In some patients, the auditory comprehension problem the test may reveal may be due to a failure to understand just the color, shape, and size of the tokens. To rule this out, the clinician may ask the patient to point to specific objects (e.g., a red token, a small token, a circle) before proceeding with the full test.

The *Auditory Comprehension Test for Sentences* (ACTS) (Shewan, 1981) helps assess vocabulary, sentence length, and syntactic complexity. Containing 21 test sentences, this is a comprehensive test of auditory comprehension of spoken sentences. The clinician reads each sentence to the patient who is required to respond to one of four pictures presented. It requires about 15 minutes to administer.

The *Functional Auditory Comprehension Task* (FACT) (LaPointe & Horner, 1978) is a measure of comprehension of more functional language than that of other tests (e.g., the Token Test). The test uses of 1-, 2-, and 3-part commands given to the patient to assess auditory comprehension at different levels of information complexity. The test contains sentences that differ in length, vocabulary level, and syntactic complexity.

The *Discourse Comprehension Test (DCT)* (Brookshire & Nichols, 1993, 1997) is designed to assess comprehension of narrated stories in contrast to the more typical words, sentences, and phrases used in many tests. The clinician plays 10 audiotaped narrated stories and asks eight questions to evaluate comprehension. The questions test the stated as well as implied story idea and story details. The test may be used with any adult with brain damage.

Tests that evaluate auditory comprehension but are not designed especially for aphasia also may be used. Some of these tests may have to be modified to suit adult aphasic patients. For example, the *Northwestern Syntax Screening Test* (Lee, 1971) and *The Test for Auditory Comprehension-Third Edition* (TACL-R) (Carrow-Woodfolk, 1999) may be administered to patients with aphasia.

Tests of Reading Skills

Comprehensive aphasia test batteries contain subtests of reading skills. Most evaluate both oral and silent reading of printed words, sentences, and paragraphs. In some tests, patients may be asked to match printed words to pictures or objects. A more difficult task for most patients is matching printed words to spoken words.

Questions may be asked to assess comprehension of orally or silently read material. In addition, a few specialized tests of reading skills may be used to make a more in-depth assessment of reading skills.

The Reading Comprehension Battery for Aphasia (RCBA) (LaPointe & Horner, 1998) is a specialized test for assessing reading skills. Ten subtests, each with 10 items, test single-word reading; functional reading of signs, menus, and labels; comprehension of printed sentences; comprehension of paragraphs; and sentence-to-picture matching. The test can help assess reading skills in any person with a diagnosed brain injury.

Because of the paucity of independent and specialized reading tests for aphasia, many clinicians use commercially available standardized reading tests. The commonly used reading test, *Gates-MacGinitie Reading Tests* (Gates, MacGinitie, Maria, et al., 2000) are designed to assess reading at primary grade levels through post high school. For patients with aphasia and other forms of neurogenic communication disorders, tests for grade 3 and higher may be useful.

Two other reading tests that may be used with appropriate modification are the *Nelson Reading Skills Test* (Hanna, Schell, & Shreiner, 1977) and the *Nelson-Denny Reading Skills Test* (Brown, Fischco, & Hanna, 1993). While the former test includes reading material from grades 3 through 9, the latter includes material from high school through college levels. Both measure reading and reading comprehension.

Tests of Writing Skills

Comprehensive test batteries of aphasia include measures of writing skills. Patients may be asked to write the alphabet, numbers, words, phrases, and sentences. They may be asked to copy printed letters, words, phrases, and sentences; numbers; geometric shapes; and self-formulated material. Patients also may be asked to write to dictation. Because most writing subtests included in aphasia diagnostic tests are adequate for assessing writing skills of patients with aphasia, most clinicians do not use independent tests of writing skills.

Psychological Tests

In addition to tests for aphasia, psychological tests, including verbal and nonverbal tests of intelligence, memory tests, cognitive skills tests, and various other assorted tests, may be administered. Selection and administration of psychological tests will depend on the theory of aphasia, assessment objectives, and treatment planning needs. Most psychological tests are administered by psychologists, however.

An Outline of Aphasia Assessment

This outline of assessment groups assessment tasks into seven major categories: I. case history; II. verbal expression; III. auditory comprehension; IV. reading skills; V. writing skills; VI. motor speech; and VII. nonverbal communicative skills.

I. Take a Detailed Case History

A detailed case history helps identify the patient's current problems and his or her premorbid communication and intellectual skills. This information is helpful in making a diagnosis and planning a treatment program.

Gather detailed information on:

- *Patient's biography.* Biographical information on the patient's age, education, occupation, oral and written language skills, and hobbies and interests will be useful in understanding the changes in the patient that are brought about by the stroke. This information also will be useful in setting certain treatment goals.

- *Current family constellation.* Information on the current living arrangements, family members who live with the patient, and others who might be able to help in supporting treatment will be especially helpful in sustaining and generalizing treatment gains in natural settings.

- *Medical history and data.* Information on the patient's health history, the potential causes and consequences of aphasia, associated diseases, current physical condition, any psychiatric complications (e.g., depression), current medications, and physical limitations or disabilities will help make a comprehensive assessment and set realistic treatment goals.

- *Behavioral observations.* Important diagnostic and treatment implications may emerge from careful and systematic observations of the patient's general and communicative behaviors. Changes in a patient's behavior over time may suggest diagnosis and treatment targets that are different from the ones initially found appropriate.

II. Assess Verbal Expression

In assessing verbal expression of patients with aphasia, measure repetition skills, naming skills, speech fluency, and syntactic and morphologic aspects of language production. Use both informal measures and standardized tests. An informal measure that will be helpful in making a variety of communicative skill analyses is a sample of the patient's conversational speech.

A. Record a Conversational Speech Sample

Record a patient's conversational speech during the initial interview designed to obtain the case history and related information. Make use of the questions designed to obtain biographic information, details on past and current health status, and information on current family constellation from the patient to accomplish this task.

Use the recorded conversational speech sample to make an analysis of sentence structures, production of grammatic morphemes, comprehension of spoken speech, speech fluency, word-finding problems, associated dysarthric features, conversational turn taking, topic maintenance, and other aspects of communication.

B. Assess Repetition Skills

To assess repetition skills, model words and sentences and ask the patient to immediately imitate (repeat) the production as accurately as possible. The patient may totally fail to repeat, repeat correctly, or repeat only a part of the modeled production. Note such errors.

1. REPETITION OF SINGLE WORDS
- Start with modeling single-syllable words with visible voiced consonants (*bed*).
- Model object names, verbs, numbers, letters, and function words for repetition.
- Model words with blends and multisyllables.

2. REPETITION OF SENTENCES
- Begin with modeling short and commonly used sentences ("Sit down").
- Model some short, but infrequently used, sentences.
- Model progressively longer sentences.

C. Assess Naming Skills

Assess two categories of naming skills: responsive naming and confrontational naming.

1. RESPONSIVE NAMING

- In assessing responsive naming, give some verbal-contextual cues. Ask direct questions that require a specific response:
- "Why do you need a heavy jacket?" "What do you do with a cup?" "What color is a banana?"

2. CONFRONTATION NAMING

- Confrontation naming provides the typical stimulus (e.g., a question or a request to name an object shown) but no other clue.
- Select a set of pictures and objects that are functional to the patient. Show each to the patient and ask, "What is this?" Record the response.
- Administer a naming test (e.g., the Boston Naming Test) or analyze responses to a naming subtest items on an aphasia diagnostic test.

D. Assess Speech Fluency

Use word fluency tasks and the recorded conversational speech sample.

To obtain a measure of word fluency, ask the patient to recall names that belong to a specific category. For instance, ask the patient to:

- "Name all the animals you can think of."
- "Name all the flowers you can think of."
- "Name all the fruits you can think of."
- "Name all the clothing items you can think of."

Analyze the conversational speech sample to assess the length of phrases and sentences; pauses, repetitions, and other kinds of dysfluencies that impair fluency; and general flow of speech.

E. Assess Automated Speech and Singing

- Ask the patient to recite the alphabet, days of the week, months of the year, and numbers.
- Ask the patient to recite prayers, poems, and nursery rhymes.
- Ask the patient to sing something or hum a tune.

F. Assess Syntactic and Morphologic Aspects of Verbal Expressions

Use the recorded conversational speech sample to understand the syntactic and morphologic aspects of the patient's language production. Take note of telegraphic speech (omission of grammatical elements) and incomplete sentences.

Administer a standardized test of syntactic and morphologic skills. Analyze subtests of aphasia diagnostic tests that may include relevant subtests.

III. Assess Auditory Comprehension of Spoken Language

Note that auditory comprehension is totally lost or totally intact in only a few, if any, aphasic patients. This skill is impaired to varying degrees in nearly all patients. Therefore, use evaluation material that varies from the simple to complex to challenge patients with mild to severe impairment.

Before attempting a complete auditory comprehension assessment, screen the client's hearing; refer patients who fail the screening to an audiologist for diagnosis. Also, evaluate right-sided visual problems; some patients ignore or do not see stimuli to the right side of the midline.

Note that generally, aphasic patients respond better to (1) personal questions than to neutral questions; (2) frequently occurring commands than to infrequent or unusual commands; (3) stories of daily events than to those with strange themes; and (4) simpler sentences than to more complex sentences.

To diagnose auditory comprehension deficits, assess responses to commands, understanding of single words, and comprehension of connected speech.

A. Assess Comprehension of Commands

Note that single words are not necessarily easy for aphasic patients to comprehend, because of lack of contextual cues. The patients may respond more accurately to some commonly used commands ("Pick up the pencil") than to single words. Therefore, begin with commands, not single words. Also, do not use gestures, as the purpose is to assess response to verbal stimuli.

- Give natural and simple commands:
  "Move your chair a little closer."
  "Close your eyes."
  "Show me the door."
  "Please, turn off the lights."
  "Please, remove your glasses."
- Give several multistep commands:
  "Please pick up the pencil and the comb and place them in the box."
  "Please place the red square first, the blue circle next, and the yellow triangle the last."

  Note whether the whole command is performed or only certain elements and, if so, which elements.

B. Assess Comprehension of Single Words

Note that the diagnostic value of comprehension of single words is that Wernicke's patients may have special problems with names of body parts. Patients with transcortical sensory aphasia may repeat a word, but may not understand the meaning of it.

Use single items ("red" or "cat") and semantic groups of items ("colors" or "animals"). Select stimulus words that vary in (1) number of syllables, (2) emotionality, (3) frequency of use, (4) semantic class, and (5) phonemic similarity.

Start with items from varied semantic groups (e.g., objects, actions, numbers, colors, and letters):

- "Point to *blocks*."
- "Point to *colors*."
- "Point to *running*."
- "Point to *letters*."
- "Point to *numbers*."

Move to specific items within semantic groups:

- "Point to the *small block*."
- "Point to *red*."
- "Point to the *boy running*."
- "Point to *B*."
- "Point to *ten*."

Write down the exact responses. Take note of the (1) speed with which the patient responds, (2) errors within and across semantic categories, (3) perseveration of responses, and (4) relative strengths and weaknesses across and within categories.

C. Assess Comprehension of Sentences and Connected Speech

Note that an assessment of comprehension of connected speech gives a more realistic picture of the patient's everyday communicative performance. Many patients understand connected speech better than single words. Both individual sentences and connected speech may be presented and responses assessed.

- Administer sentence comprehension subtests that are found in most diagnostic tests. Note that the Token Test described previously helps assess auditory comprehension of sentences.

- Ask several questions to which the patient responds either yes or no. For instance, ask such questions as "Do you live in a city?" "Does it rain here in July?" "Do you eat lunch at 7 a.m.?" and "Do you live with your son?"

- Tell a brief story and then question the patient about it.

- Tell a unique story that will be new to most patients.

- Tell stories that do not offer a special advantage to the patients. (Do not summarize *ET* to Steven Spielberg.)

- Select stories with some humor and emotionality.

- Ask both "yes" and "no" questions to assess comprehension.

- Ask questions to assess comprehension of both the main ideas and specific details, including the characters, their actions, chronological order of events, and the moral of the story.

IV. Assess Reading Skills

The depth of assessment of reading skills will depend on the patient's premorbid education and literacy skills and the current need for regaining and maintaining advanced literacy skills. If treatment is expected to include reading skills, the clinician should assess reading and reading comprehension in some detail.

A. Assess Oral Reading Skills

- Administer subtests of reading skills that are a part of diagnostic tests.
- Select client-specific reading materials that vary in length and complexity. Have the client read them aloud.
- Analyze reading errors, including omission of words, paraphasic reading, slow rate, unwillingness to read, and struggle while reading.

B. Assess Reading Comprehension

- Administer reading comprehension subtests of diagnostic tests.
- Ask the patient to match single printed words to pictures.
- Ask the patient to match printed words with spoken words.
- Ask the patient to cross out words that do not belong in a list.
- Ask the patient to complete a printed incomplete sentence. For example, ask the patient to read the printed incomplete sentence "We wear hats on our . . ." and complete it with the verbal response "head."
- Ask the patient to read complex printed material and underline key words and phrases.
- Ask the patient to read a story and answer questions about it.

V. Assess Writing

The need for an in-depth assessment of writing skills depends on the premorbid literacy skills and the current demands made on the patient.

A. Assess Graphomotor Skills (Letter Formation)

- Take note of the hand used in writing before the onset of aphasia and at the time of testing.
- Administer independent writing tests or writing subtests of diagnostic tests.
- Ask the patient to copy letters and words.

- Ask the patient to write letters and words to dictation.
- Analyze such errors as a failure to use the upper- and lowercase letters, poor letter formation, illegible letters, failure to produce script or printed letters, and spacing between letters.

B. Assess General Writing Skills

- Administer the writing subtests of a standardized diagnostic test.
- Ask the patient to write a paragraph on his or her own on a given topic (propositional writing).
- Ask the patient to write a few numbers, days of the week, months in a year, and so forth to assess automatically sequenced writing.
- Have the patient complete a confrontation writing task. For example, while showing some pictures, ask the patient to "Write the names of these pictures."
- Dictate a paragraph to the patient to assess writing to dictation.
- Ask the patient to write a story about a picture shown to assess narrative writing.
- Obtain a sample of premorbid writing for comparison.
- Analyze the overall quality of writing, errors in word arrangement, use of morphologic features, omission of words and phrases, and telegraphic writing.

VI. Assess Motor Speech Skills

Because aphasia may coexist with motor speech disorders, it is important to assess all patients with aphasia for apraxia of speech and dysarthria.

Make a clinical judgment about the need to administer standardized tests for apraxia and dysarthria. In most cases, a thorough orofacial examination and an analysis of the conversational speech may be sufficient to judge speech intelligibility and acceptability of articulatory performance.

Administer standardized tests if judged necessary, and combine them with client-specific procedures to assess apraxic and dysarthric symptoms. Consult sources on diagnosis of motor speech disorders for details (Duffy, 1995; Freed, 2000; Hegde, 2001a).

VII. Assess Nonverbal Communicative Skills

The need to assess nonverbal skills will vary across patients. Patients with severe aphasia who have limited verbal expression (e.g., those with global aphasia) will need this assessment the most. A patient who may need nonverbal skill training to achieve functional communication also needs nonverbal communication assessment.

In addition, assess gestures and pantomime. Take note of the client's use of common gestures (such as hand movements), facial expressions, variations in intonation, and such other devices during conversation.

Demonstrate a few common gestures (e.g., drinking from a cup, writing with a pen, cutting with a pair of scissors) to evaluate the patient's understanding of gestures.

Demonstrate a few formal signs, such as those in AMERIND (Skelly, 1979), to evaluate the patient's understanding. The same signs may be used later in treatment.

Assessment of Clients from Varied Ethnocultural Backgrounds

Assessment of clients who are of minority ethnocultural background poses challenges to a clinician of any ethnocultural background. Most standardized tests have not included a representative number of persons from ethnocultural minority groups in their standardization sample. In addition, certain tests may be heavily culturally biased. Therefore, clinicians need to be cautious in selecting assessment tools. A few sources offer suggestions based on clinical experience and knowledge of different ethnocultural groups; all experts recognize the need for more careful research into assessment tools that produce reliable and valid information when used with specific ethnocultural individuals (Payne, 1997; Tonkovich, 2002; Wallace, 1996). Most suggestions available in the literature are applicable to all clients with varied ethnocultural background, not just those with neurogenic language disorders (Hegde & Davis, 2005).

Some of the suggestions clinicians should consider in working with clients of varied ethnocultural background include:

- Adhere to the philosophy of having a client-specific approach to assessment (and treatment). Design assessment procedures that are specific to a patient's cultural and linguistic background.
- Select only those assessment tools that have included persons from the client's ethnocultural group in the standardization sample.
- If a test is known to be culturally biased or you think it might be, do not use it with individuals who might be negatively affected by it.
- If the use of a standardized instrument is necessary, although it may not be totally appropriate for a given client because of its demonstrated limits in reliability, validity, and comprehensiveness, then interpret the data more cautiously. Do not rush to judgments based on the test norms. Instead, analyze the client's performance in light of his or her ethnocultural background.
- Use a content-open assessment outline, such as the one described in the previous section; note that such outlines specify areas or skills to be assessed and give much freedom to develop stimulus materials and specific assessment items. Develop individual assessment stimuli and items that are appropriate to the client and his or her cultural background.
- Avoid multicultural stereotypes. Do not automatically assume that clients of a different ethnocultural background necessarily need unique procedures or that they do not have English proficiency. Through interviews and behavioral observations, case history, information about education and occupation, and evidence of acculturation, evaluate the need for unique procedures. Do not assume that all

white clients speak English; your client may be a recent immigrant from Portugal or Serbia.

- Take note that knowledge of accessibility to health care and rehabilitation services is a significant ethnocultural issue. Therefore, during the clinical interview, investigate the client's and family members' knowledge of health care facilities in the community, need for additional services, and availability and access to such services.

- Investigate also whether the services you recommend are affordable to the client and family, whether the family has transportation to clinical facilities, and whether a family member can accompany the client to clinical facilities.

- Investigate whether the clients and their family members share your sense of time and appointment schedules. If not, modify their understanding, change your schedule, or work on a combination of the two.

- Take note that while working with certain ethnocultural groups, beliefs about health, disease, disability, disorders, and treatability of such clinical conditions may have to be explored, because such beliefs affect motivation to seek and sustain services.

- Informally assess the family members' language skills, cultural dispositions toward communication, and family communication patterns so that the client's communicative deficits can be placed in his or her cultural milieu.

- Consult with a speech-language pathologist who belongs to the client's ethnocultural background.

- As a member of a multidisciplinary team of specialists, work with other professionals to educate them about ethnocultural differences and the need to develop client-specific procedures.

- As the sources specific to aphasia and other adult language disorders are limited, consult various general sources on assessment and treatment of communication disorders in ethnoculturally varied populations (Battle, 2002; Hegde & Davis, 2005; Kaiser, 1995; Lubinski & Frattali, 1994; Payne, 1997; Screen & Anderson, 1994).

Differential Diagnosis

Aphasia may be confused with other neurogenic communication problems, including dementia, language of confusion, right hemisphere syndrome, apraxia of speech, and dysarthria. Aphasia also needs to be distinguished from some psychiatric problems, notably schizophrenia. Additionally, mild forms of aphasia need to be distinguished from normal language.

Principles of Differential Diagnosis

- The patient's history and the results of medical (including neurological) examinations are essential to make a differential diagnosis.
- Detailed, adequate, reliable sampling of verbal and nonverbal communicative behaviors is necessary, because diagnosis or differential diagnosis should be based on systematic observations or reliable measurement of behaviors.
- Disturbed language is not the same as disturbed communication. Some persons with little language may communicate much (e.g., patients with Broca's aphasia), while others with much language may communicate little (e.g., patients with Wernicke's aphasia).
- Within the same subtype of aphasia, individual patients differ markedly. Therefore, individual differences are as important as common symptoms.
- A score or a number on a rating scale does not describe a behavior. In many cases, a patient's communication in everyday situations may be better than what the test results and rating scales indicate.
- Symptoms of aphasic patients change over time, so repeated assessment across time or periodic probes are important.
- Unless a single symptom is diagnostic, the diagnosis or differential diagnosis is made on the basis of a pattern of multiple symptoms.
- Patients who are diagnosed with different types of aphasia share many common behaviors.

- Aphasic patients share a few or several symptoms with neurologically involved patients who have other forms of communicative problems (e.g., dementia).
- Aphasia may coexist with other communicative disorders and other neurological diseases (e.g., dysarthria, apraxia, and dementia).

An Important Reminder

The objectives of assessment and differential diagnosis are to select the most appropriate target behaviors and suitable treatment procedures for a given client.

Whether selected target behaviors improve the communicative skills of a patient in everyday situations is an important question to be answered.

In some cases, differential diagnosis may have to be postponed. In others, differential diagnosis may remain doubtful forever.

In still others, what appeared to be a firm diagnosis may change as the patient recovers from the initial symptoms.

The following tables offer guidelines to help make differential diagnosis:

Table 8-3   Aphasic or normal language?
Table 8-4   If aphasia, what type?
Table 8-5   Aphasia or dementia?
Table 8-6   Aphasia or the language of confusion?
Table 8-7   Aphasia or schizophrenia?
Table 8-8   Aphasia or right hemisphere problems?
Table 8-9   Aphasia or apraxia of speech?
Table 8-10 Aphasia or dysarthria?

TABLE 8-3 Aphasia or normal language?

In general, mild aphasia is the most difficult to distinguish from normal language. If a patient appears to have language deficits that seem to be aphasic in nature, but without neurological or other kinds of evidence supporting aphasia, look closely at the patient's premorbid background.

Aphasia	Deficits Similar to Aphasia but Normal Language
Positive history of central neuropathology	Negative history of central neuropathology
Prior history of normal language (if language skills were limited, then other factors should support a diagnosis of aphasia)	Prior history of limited language skills (limited literacy)
Lack of education does not explain the problems (if the education or level of literacy was limited, then other factors should support a diagnosis of aphasia)	Lack of education (limited literacy) explains the problems
Current environment could not explain the problem	Current environment could explain the problem
Sudden onset	Lifelong problem

Note: An impoverished current environment may explain deficient language in some older individuals. Older individuals who live in socially isolated situations or in certain extended care facilities with limited opportunities for communication may have depressed language performance. Some nursing homes may be described as communication-impaired environments (Lubinski, 1981). Therefore, along with the patient's medical conditions, language history, and status at time of assessment, living conditions help in making a differential diagnosis.

TABLE 8-4   If aphasia, what type?

Overlap of symptoms makes it difficult to arrive at a differential diagnosis of aphasia type. The following guidelines may be used to diagnose a particular type of aphasia.

Type	Main Features	Distinguishing Features
Broca's aphasia	Nonfluent, effortful, agrammatic, slow, sparse speech; impaired naming and repetition; mild comprehension problems; some articulation problems; impaired reading and writing	Nonfluent, agrammatic, sparse speech with relatively good comprehension
Transcortical motor aphasia	Initial mutism; nonfluent, sparse, echolalic speech with incomplete sentences; mild naming problems; mild comprehension problems; impaired reading and writing	Good repetition, echolalia, and articulation; otherwise similar to Broca's aphasia
Mixed transcortical aphasia	Nonfluent, echolalic, sparse, agrammatic telegraphic, speech; impaired naming and comprehension; reading and writing problems	Good repetition, echolalia, and articulation; a nonfluent aphasia with poor auditory comprehension
Global aphasia	Extremely limited nonfluent speech, all aspects of communication severely impaired	Generalized communication deficit
Wernicke's aphasia	Severely impaired auditory comprehension; excessively fluent, paragrammatic, pseudogrammatic, paraphasic, empty speech; severe naming problems; impaired repetition; good articulation; impaired reading and writing	Excessive fluency, empty speech, para- and pseudogrammatism
Transcortical sensory aphasia	Impaired auditory comprehension; fluent, paraphasic, empty speech; echolalic speech; good grammar, articulation, and reading aloud; impaired naming and writing	Echolalic speech with impaired auditory comprehension
Conduction aphasia	Fluent speech full of pauses and paraphasia; severely impaired repetition; impaired naming; good grammar, articulation, auditory comprehension; impaired reading and writing	Severely impaired repetition with good auditory comprehension
Anomic aphasia	Severe naming problems; highly paraphasic speech, with good articulation, repetition, reading and writing skills; mild auditory impairment	All aspects of communication better preserved than the naming deficit, which is severe

Note: In addition to the communication deficits listed for each type, use the case history and medical information (including neurological, radiological, and scanning data) to make a firm diagnosis.

TABLE 8-5 Aphasia or dementia?

While most forms of dementia are irreversible, chronic, and degenerative, some forms are reversible. See Chapters 14, 15, and 16 for details on dementias, their assessment, and diagnosis.

Aphasia	Dementia
Sudden onset	Slow onset
Damage in the left hemisphere Focal brain lesions	Bilateral brain damage Diffuse brain damage
Mood is usually appropriate, though depressed or frustrated at times	May be moody, withdrawn, agitated
Nonverbal cognitive functions are mostly intact	Mild to severely impaired cognition
Most memory functions are typically intact	Memory is impaired to various degrees, often severely
Generally relevant, socially appropriate, and organized	Often irrelevant, socially inappropriate, and disorganized
Semantic, syntactic, and phonologic performance simultaneously impaired	Progression of deterioration from semantic to syntactic to phonologic performance
Fluent or nonfluent	Fluent until dementia worsens
Generally stable, unless in the case of multiple strokes	Generally progressive, unless in the case of reversible dementia

Caution: Aphasia and dementia may coexist. An aphasic patient may develop a neurological disease resulting in dementia (Alzheimer's disease). A patient with dementia may have a stroke, resulting in aphasia. Also, in some early stages of dementia, the diffuse and bilateral damage may not be evident on neurodiagnostic tests (e.g., brain imaging).

TABLE 8-6 Aphasia or the language of confusion?

Aphasia	Language of Confusion
Left hemisphere damage, focal; often induced by CVA	Bilateral damage, diffused; often induced by trauma
Speech is often relevant	Typically irrelevant
No confabulation	Confabulation
Syntactic difficulties	Little or no syntactic difficulties
No disorientation except for the first few hours or days after a stroke	Disoriented to time, place, and persons
Cognitive deficits are not typical	Cognitive deficits are typical
History suggests stroke	History suggests brain trauma
Communication better than demonstrated language skills	Communication worse than demonstrated language skills
No significant behavioral (personality) change	Significant behavioral (personality) change

Caution: A patient with traumatic brain injury may suffer focal left hemisphere damage. In this case, confusion may coexist with aphasia.

TABLE 8-7 Aphasia or schizophrenia?

Schizophrenia is a behavioral (psychiatric) disorder. Its causes are not well understood, although biochemical and genetic factors are strongly suggested. It is characterized by significant thought disorders, affective disturbances, a dissociation from reality, and hallucinations and delusions. None of these characterize aphasia. Schizophrenia is not characterized by focal brain injury, but aphasia is.

Aphasia	Schizophrenia
A neurologically based language disorder with focal brain pathology	A profound psychiatric disorder with possibly biochemical and genetic etiology
Sudden onset	Gradual onset
Typically, late onset (adult or old age)	Typically, early onset (adolescent or early adulthood)
No disorders of perception and thinking; no irrational, disorganized, and bizarre thinking; no delusions	Disorders of perception and thinking; irrational, disorganized, and bizarre thinking; presence of delusions
No abnormal or bizarre sensations	Presence of abnormal and bizarre sensations (hallucinations)
No significant and sustained social withdrawal	Significant and sustained social withdrawal
Left hemisphere damage, often focal and of recent origin	No evidence of focal left hemisphere damage; some evidence of enlarged third and lateral ventricles and degeneration of brain tissue, but none of recent origin
No confabulation, generally relevant and socially appropriate speech	Confabulation, typically irrelevant and socially inappropriate speech
Deficits in auditory comprehension	No deficits in auditory comprehension (may be inattentive)
Reading and writing affected	Reading and writing may not be affected
Normal emotional responses	Inappropriate emotional responses
Generally in touch with reality	Generally disassociated from reality
Behavior (personality) changes not characteristic; no grossly disorganized behavior	Behavior (personality) changes and grossly disorganized behavior are characteristic
Impaired interpersonal relations are not typical	Impaired interpersonal relations are typical
Catatonia (abnormal postures) is not characteristic	Catatonia is characteristic of some patients

Caution: Aphasia and schizophrenia may coexist; the most difficult differential diagnosis may be schizophrenia with Wernicke's aphasia.

TABLE 8-8 Aphasia or right hemisphere problems?

Lesions in the right hemisphere produce a pattern of communication and behavior deficits that share a few common symptoms with aphasia. See Chapters 10 and 11 for details on right hemisphere syndrome.

Aphasia	Right Hemisphere Problems
More severe problems in naming, fluency, auditory comprehension, reading, and writing	Only mild problems
No left-sided neglect	Left-sided neglect
No denial of illness	Denial of illness and lack of insight into their problems
Speech is generally relevant	Speech is often irrelevant, excessive, rambling
Generally good expression of emotion and understanding of emotional expressions of others	Difficulty expressing their own emotions and lack of appreciation of emotions expressed by others
Generally oriented to space and surroundings	Disorientation to space and surroundings
Recognizes familiar faces	May not recognize familiar faces
May simplify drawings	Rotation and left-sided neglect
Some prosodic defect	More pronounced prosodic defect
Appropriate humor	Inappropriate humor
May retell the essence of a story	May retell only nonessential, isolated details (no integration)
May understand implied meanings of statements	Understands only literal meanings
Pragmatic impairments less striking	Pragmatic impairments more striking (eye contact, topic maintenance, etc.)
Although limited in language skills, communication can often be good	Although possessing good language skills, communication can be very poor
Pure linguistic deficits are dominant	Attentional and perceptual deficits more dominant than pure linguistic deficits

Note: Right hemisphere damage in those few individuals whose right hemisphere is dominant for language results in aphasia. The causes of right hemisphere damage may be the same as those of left hemisphere damage.

TABLE 8-9 Aphasia or apraxia of speech?

Apraxia of speech is a motor speech disorder in which motor planning of speech movements is impaired, even though there is no evidence of muscular weakness, sensory loss, or paralysis. Apraxia of speech and Broca's aphasia may coexist. Pure apraxia is rare. It often is associated with Broca's aphasia. Description of Broca's aphasia is hard to distinguish from the descriptions of apraxia of speech. Diagnosis of apraxia of speech in Broca's aphasia may be postponed until the patient begins to produce enough speech to reveal apraxia.

Aphasia Without Apraxia of Speech	Apraxia of Speech Without Aphasia
Neurogenic language problem	Neurogenic speech problem
More often associated with temporal or temporoparietal lesions	More often associated with posterior, frontal, or insular lesions
Right hemiparesis infrequent	Right hemiparesis frequent
Agrammatism and paraphasia often present	Agrammatism and paraphasia are generally absent
Trial-and-error, groping articulatory movements are not significant	Trial-and-error, groping articulatory movements are significant
Misarticulations less variable, more consistent	Misarticulations more variable, more inconsistent
Phonologic problems of fluently aphasic patients may be unpredictable and not resemble the target sounds/words	Phonologic problems of apraxic patients are predictable and approximations of target sounds/words
Articulatory errors unaffected by complexity of productions	Articulatory errors significantly affected by complexity of productions
Lack of attempts at self-correction, especially in fluent aphasia	Repeated and failed attempts at self-correction
Some impairment in auditory comprehension	Generally, no impairment in auditory comprehension
Prosodic problems not dominant	Prosodic problems dominant
Difficulty in initiating utterances is less obvious	Difficulty in initiating utterances is more obvious
Omission of function words	No significant tendency to omit function words
Word-finding problems	No word-finding problems, although articulatory groping can make it look like such problems
Reading comprehension deficits	No reading comprehension deficits
Severe aphasia may mask apraxia	Does not mask aphasia
Limb or oral apraxia not dominant	Limb or oral apraxia or both may be dominant

TABLE 8-10 Aphasia or dysarthria?

Dysarthria is a group of motor speech disorders due to poor muscle control caused by damage to central or peripheral nerves that supply muscles involved in speech production. Frequently, aphasia and dysarthria may coexist. Subcortical lesions that produce aphasia are likely to be associated with dysarthria. Also, patients who first suffer a left hemisphere stroke and then a right hemisphere stroke may exhibit spastic dysarthria, because of bilateral upper motor neuron damage.

Aphasia without Dysarthria	Dysarthria without Aphasia
Neurogenic language problem	Neurogenic speech problem
Main difficulty is language formulation, expression, and comprehension	Main difficulty is speech production
Lesions in the central nervous system (language-dominant hemisphere)	Lesions in the central nervous system, peripheral system, or both
Normal orofacial mechanism except in cases of facial paralysis	Weakness, paralysis, incoordination of orofacial muscles a significant factor
The language problems are not due to muscle weakness	The speech problems are due to muscle weakness
Significant word-finding problems	No significant word-finding problems
Mild to severe auditory comprehension problems	No significant auditory comprehension problems
No consistent misarticulations	Consistent misarticulations
Intelligibility of speech not clearly related to the rate of speech	Intelligibility clearly related to the rate of speech
No respiratory problems associated with speech production	Respiratory problems associated with speech production
Phonatory problems not significant	Phonatory problems may be significant
Resonance disorders not significant	Resonance disorders significant
Prosodic disorders not dominant	Prosodic disorders may be dominant
Abnormal voice quality not significant	Abnormal voice quality may be significant
Abnormal stress not significant	Abnormal stress may be significant
Reading problems are often present	Reading problems are not typical
Writing problems are often present	Writing problems are not typical

Note: There are several types of dysarthria; all of the distinguishing features just listed do not apply to all cases of dysarthria.

Suggested Readings

Read the following for additional information on assessment and differential diagnosis of aphasia:

Davis, G. A. (2000). *Aphasiology: Disorders and clinical practice.* Needham Heights, MA: Allyn & Bacon.

Golper, L. A. (1996). Language assessment. In G. L. Wallace (Ed.), *Adult aphasia rehabilitation* (pp. 57–86). Boston: Butterworth-Heinemann.

Holland, A. (1996). Pragmatic assessment and treatment for aphasia. In G. L. Wallace (Ed.), *Adult aphasia rehabilitation* (pp. 161–173). Boston: Butterworth-Heinemann.

Murry, L. L., & Chapey, R. (2001). Assessment of language disorders in adults. In R. Chapey (Ed.), *Language intervention strategies in adult aphasia* (pp. 55–118). Baltimore, MD: Williams & Wilkins.

Spreen, O., & Risser, A. (1998). Assessment of aphasia. In M. T. Sarno (Ed.), *Acquired aphasia* (3rd ed., pp. 71–156). New York: Academic Press.

TREATMENT OF APHASIA

Chapter Outline

- Is Aphasia Treatment Effective?
- Variables That Affect Treatment Outcome
- Pharmacological Treatment for Aphasia
- Principles of Language Treatment for Aphasia
- Ethnocultural Considerations in Treatment
- General Treatment Targets
- Treatment of Auditory Comprehension Problems
- Treatment of Verbal Expression
- Social Approaches to Aphasia Rehabilitation
- Treatment of Reading Problems
- Treatment of Writing Problems
- Group Treatment for People with Aphasia
- Augmentative and Alternative Communication for Patients with Aphasia

Learning Objectives

After reading this chapter, the student will:

- Distinguish between improvement under treatment versus effectiveness of treatment techniques.
- Summarize the various medical treatments for stroke patients.
- Describe how treatment needs to be modified for clients of varied ethnocultural backgrounds.
- Specify the target skills and treatment procedures for all forms of communication deficits for patients with aphasia.
- Compare traditional and social approaches to the rehabilitation of patients with aphasia.
- Evaluate group treatment procedures offered to patients with aphasia.
- Describe the need and varieties of augmentative and alternative communication strategies for patients with aphasia.

Is Aphasia Treatment Effective?

Historically, there have been questions about the efficacy of language treatment for aphasia. Demonstrating treatment *effectiveness* is different from documenting *improvement* under treatment (Hegde, 2003). While routine clinical treatment and case studies that document positive changes may claim improvement in clients, only controlled experimental treatment efficacy studies can claim effectiveness.

A complicating factor in claiming effectiveness for treatment procedures in general and those for aphasia in particular is that patients improve to an extent without professional help. Such an improvement, called *spontaneous recovery*, must be ruled out in a study designed to show effectiveness for a treatment procedure. Language skills of patients with aphasia may improve because of significant improvement in the neuropathology underlying the aphasia. Separating spontaneous improvement from treatment effects has been a challenge for clinical scientists (Benson & Ardila, 1996).

Treatment efficacy studies in the past have not always produced consistent results, raising questions about language treatment efficacy (David, Enderby, & Bainton, 1982). However, such results may be due to ineffective treatments, inefficiently implanted treatments, poorly designed studies, or all three of them. More effective treatment procedures, implemented more competently and evaluated with better research designs, may have produced more positive and more convincing results.

Aphasia treatment research has improved in recent decades. Single-subject experimental studies have increased in recent years and have generally produced data to support aphasia treatment (Robey, Schultz, Crawford, & Sinner, 1999). Even historically, better designed and implemented treatment studies (e.g., Basso, Capitani, & Vignolo, 1979) had produced more favorable results than poorly designed studies (e.g., Lincoln, Mulley, Jones, et al., 1984). Because of continued and better controlled research in recent years, there is now evidence that aphasia treatment is effective.

More-or-less controlled group design studies (with or without randomization) have demonstrated the usefulness of systematic treatment. In his two meta-analyses of treatment efficacy studies, Robey (1994, 1998) reviewed a total of 76 group design studies with no random selection or assignment of participants. He concluded that patients who receive treatment attain better communication skills than those who do not. In another review of single-subject treatment efficacy research on aphasia, Robey, Schultz, Crawford, and Sinner (1999) reviewed 63 studies and concluded that various forms of treatments produced clinically important outcomes for patients. Generally, in all three reviews, treatment received especially during the acute stage (as soon after the stroke as possible) produced the greatest gains. Even the patients who received treatment beyond the acute stage showed improvement, although to a lesser extent. Therefore, many clinicians conclude that aphasia treatment is effective and that all patients should be offered it (Basso, 2003; Brookshire, 2003; Davis, 2000; Helm-Estabrooks & Albert, 2004; Helm-Estabrooks & Holland, 1998; Holland, Fromm, DeRuyter, & Stein, 1996; LaPointe, 2005; Rosenbek et al., 1989).

Although long-term follow-up studies on the effects of treatment are few, available evidence suggests that treatment produces a certain degree of lasting effects. Some studies report that treatment effects last over time. For instance, a study of people with aphasia done 18 months after dismissal from treatment (Collins & Wertz, 1983) and another study (Aten et al., 1991) done 7 years after treatment both reported good maintenance of treatment effects. It is likely that poor maintenance, although not uncommon, may be due to ineffective treatments, lack of sustained environmental support (e.g., continued cueing or reinforcement from family members), extinguished self-management skills, deterioration in the health status of the clients (especially additional multiple strokes), or a combination of any and all of these factors.

Variables That Affect Treatment Outcome

Part of the difficulty in determining treatment outcome is that many variables affect it and controlling for them is difficult. Experienced clinicians report that several variables seem to limit or enhance the chances of significant recovery with treatment. Only a few variables thought to be related to good outcome are based on treatment data; most are based on clinical judgments. Therefore, the list of variables that follows should be considered tentative:

- *Age of patients.* Younger patients may improve more than older patients.
- *Premorbid language skills and literacy.* Patients with higher premorbid language and literacy skills may improve better than those with limited premorbid skills.
- *Education and occupation.* Patients with a higher level of education and those who have faced greater occupational demand for language use may improve better than those without such education and occupational demand.
- *Nature of neuropathology (extent and location of lesions).* Patients with smaller lesions and those with no repeated infarcts may improve better than those with larger lesions and repeated infarcts.
- *Medical, neurological, and behavioral status.* Patients with relatively healthy status improve better than those with compromised status.
- *Hearing ability.* With certain kinds of treatments, especially those emphasizing auditory stimulation, patients with better hearing acuity improve more than those with reduced hearing acuity.
- *Visual status.* With certain kinds of treatment, especially those emphasizing visual stimulation, patients with normal or well-corrected vision may improve better than those with significant visual impairment.
- *Motor skills.* Patients with better motor skills may improve more than those with paralysis and paresis.
- *Severity of aphasia.* Patients with less severe aphasia improve more than those with more severe aphasia.
- *Timing of treatment initiation.* Patients who receive early treatment may improve more than those whose treatment is significantly

delayed (Robey, 1994, 1998), although all patients may benefit from treatment.

- *Treatment technique.* Obviously, only the effective techniques are likely to produce positive outcomes.

- *Accuracy of treatment application.* Only those patients who receive an accurate application of an effective treatment are likely to improve.

- *The length of treatment.* Generally and within certain limits, longer treatments produce greater improvement than brief treatments; however, widely spaced and brief treatment sessions offered over a longer duration may be less effective than intense and massed therapy given over a shorter duration (Bhogal, Teasell, Foley, & Speechley, 2003).

- *Intensity of treatment.* Generally and within certain limits, more intensive treatments produce better results than less intensive treatments. Treatment offered for 8 hours a week for about 12 weeks may produce better outcome than treatment offered less often and for shorter duration (Bhogal, Teasell, & Speechley, 2003). Possibly, even those with chronic aphasia gain from intensive treatment in which the skill practice is massed over a short duration (Pulvermuller et al., 2001).

- *Family involvement.* Patients whose family members participate in treatment and learn to help the patient in natural communication contexts improve better than those who do not receive such help from their family members.

- *Improvement or deterioration in general health during the course of treatment.* Patients who sustain their health during treatment improve more than those whose health deteriorates in the same period.

- *Spontaneous recovery.* Treatment improvement tends to be combined with spontaneous improvement, especially during the first 6 months although in some cases recovery may be noted up to 12 months postonset.

Limitations of Research Studies

- Lack of control of variables that affect treatment outcome.

- Questionable internal validity of research studies (did the treatment produce the changes?).
- Poor description of patients, individual skill level before and after treatment, and vague information on the health status (especially in studies involving group designs).
- Poor description of treatment procedures (especially in studies involving group designs).

Pharmacological Treatment for Aphasia

Various pharmacological treatments have been tried alone and in combination with behavioral treatment for aphasia (MlCoch & Metter, 2001). In the acute stage (a period soon after the stroke), medical treatment is urgently needed to improve the physical condition of the patient by enhancing the blood supply to the affected region of the brain. The sooner the blood supply is restored or significantly improved, the better the prognosis for the patient. Several drug treatments are available for patients who already have had a stroke ("completed stroke") (Greenberg, Aminoff, & Simon, 2002; MlCoch & Metter, 2001):

- *Intravenous thrombolytic therapy.* For the treatment of acute ischemic strokes, a drug known as recombinant tissue plasminogen activator (t-PA) has been demonstrated to be effective in minimizing subsequent disability and reducing the chances of death. To work well, the drug should be administered within 3 hours of the ischemic stroke onset, highlighting the importance of awareness of early signs on the part of the patient and the family and getting urgent medical attention. A potential risk of t-PA treatment is hemorrhage.
- *Antiplatelet agents.* Drugs that prevent the formation of blood **platelets** that play a role in coagulation (clotting) of the blood are effective in reducing the chances of major strokes in people who have had transient ischemic attacks. Antiplatelet agents include such nonprescription drugs as aspirin and prescription drugs as ticlopidine. If taken regularly, a low-dose aspirin (81 mg) is also

known to reduce the chances of ischemic strokes in healthy adults.

- *Anticoagulation agents.* These drugs also prevent blood clotting but are useful for patients whose stroke is due to cardiac embolus but not for patients with other kinds of stroke (Greenberg, Aminoff, & Simon, 2002). Drugs in this class include heparin and warfarin.

- *Carotid endarterectomy.* When a stroke is due to the formation of thrombus in the common or internal carotid artery, a surgical procedure called endarterectomy is known to significantly reduce the chances of a subsequent stroke (up to a 50 percent reduction). In this procedure, the thrombus is surgically removed.

Drug therapy is important in improving the general health of the patient. Nonetheless, drug therapy alone has not produced clinically significant improvements in communication skills of stroke patients. However, when combined with behavioral language treatment, some drugs (e.g., dextroamphetamine, piracetam) have produced promising—though not clinically significant—results that need to be researched further (Greener, Enderby, & Whurr, 2001; Huber, 1999; Kessler, Thiel, Karbe, & Heiss, 2000; Walker-Batson et al., 2001). It is likely that in the near future, better drug formulations will help enhance the behavioral treatment methods.

No drug has produced results comparable to those produced by intensive behavioral language treatment in improving communication skills. Further research may show, however, that the effects of language treatment may be enhanced by certain drugs that are neuroprotective and increase the rate of neural transmission.

Principles of Language Treatment for Aphasia

The following principles are basic to treating any disorder of communication, including those associated with aphasia:

- Systematic analysis of the client's intact skills and deficiencies.

- An understanding of the client's family and family communication patterns; the presence or absence of family support the client receives.

- An understanding of the client's and the family members' expectation about treatment; the social and occupation demands the client faces.

- Mobilizing family and social support systems to help improve the overall functional improvement in the client's life and communication patterns.

- Selection of client-specific and personally meaningful target behaviors that, when taught, provide the greatest improvement in functional communication in natural settings and presumably improves the client's quality of life in a global sense.

- Sequencing target behaviors appropriately to ensure a patient's success in treatment (easier initial targets and progressively more difficult ones).

- Offering as intensive a treatment regimen as possible, acceptable to the patient and the family, and feasible in view of the patient's general health and motivation.

- Providing the maximum amount of stimulus control in the beginning, including instructions, modeling, pictures, objects, role playing, and other events that help establish the target language skills.

- Reducing the clinically manipulated stimulus control (e.g., fading, modeling, stimulus pictures) in gradual steps so that the target language skills are produced in response to more natural stimulus events.

- Providing immediate, response-contingent, positive feedback to the client to increase the target language skills and to maintain them at a minimum of 80 percent accuracy.

- Providing immediate corrective feedback for incorrect responses to reduce their frequency.

- Arranging naturally occurring consequences for the patient's attempts to strengthen those attempts in later stages of treatment (e.g., handing an object when a request is made, as against verbal praise for making a good request).

- Training clients in self-monitoring skills to sustain the treatment gains.
- Training significant others to evoke, prompt, support, reinforce, and maintain appropriate communicative behaviors of the client in natural and functional contexts.
- Creating a family and social support system so the client's residual deficits do not produce undue hindrance for the client in personal, social, and communicative situations.
- A follow-up schedule that allows periodic monitoring of the client's communicative behaviors and family and social support systems with a view to offer booster therapy when needed.

Special Considerations in Treating Patients with Aphasia

In many cases, both the patient and his or her family need to learn to live with aphasia. This means that:

- The family members should be counseled and educated to help them cope with the residual deficits.
- Some compensatory communicative strategies should be taught (e.g., a few functional gestures, carrying a notebook to write crucial words when oral communication fails). In some cases, a more extensive approach involving augmentative and alternative communication, described in a later section, may be needed.
- A realistic prognosis that modifies the patient's and the family members' expectations should be given.
- Treatment should be structured and the target behaviors should be repeatedly practiced because intensive and massed therapy is more effective than sporadic therapy with widely spaced treatment trials.
- Treatment should be client-specific; a client's performance should be the guiding principle in modifying partially effective techniques to enhance their effectiveness and in abandoning ineffective ones.

- Treatment in many rehabilitation settings is team-based. Often, the speech-language pathologist (SLP) may work closely with an occupational therapist (OT), a physical therapist (PT), a recreational therapist (RT), or with all of them. The speech-language pathologist may coordinate both the treatment target skills and treatment activities with these other therapists. **Recreation therapists** are specialists who manage the daily activities of patients in rehabilitation settings. A group recreational activity conducted by an RT may be the context to encourage social conversation skills. **Occupational therapists** are most concerned with daily living activities, including self-care (cooking, bathing, dressing, driving), safety, and such other functional skills that also provide an excellent context for communication retraining. For instance, while teaching cooking in a safe manner, both the OT and the SLP may have the patient name the ingredients. Finally, **physical therapists** are mostly concerned with improving the physical status of the patient by implementing various physical exercise and other programs to enhance the physical strength, endurance, range of motion, and general mobility and balance. Such activities as walking in the hallway or carrying an object across a room that a PT may have targeted for treatment may also provide opportunities for the SLP to teach basic conversational skills.
- The clinician should expect to make a judgment about when it is not useful or ethical to continue the treatment.

Some patients who recover neurologically may exhibit symptoms that indicate poor prognosis for recovery of language functions with or without language treatment. Neurological recovery is essentially complete during the 4th through 6th week in the cases of occlusive stroke. It is essentially complete by 3 to 6 months in the case of hemorrhagic strokes and traumatic brain injury.

Generally speaking, globally aphasic patients with severely depressed language in all aspects have been considered poor candidates for language treatment. More specifically, patients who have *neuro-*

logically recovered but still exhibit the following characteristics may not benefit from treatment (Brookshire, 2003):

- Severe auditory comprehension problems coupled with verbal stereotypes (such repetitive utterances as *"me-me-me"* or *"oh boy, oh boy, oh boy"*).
- Failure to match identical stimuli (matching identical objects or matching pictures and objects).
- Indiscriminate yes/no responses.
- Jargon and empty speech without self-correction.

If the resources permit, the best strategy to determine candidacy for treatment is to offer a period of trial treatment to evaluate whether it is worthwhile to continue. Although expensive, this strategy allows for a decision to be made on the basis of client-specific data.

Clinicians should note, however, that persistent treatment research involving patients who exhibit negative prognostic symptoms may show partial success. Such research efforts have been made (Brookshire, 2003). Negative prognostic outlook should always be scrutinized in light of more effective or newer treatment options that may be researched.

Ethnocultural Considerations in Treatment

Ethnocultural research and writing in speech-language pathology have mostly been concerned with assessment of clients with varied cultural or ethnic backgrounds. Empirical research on treatment techniques designed to find the most and the least effective techniques with specific ethnocultural groups is extremely limited. Therefore, it is not possible to suggest specific treatment techniques that are most suitable to individual clients of varied ethnocultural backgrounds.

Clinicians should design treatment programs based on their knowledge of the ethnocultural background of a client. Suggestions of the following kind may be useful in planning and implementing treatment techniques for varied clients:

- The clinician should gain an understanding of a client's ethnocultural background, including the premorbid first and second language, if relevant.
- The clinician should understand the family constellation and family communication patterns that may help select treatment targets (e.g., living in an extended family; the client's role in educating and raising grandchildren).
- The clinician should understand the family resources, accessibility and affordability of clinical services, and public or private support available for extended treatment sessions.
- The clinician should explore whether the client and the family can arrange for and afford transportation for regular treatment sessions and whether they can keep their appointments.
- The clinician should select treatment targets with the help of the client and family members, although this is a good policy with all clients, not just ethnoculturally different ones; the clinician should evaluate all standard techniques for their suitability for an individual client (e.g., does the client need treatment for reading or writing skills?).
- The clinicians should select treatment stimuli that are a part of the client's environment (e.g., stimuli used in treating an elderly Hmong patient may be different from those used in treating a white American).
- Because of lack of research on treatment, clinicians should carefully document the procedures and their effects in all sessions. Such documentation will help assess whether a client of a particular ethnocultural background is improving or not with the technique. If there is no improvement with techniques that are known to be effective with other populations, then the clinician may have found something useful; at least, the clinician can effect timely modifications in the technique.

- Clinicians who treat ethnoculturally different clients should consider publishing case studies in professional journals to promote a better understanding of treatment techniques that work with certain clients, those that do not, and those modifications that will improve the effectiveness of standard techniques.

General Treatment Targets

The many communication skills targeted in treatment of patients with aphasia can be subsumed under four main categories:

- Auditory comprehension of spoken language
- Verbal expression
- Reading skills
- Writing skills

Treatment of Auditory Comprehension Problems

In most cases, it is necessary to treat auditory comprehension problems. In some cases, as in patients with Wernicke's aphasia, it might be the primary goal. Clinicians should note that auditory comprehension problems are not as readily apparent as production problems. At one time, people with what clinicians now call *Wernicke's aphasia* were thought to be psychiatric patients, because their speech often did not make sense. Also, some production problems may be due to comprehension problems. Therefore, treatment that improves auditory comprehension also can help improve language production.

Prognostic Indicators for Auditory Comprehension

Note that lesions *within* and *outside* the posterior superior temporal lobe (PST) can cause auditory comprehension problems. A lesion in the PST suggests poor prognosis for auditory comprehension and slower recovery. A lesion outside the PST suggests good prognosis and faster recovery.

The Nature of Auditory Comprehension Deficits

Different aphasic patients may have different patterns of auditory comprehension problems. Rosenbek et al. (1989) list the following patterns:

- *Slow rise time.* The patient does not comprehend the first few words but comprehends the rest.
- *Noise buildup.* The patient comprehends the first few words but fails to comprehend as the message gets longer or more complex.
- *Information processing lag.* The patient comprehends the first and the last few words better than the other words in a message.
- *Intermittent auditory imperception.* The patient comprehends some but not all with no pattern (fading in and out).
- *Capacity deficit.* The patient comprehends only a limited number of units.
- *Retention deficit.* The patient's correct responses decrease when asked to delay a response after stimulus presentation.

Factors That Promote Auditory Comprehension

The clinician should exploit factors that seem to promote auditory comprehension by building such factors as the following into the treatment program:

- Patients *comprehend more frequently used words better* than less frequently used words. Therefore, in treatment, include more frequently used words.
- Patients *comprehend nouns better* than verbs, adjectives, and adverbs. Therefore, initially use nouns; later use the more difficult words.
- Patients *comprehend picturable verbs better* than nonpicturable verbs. Therefore, show pictures of actions in teaching comprehension of verbs. For example, such verbs as *walking* or *eating* are more easily represented through pictures than *listening* or *thinking*.
- Patients *do better when pictures used are unambiguous.* Therefore, make sure the stimuli

used are unambiguous. For example, photographs of objects may be more unambiguous than poor line drawings.

- Patients *comprehend shorter sentences better* than longer sentences. Therefore, use shorter sentences initially and increase the length gradually.

- Patients *comprehend syntactically simpler sentences better* than more complex sentences. Therefore, use simpler sentences initially and gradually increase the complexity.

- Patients *comprehend active sentences better* than passive sentences. Therefore, use active sentences.

- Patients *comprehend personally relevant sentences better* than those that are not relevant to them. Use sentences that are relevant, meaningful, and interesting to the patients. Let these sentences refer to the patient's personal life experiences, not to bookish information.

- Patients *comprehend better when the speakers reduce their rate of speech and insert pauses.* Therefore, present verbal stimuli at a rate slightly slower than normal and with frequent pauses. The rate you use should be client-specific.

- Patients *comprehend better when the speaker stresses* the important words in a sentence (e.g., the clinician might stress the italicized key words in the request, "Show me the *man* is *walking*"). Their comprehension improves further if a slow rate is combined with stress on target words or phonemes.

- Patients *comprehend better when there is no background noise* or when taped stimuli, if used, are clear and not distorted. Make sure the therapeutic environment is quiet and that taped messages are high fidelity.

- Patients *comprehend better when the message is redundant.* Generally, redundancy improves with context. For instance, an isolated sentence may be more difficult than a sentence that is preceded by other sentences, pictures, or other forms of stimuli. For the same reason, some patients may comprehend connected speech better than isolated words or sentences. Therefore, in treatment, always present contextual information.

- Patients *comprehend better when verbal stimuli are repeated.* Therefore, repeat such verbal stimuli as "Show me the . . ." or "What is this?" type of requests when the initial request fails to evoke a response.
- Patients *comprehend better if the number of choices presented is limited.* Therefore, when asking the patients to point to objects or pictures, initially do not display too many items. Increase the number gradually as the patient's success rate improves.
- Patients *comprehend better when auditory stimuli are accompanied by appropriate visual stimuli.* Therefore, use visual cues that facilitate auditory comprehension. For example, in treating comprehension of such a question as "Did you drive to the clinic today?" the clinician may gesture a steering wheel movement or may show the picture of a car.
- Patients *comprehend better if the speaker's face is visible.* Therefore, make sure that the seating arrangement in treatment is appropriate.
- Patients *comprehend better if an alerting stimulus is presented* before a message is delivered. For instance, before presenting a picture or a message, the patient may be told: "Mrs. White, look at this one!" "Mr. Green, here it comes!" "Ready!" "Listen!" Alerting stimuli must be given 1 to 3 seconds before the target message or stimulus is presented.

Factors That Are Ineffective or Detrimental to Auditory Comprehension

Among the variables that do not help or even adversely affect auditory comprehension are:

- *Increased vocal intensity.* Louder speech does not help.
- *Telephone presentation.* Some patients do worse in telephone conversations.
- *Audio and videotape stimulus presentations.* These do not make a difference.

Finally and most importantly, clinicians should remember that persons with aphasia vary, and the generalities of the kind summarized here apply only to groups of patients, not every single patient.

Some patients do not benefit from a particular strategy that works with most patients. For instance, some may not benefit from slower rate or contextual cues.

Clinicians should determine the suitability of each strategy for each patient. Objective, continuous measurement of target behaviors under treatment will help make prudent judgments about the suitability of selected treatment techniques.

Sequence of Auditory Comprehension Treatment

To correctly sequence the auditory comprehension treatment, the clinician should first determine the current auditory comprehension skills:

- Start treatment at a level appropriate for the current level of auditory skills of each patient.
- Note that the more severe the deficit, the lower the response topography. For instance, for patients with severe deficits, the treatment is begun with comprehension of single words. If the deficits are moderate to mild, the beginning level of response topography may be phrases, sentences, or discourse.

Comprehension of Single Words

If assessment shows the client needs treatment at the level of single-word comprehension, begin treatment at this level. Typical target responses and treatment procedures at the single-word level include:

- *Target response: Pointing to specific stimulus items.* Pointing to body parts, objects, pictures of objects, clothing items, food items, and other personally relevant items.
  - *Basic treatment procedure.* Name a body part and ask the client to point to it. Select several pictures or objects, place them in front of the client, and ask the client to point to a specific item. Repeat trials on which the client is successful. Present all items at least once.

- *Target response: Pointing to action pictures.*
  - *Basic treatment procedure.* Place an array of action pictures in front of the client. Name an action and ask the patient to point to the correct picture (e.g., "show me the man who is *walking*"). Present all selected items at least once. Repeat the items the client correctly identifies.

Comprehension of Spoken Sentences

For patients who comprehend single words either at baseline or because of treatment, the next level of treatment is for spoken sentences. Typically, three specific tasks are targeted: comprehending spoken questions, following spoken directions, and verifying sentences. Typical target responses and treatment procedures at the sentence level include the following:

- *Target response: Comprehension of spoken questions.* Begin with yes/no questions and open-ended questions; move from simpler to more complex questions. The patient's acceptable response may be verbal ("yes" or "no") or nonverbal (e.g., a head shake).
  - *Basic treatment procedure.* Ask a variety of questions about the patient's family and personal life (e.g., "Do you have a daughter?" "Do you live in the country?"), about general knowledge (e.g., "Is San Francisco in Nevada?"), about discrimination of word classes ("Is dog an animal?"), and about phonemic discrimination ("Do you wear a hat and a bat?").
- *Target response: Following spoken directions.* Specific targets include pointing to stimuli in sequence and manipulating objects according to the given directions.
  - *Basic treatment procedure.* Select common but functional pictures and objects. Initially, present a pair of stimuli (e.g., a piece of paper and a pen) and give a simple sequential direction for the client to follow (e.g., "point to the paper and then the pen"). If the client has a problem identifying the two objects involved, provide a few trials on which you ask the client to point to each of the objects separately. When success is demonstrated, re-present the se-

quential directions. When the client can correctly follow two-sequence directions, present progressively more complex directions (e.g., "point to the paper, the pen, and the eraser"; "touch the ball, the spoon, and the cup and then give me the ball").

Place manipulable objects on the table (e.g., a small ball and a box) and give directions that involve object manipulation (e.g., "put the ball in the box"). Give progressively more complex directions (e.g., "put the ball in the box and pick up the pencil from the box and put it on the table").

- *Target response: Sentence verification.* The client determines whether a spoken sentence is true or false. The client also may match a picture to the spoken sentence ("The woman is riding the bicycle") or may say "yes" or "no" to such questions as "Is a plant bigger than a tree?"

  - *Basic treatment procedure.* Show a picture (e.g., a woman riding a bicycle) and a foil (e.g., a woman driving a car or a woman walking). Say the target sentence (e.g., "The woman is riding a bicycle") and ask if the picture shows what the sentence means; on some trials, present a foil that does not match.

    In a variation of the procedure called *match-to-sample,* show the target picture and its foils simultaneously or printed on the same page (e.g., pictures of a dog chasing a man, a man chasing a dog, a boy chasing a dog, and a dog chasing a boy); ask the client to point to the correct picture as you orally present a sentence (e.g., "The man is chasing the dog").

Discourse Comprehension

This involves a complex and naturalistic response topography. Training at this level includes such pragmatic skills as understanding narrative stories and answering questions in a conversational format.

- *Target response: Understanding narratives.* Collect a few short, simple, and interesting stories (or use the *Discourse Comprehension Test* by Brookshire & Nichols, 1993).

- *Basic treatment procedure.* Read the story aloud to the client and then ask specific questions about the *main idea, stated details,* and *implied details.* Implied details require an inference (e.g., when the story is about a *family man,* the implied detail may be that he has a wife or a child).

- *Target response: Understanding questions in a conversational format.* Start with simple yes/no questions in a conversational format and ask progressively more complex questions that require more elaborate responses.

  - *Basic treatment procedure.* Engage the client in conversational speech. Ask personally relevant questions (e.g., "Do you watch football games on TV?" "Did you go to the zoo yesterday?" "Do you live in Fresno?"). Accept appropriate verbal or nonverbal response as the target is correct comprehension of questions.

    Treat comprehension of more complex questions by progressively asking questions that require more elaborate answers (e.g., "What did you do this weekend?" or "Did someone visit you last Sunday?").

Note that when a clinician moves to complex levels of auditory comprehension training, verbal expression also is simultaneously trained. Some form of verbal expression may be required to suggest correct comprehension of complex verbal material.

Treatment of Verbal Expression

Clinicians spend a major portion of their treatment time on verbal expression. Several aspects of verbal expression are typically targeted. As is typical in treating most clients, treatment begins at the most simple level of verbal expression and progresses to more complex levels, including conversational speech.

Treatment of Naming

A difficulty in finding the right words at the right time is a pervasive problem in patients with aphasia.

A significant improvement in naming helps the patient with aphasia achieve much more fluent and effective social communication. Therefore, naming is a major speech production target for most patients with aphasia; much of aphasia treatment research is about treating naming disorders.

Several researched techniques are available to retrain naming skills; but generally, most depend on matching stimuli (e.g., matching pictures with printed or spoken words) or prompting the correct word with phonologic or semantic cues. These techniques have been effective to varying degrees (Hickin et al., 2002; Nickels, 2002).

Treatment of naming depends on the type of error the patient makes. Research has shown that patients with anterior lesions (mostly those who exhibit Broca's aphasia) and those with posterior lesions (those who exhibit Wernicke's and anomic aphasias) tend to have different kinds of naming problems. Therefore, selected treatment procedure should be appropriate for these problems, although selection of client-specific treatment remains a difficult task (Nickels & Best, 1996a, 1996b). An initial period of experimentation with different techniques is still the best course of treatment selection for most patients.

Types of Naming Problems

Benson and Ardila (1996) have given a detailed classification of naming problems in patients with aphasia. This classification is based mostly on Benson's (1979a) descriptions of varied naming deficits found in his patients with aphasia.

- *Word production anomia.* Damage to the frontal lobe, including Broca's area, areas above or in front of Broca's area, and the supplementary motor area in the left hemisphere, causes this type of anomia. The anomia itself results from motor problems that are consequences of such anterior lesions. Word production anomia is further classified into several subtypes:
  - *Prefrontal anomia* is commonly found in prefrontal lesions that result in transcortical motor aphasia. The typical problem is (a) *fragmentation* or whole-part errors

(e.g., calling a refrigerator "kitchen" because no attention is paid to the specific part of a picture); (b) incorrect *perseveration* of a previously correctly produced name; or (c) *extravagant verbal paraphasia* based on free association of ideas or words (e.g., naming a blue sofa "sky").

- *Articulatory initiation anomia* is associated especially with supplementary motor lesions. It also is found in transcortical motor aphasia and Broca's aphasia. The naming problem is a result of the patient having extreme difficulty in initiating articulatory gestures to produce words and phrases.

- *Articulatory reduction anomia* is found mostly in Broca's aphasia. Reduced articulatory competency results in naming problems characterized by deletion of syllables in clusters and phonetic assimilation (repetition of a phoneme in a subsequent syllable and production of a phoneme that is a part of a word yet to be produced, sometimes called *phonemic anticipation*).

- *Paraphasic anomia* is often found in conduction aphasia. It is characterized by literal paraphasia in which phonemes of a word are substituted. Cueing may not help.

- *Phonemic disintegration anomia* is found in some patients with Wernicke's aphasia. This kind of anomia results in jargon because of phonemic paraphasias. Cueing has little effect on this type of naming problem.

- *Word selection anomia.* The typical lesions that cause this type of anomia are in the posterior inferior portion of the temporal lobe. This is true anomia. Patients can describe, gesture, write, and draw to suggest a word they cannot say. They can correctly recognize the name when given or even promptly and correctly point to objects named, but they cannot name it. This problem can exist when most other language functions are near-normal. Circumlocutions and pauses because of naming problems may be evident.

- *Semantic anomia.* Often associated with transcortical sensory aphasia (TSA), patients with semantic anomia do not recognize the words they cannot produce. Patients can neither say the word nor point to the object when named; they even fail to experience the familiar tip-of-the-tongue phenomenon. The patient can repeat the word without understanding its meaning. The lesion usually is in the parietal-occipital area, especially the angular gyrus. In this case, even word recognition may have to be trained.

- *Disconnection anomias.* A few forms of anomia are thought be a result of disconnection of specific neural pathways.

  - *Category-specific anomia* is a problem in which the patient has a disproportionately greater difficulty naming words of a certain category. Some patients have excessive difficulty in naming body parts, others in naming animals or vegetables. For example, patients with medial occipital lesions show a debilitating color naming problem (color anomia), though they can much more easily name objects or body parts. Color perception is normal; they can correctly categorize colors and produce color words in spontaneous speech.

  - *Modality-specific anomia* is difficulty in naming an object presented through a certain sensory modality with the same object readily named when presented in another modality. *Tactile anomia* is difficulty naming objects held in hand with no difficulty in naming the same item when it is shown. Some patients cannot name foods whose taste they can discern, and others cannot name odors associated with substances they can name (e.g., *flower, bacon*). A modality-specific naming problem is typically described as *agnosia*. See Chapter 4 for a description of agnosias.

  - *Callosal anomia* is naming difficulty following surgical severance of the corpus callosum, resulting in disconnected hemispheres. The patient cannot name objects held in the nonpreferred left hand but soon thereafter can select the same object among an array of objects by left-hand palpitation. Disconnection between the hemispheres prevents naming because the palpated sensory information, although correctly interpreted, does not evoke a name from the left hemisphere.

Most patients with aphasia may show a combination of naming problems. In some cases, the difficulty may not be easily classified. Most patients exhibit certain consequences of their naming problems. For example, some show a *delayed response:* The patient may "buy" time for the response to be triggered. Some *self-correct* their mistakes, while others apparently are unaware of their problems. The clinician should analyze each patient's difficulty in planning treatment.

Use of Stimuli That Facilitate Correct Naming

In treating naming problems, recall that certain stimuli facilitate a correct response. To recapitulate, for most aphasic patients:

- High frequency words are easier than low frequency words.
- Names of manipulable objects (e.g., a ball that can be held, bounced, or thrown; a piece of paper that can be folded or written on) are easier than those that are not (e.g., a sofa or a refrigerator, which cannot be manipulated).
- Objects may be easier than pictures.
- Realistic drawings are easier than distorted or poorly drawn stimuli.
- Phonemic cueing makes it easier for Broca's patients and those who have mild to moderate naming problems, but not for Wernicke's patients.
- Self-regulation of stimulus presentation is better than machine-spaced presentation.
- Extra time given for naming improves performance.
- Longer stimulus exposure time (30 seconds or more) leads to better performance.
- Visual and auditory presentation of stimuli (e.g., seeing the object and hearing the name) is better than just the visual presentation.

- Movement from easier to difficult task is better than vice versa.

Naming: Treatment Targets and Techniques

Confrontation naming. A frequently used procedure is to place pictures or objects in front of the patient and ask "What is this?"

This procedure may not help produce functional communicative behaviors, because the targets are not useful in nonclinical settings. Adults are rarely asked to name pictures or objects. However, such naming tasks may facilitate spontaneous production of nouns in conversational speech produced in natural settings. Unfortunately, there is little research on generalization of naming skills established in clinical settings to such spontaneous speech. Generalization data do suggest, however, that when a number of nouns are trained, untrained nouns may be produced when patients are shown pictures or objects (Nickels, 2002; Freed, Celery, & Marshall, 2004). Again, such generalized production in relation to pictures and objects is of limited functional value to most people. A study has shown that although clients may generalize word productions, they may still fail to produce them during discourse (Boyle, 2004).

Use of cueing hierarchies. A patient who cannot name in natural stimulus contexts needs additional stimuli that might help evoke the response. These additional stimuli are called *cues*. Various cueing hierarchies may be described as phonologic (or phonetic in some studies), semantic (based on word meanings, words of similar or different meanings), orthographic (printed words, letters), pictorial (pictures of objects to be named), auditory (hearing a word and saying it), and written (writing or copying a word and then saying it). See Nickels (2002) for an excellent review of studies on varied forms of cues.

The basic logic and procedure of cueing hierarchies are simple:

- Find a stimulus or a cue that evokes the response. The stimulus may be visual (a picture or a printed word); auditory ("it makes a mew sound"); phonetic ("It starts with a *p*" [for *pen*]); syllabic ("it starts with *stoo*" [for *stool*]; semantic, which is related to meaning

("You wear it on your head"); an incomplete sentence (e.g., "These are two . . ."; "the word starts with *spoo* . . ." [for *spoon*]).

- Let the client, family members, or both suggest cues that are specific to their personal experiences. Such cues are better than standard phonological (e.g., "the word starts with a *d*" or "the word has three letters in it" for *dog*) or semantic cues ("You use it to hit a nail" for *hammer*). Instead, when allowed to choose a cue for *hammer*, the patient may suggest a cue that is personal: "I once hit my finger with it" (Freed, Celery, & Marshall, 2004).

- Use a stronger stimulus or cue only when weaker stimuli do not evoke the response. For example, presenting a picture and asking "What is this?" uses a weaker stimulus than asking the question and saying "It starts with *spoo*. . . ."

- Start with a minimum number of cues and add cues only when necessary. If only pictures will do, do not add a phonetic cue or a syllabic cue or any other cue. If pictures do not evoke the response, add only one other cue. Thus, add one cue at a time and only when needed.

- Fade the special stimuli, so that natural stimuli eventually evoke the response. Phonetic and syllabic cues, incomplete sentences, and cues based on use are not natural stimuli that evoke responses. Questions are more natural in conversational situations (e.g., "What is this?" "What is that?"). Unnatural stimuli, when used because of necessity, should be faded. Natural objects, conversational contexts, and so forth should replace them.

Essentially, all cues given in treatment sessions should be seen as devices to initially evoke a response. The cues should be followed by procedures in which the client manages to generate his or her own responses in naturalistic settings.

Target Word Selection

Target words selected for treatment should be client-specific and functional. It is not useful to drill a client on words that he or she is unlikely to use in naturalistic contexts. An earlier example, *hammer,* may be a good choice for someone who regularly uses one; it is a poor choice for someone who has never touched one. Therefore, in developing a list of target words, the clinician should first talk to the client and his or her family members. The client's interests, hobbies, occupation (especially if the client is expected to return to it), food items, clothing items, favorite television shows, and pets are important sources of target words. Similarly, names of family members, their occupations and activities, and the towns in which different family members live provide varied and useful target words. In many cases, the names of the client's family physician, relevant hospital and other health care institutions, and medications taken regularly may also help generate a client-specific and functional list of words. The patient's address, home number, telephone number, and such other personal information items as target behaviors may also serve the client well.

Once a functional list of words is developed, the clinician can discuss with the client and his or her family members (or other caregivers) to develop a personalized cueing hierarchy. The following general cueing hierarchies may be modified to implement a naming treatment program.

MODELING

Modeling is probably the most frequently used special stimulus in the treatment of communication disorders. Technically, modeling is not a cue, because it displays the correct response completely. Nonetheless, some cue-based training of words may start with modeling. The full model is then reduced in some way to turn it into a *cue,* which hints a response but does not fully display it. Thus, modeling may be the first element in a hierarchy of cues presented to clients. A clinician's production of a correct response that may lead to imitation by the client is called **modeling.** To use this procedure, present a picture or an object, ask the question, immediately model the response, and let the patient imitate (e.g., the clinician asks "What is this?" and immediately models by saying "say *ball*"; the client imitates by saying "ball"). When the client has imitated the modeled response a few times, transform the model into a cue.

CUEING THE CORRECT RESPONSE

Although all cues are preferably based on the client's personal experiences (Freed, Celery, & Marshall, 2004), one or the other format in which those cues are presented may be more or less effective with given clients. Therefore, the clinician should be aware of the different formats in which a cue may be presented. For instance:

- *Partial sentences as cues.* This method uses the power of the previous elements of a stimulus chain to evoke a subsequent element of the chain. The procedure evokes *intraverbal control,* in which previous words are stimuli for subsequent words. The target word is the final word in a sentence, and the clinician produces as many words as necessary to trigger that word.

  1. **The clinician:** "You write with a ballpoint _____?"
     The patient: "Pen."
  2. **The clinician:** "You write with a _____?"
     The patient: "Pen."

  Note that the preceding two examples are standard cues, while the following two are personalized cues:

  3. **The clinician:** "A blue Parker that was your birthday gift _____?"
     The patient: "Pen."
  4. **The clinician:** "You have one with pink flowers _____?"
     The patient: "Dress."

- *Phonetic cues.* The clinician produces the first letter of the word or the sound. There is controversial evidence on the effectiveness of phonetic cues. Sometimes they are criticized as being less effective than semantic cues, although some evidence suggests that the difference between the semantic and phonetic cues has been exaggerated (Doesborgh et al., 2004; Nickels, 2002). Therefore, the clinician may have to experiment to see if phonetic cues work for given clients. Note that the first example is purely phonetic and the second is personalized-phonetic:

  1. **The clinician:** "You write with a— (pause)—the word starts with a p_____."
     The patient: "Pen."

2. **The clinician:** "It's your blue Parker birthday gift—(pause)—it starts with a *p*—."
The patient: "Pen."

- *Partial words as cues.* Within a sentence completion task, the clinician may produce a syllable if the sound cue is not effective and may combine it with a personalized element.

    1. **The clinician:** "This is a spoo _____."
    The patient: "Spoon."
    2. **The clinician:** "You use this to eat your mushroom soup. This is a spoo _____."
    The patient: "Spoon."

- *Silent phonetic cues.* The clinician may evoke a name through sentence completion by giving cues of articulatory posture without vocalization.

    The clinician: "This is a (p)." The clinician shows a silent articulator posture for the initial sound in *pen.*
    The patient: "Pen."

- *Functional descriptions as cues.* A description of the use of an object may help evoke a naming response. The first is a generic cue, the second is personalized:

    1. **The clinician:** "This is a round object that you roll or kick. What do you call it?"
    The patient: "Ball."
    2. **The clinician:** "This is a round object you are fond of playing with your grandson. What do you call it?"
    The patient: "Ball."

- *Activity and time as cues.* The clinician may describe an activity and its typical time of performance generically to evoke a word (1) or make it personalized (2).

    1. **The clinician:** " What is this? This is something you eat at lunch time."
    The patient: "Hamburger."
    2. **The clinician:** "What is this? This is what you like to eat at lunch time."
    The patient: "Eggplant sandwich."

- *Description and demonstration of an action.* This is followed by a request to give the target name:

    The clinician: "You use this to write" (demonstrates writing). "What is this?"
    The patient: "Pen."

- *Patient's description as stimuli for naming.* The clinician may evoke a name first by having the client say what an object is used for and then name it. See how it can be personalized in the second example.
  1. **The clinician:** "Tell me what you use this for and then tell me its name."
     The patient: "I use it to write. It is a pen."
  2. **The clinician:** "Tell me what you use this birthday gift of yours for and then tell me its name."
     The patient: "I use it to write. It is a pen."

Alternately, the clinician may first ask the patient to describe the function and then ask to name it.

The clinician: "What is this used for?" or "What is this birthday gift of yours used for?"
The patient: "To write."
The clinician: "What do you call it?"
The patient: "Pen."

- *Patient's demonstration of function as a cue.* The clinician may evoke a name by first having the patient demonstrate the function of an object and then name it.

The clinician: "Show me how you use this and then tell me the name."
The patient: Demonstrates the action of drinking and then says "cup."
Alternately, the clinician first asks for demonstration and then for the name.

- *Pairing an object or a picture with its printed name.* An object or a picture of an object and its printed name may be presented simultaneously and the patient may be asked to name it. This is one of the most researched cues for teaching naming in patients with aphasia (Nickels, 2002). Printed letters of the target word may also be used in this format.

The clinician: Presents a book (or the picture of a book) and the printed word *book* (or the letter B) and then asks the patient, "What is this?"
The patient: "Book."

- *Patient's spelling as a cue.* The patient may be asked to spell a word orally and then name the object.

The clinician: "Spell this word for me and then say it."
The patient: "b-o-o-k. Book."

- *Patient's spelling and writing as cue.* The patient may be asked to spell a word, write it, and then say it.

  The clinician: "Spell this word, write it, and then say it."

  The patient: "B-o-o-k." The patient writes it and then says "book."

- *Presentation of associated sound as a cue.* The patient may be asked to name a stimulus soon after presenting the typical sound associated with it.

  The clinician: Presents the picture of a dog and says "arf-arf." Then asks, "what is this?"

  The patient: "Dog."

- *Use of rhyming words as cues.* The clinician may present a word that rhymes with the target word (Spencer et al., 2000).

  The clinician: "What is this? It rhymes with *hog.*"

  The patient: "Dog."

- *Use of words of a generic class, synonyms, antonyms, or typically associated words, or a superordinate to evoke a name.* Such words may prompt the client to say the target word (McNeil et al., 1997).

  The clinician may say "woman" (a generic word) to evoke the word "wife."

  The clinician may say "dwelling" (a synonym) to evoke the word "house."

  The clinician may say "woman" (an antonym) to evoke the word "man."

  The clinician may say "plate" (an associated word) to evoke the target word "cup."

In all procedures, the clinician should appropriately reinforce correct responses and use corrective feedback (saying "no" or "wrong") as found necessary. The use of corrective feedback can be minimized by carefully selecting target behaviors, simplifying them within a shaping procedure, and selecting stimuli that are effective in evoking the responses. When a response is effectively evoked, repeated trials are necessary to stabilize the response. Gradually, the clinician should shift to more naturalistic evoking stimuli.

FADING THE CUES

Cues should be faded in the treatment sessions so that the client can maintain the naming and other language skills in natural settings. Even the most effective and subtle therapeutic cue may be unnatural or unavailable in the natural setting. If the control over the response is not shifted over to the natural events (and self-monitoring), the response maintenance may be poor.

Most naming treatment research studies have failed to shift the stimulus control to natural events. The experimenters may probe to see if the client would name the same treated stimuli or similar untrained (novel) stimuli in nonclinical settings. If the client did name the treated and novel stimuli in nonclinical settings, the treatment is considered a success. It is a success, but only to an extent. The ultimate success is achieved only when the client is observed to produce the treated words and related untreated words without external cues and in social conversations. On both of these accounts, aphasia naming treatment research falls short.

Fading is a procedure in which special stimuli are withdrawn gradually, not abruptly. A stimulus may be faded by reducing its length, intensity, frequency, and modality. Although little controlled aphasia treatment research has given specific guidelines on fading the cues, the following are extrapolated from fading in behavioral research:

- Fade the cues in various ways.
  - Fade the length of the cues. For example, fade the number of words given in a sentence completion task. For instance, following the question "What is this?" the clinician may have modeled "You write with a . . ." to evoke the word *pen*. This cue may be progressively reduced in successive steps: "You write with . . .;" "You write . . ." and "You . . ." (with an expectant look while showing a pen).
- Fade the vocal intensity of a cue. In progressive steps, give the cue in softer voice until it is barely audible; eventually, just lip the cue words (silent articulatory movements without auditory cues). Finally, reduce and withdraw the silent articulatory cues.
- Fade the frequency of a cue. Initially cue every time you evoke a naming response. As the patient makes progress, reduce the frequency of cueing. Omit cueing on certain trials. Eventually, stop cueing to see if the re-

sponse is maintained. Reinstate cueing as found necessary, but only to fade again.

- Fade multiple cues to single and no cues. For instance, when using the spell it–write it–say it procedure, fade "spell it" and then fade "write it" and finally fade "say it" by asking the questions, "What is this?" Similarly, when an object is initially paired with a picture and a printed word, fade the picture, then the printed word, and finally maybe even the object to evoke the name in conversational speech without any concrete stimuli.

- Fade a verbal cue into a gestural cue (modality change). For instance, when the phrase "You drink with it. What is it?" has been an effective cue for the word "cup," fade the verbal cue into a gestural cue (e.g., the gesture of drinking from a cup). Reduce the gesture's magnitude until it is minute and eventually nonexistent.

- Teach family members the various ways of fading a cue so that they may become accustomed to using this strategy at home.

Teaching Self-Cueing in Natural Settings

Unless the client is taught to self-manage his or her naming deficits, treatment gains may not be maintained in natural settings. Even with effective fading of cueing, the client may need to cue himself or herself in natural settings. Therefore, teaching self-cueing in natural settings is an important strategy in promoting maintenance of naming skills.

The client should learn to use the cues that were effective in word generation. For example, a synonym, an antonym, an object, or a related word may prove to be effective for a given client. The client then should be reinforced for *generating those cues himself or herself* in the clinic session. If the client can say "wife" when the clinician supplies the word "husband," then the client can say the antonym first to generate the target word. The client may be taught to think or even verbalize, "Well, I am thinking of the word that is opposite *husband—wife.*"

The client who learns to generate his or her own cues in the clinic should be encouraged to do so in natural conversations outside the clinic. To say that "I want an eggplant sandwich," the client may be taught to think or silently verbalize, *it is my favorite lunch item* or anything similar to the cue that was used in treatment.

In stabilizing self-cueing outside the clinic, the clinician needs to train a family member to first provide a cue and then fade it. The family member can reinforce self-cueing and help document its success.

As the client's word retrieval problems come under significant control, the clinician should target expansion of words into phrases, sentences, narrative speech, and finally, conversational speech. The final goal of treatment is *functional communication* in natural settings. To the extent possible, the person with aphasia should be an effective partner in social communication.

Expansion of Verbal Expressions

Achievement of effective social communication begins with an effort to expand the verbal expressions in the clinic. These expansions have to be extended to natural settings, and additional social discourse skills will then have to be retained.

In expanding words and phrases into functional expressions, the clinician should select expressions that are:

- Most useful for the client and his or her caregivers or family
- Most useful in expressing the client's personal experiences, bodily needs, emotions, and thoughts
- Most effective in social conversational contexts
- Effective in meeting the social and occupational demands the client may face

The clinician should design client-specific treatment programs in which progressively longer utterances are shaped. The clinician should (a) start with what the client can say, perhaps a few words; (b) add additional words to create phrases or simple sentences; and (c) expand simple sentences into longer, more complex, and varied sentence forms.

In Teaching Sentence Productions, the Clinician May:

- Model sentences initially to encourage the client to imitate them (e.g., while showing a picture, the clinician asks "What is the man doing here? Say *he is chopping wood*"; the client imitates the sentence and receives positive reinforcement).

- Ask questions to evoke specific, functional sentences (e.g., the clinician shows the picture and asks the same question but does not model the response; the clinician may prompt the response by saying "*he is chopping____*").

- Fade the prompts and only ask the question to evoke the response.

In Teaching Connected Speech and Conversational Skills, the Clinician May:

- Show action-filled pictures and ask the client to describe them; select pictures depicting scenes that are of interest to the client and appropriate to the client's ethnocultural background.

- Select words useful to the client and ask him or her to make sentences using those words. Have the client, family members, and other caregivers help select the target words. Ask the client to make different kinds of sentences for each word.

- Tell short stories and ask questions about them or ask the client to retell the story.

- Show sequenced pictures that tell a story and ask the client to construct one.

- During storytelling, ask the client to say more on a topic or elaborate on the response (e.g., "Tell me more about how that character feels." "What is the moral of this story?").

- Ask the client to describe how certain tasks are completed (e.g., "How do you make apple pies?" "How do you make soup?" "How do you change a flat tire?").

- Loosen the structure of treatment sessions by engaging the client in more natural conversations.

- Evoke more natural conversational speech by introducing topics for dialogue, instead of asking questions. For instance, say, "Tell me about your favorite TV shows you watch regularly." When the client begins to talk about the shows, offer comments, express your own preferences, request more details, and invite criticisms and comments to keep the conversation as natural as possible. Other topics related to interests, hobbies, the client's jobs, and past or planned vacations afford opportunities to introduce topics of conversation.

- Briefly talk about your own personal experiences (e.g., a vacation you recently took), interests, and hobbies to see if the client would then initiate conversation on similar topics stemming from his or her own experience.

- Prompt the client to initiate a topic of conversation without you suggesting topics. For example, ask: "What shall we talk about today?" "Do you have something to tell me today?" "Do you have a topic of discussion?" Questions such as these may help the client take a lead in conversation. Generously reinforce any lead the client takes and encourage the client to do the same on future sessions.

- Have a family member, caregiver, volunteer, or another clinician participate in as many conversational treatment sessions as possible. Train them to let the client take a lead in choosing the topic of conversation. Using the suggestions offered in the following section on social approach to rehabilitation, train conversational partners to adapt to the needs of the person with aphasia and support that person's communicative attempts.

The clinician may use one of several published treatment programs to treat sentence structures, elaboration of speech and language skills, and functional communication. A few examples:

- *Promoting Aphasics' Communicative Effectiveness (PACE)*, developed by Davis and Wilcox (1981), lets the clinician train conversational exchanges between two persons. The clinician and the client exchange the roles of listener and speaker. The emphasis is on communication, not necessarily grammatically correct forms of expression.

- The *Helm Elicited Language Program for Syntax Stimulation* (Helm-Estabrooks,

1981) uses a story completion format in which the clinician tells a short story and lets the client answer questions or tells an incomplete story and lets the client complete it. The program helps target eight types of sentences, including *what, who, when,* and *where* questions; declaratives; comparatives; and yes/no questions. Some clinical case studies support the claim that the clients improve with this method (Helm-Estabrooks, Fitzpatrick, & Baresi, 1982). A controlled study has demonstrated that the procedure may promote somewhat limited generalization across sets of novel stimuli, variable maintenance, and limited judged adequacy of verbal responses of treated individuals (Doyle, Goldstein, & Bourgeois, 1987).

- *Response Elaboration Training (RET)* is designed to increase the length and information content of persons with nonfluent aphasia. Researched by Kearns and his colleagues, RET uses a loose training format known to promote better generalization of clinically established skills to natural settings (Kearns & Potechin-Scher, 1989). The method does not demand complex or compound sentence productions; instead, it emphasizes effective communication while supporting expanded sentence productions. A noteworthy feature of this approach is to promote patient-initiated language productions. The patient is encouraged to "talk about anything" that treatment stimuli may prompt, instead of asking specific, structured questions. Patients are discouraged from naming or simply describing treatment stimuli; they have to talk about it in a more natural and elaborated manner, drawing upon their personal experiences and world knowledge. Such well-researched behavioral techniques as modeling, prompting, and reinforcing responses that offer more information (instead of grammaticality) are a part of this procedure. The method has received experimental support.

- *A Program of Changing Criteria,* described by Rosenbek, LaPointe, and Wertz (1989), also helps promote longer and expanded productions, starting with simple one- or two-word utterances. Changing criteria involve a series of rules the performance must meet. For example, in the beginning, a client's one- or two-word productions may be accepted (the initial criterion of performance). But the subsequent criteria may involve progressively longer or more complex productions; each criterion is applied at one time, the responses are stabilized, and the performance bar is raised for the next criterion. When applied systematically and performance data are collected in detail, the changing criteria themselves help establish the treatment effects by showing that the client's performance changed only when a new criterion went into effect (Hegde, 2003).

Social Approaches to Aphasia Rehabilitation

As Simmons-Mackie (2001), Lyon (1998), and others point out, aphasia treatment was historically concerned with teaching specific words, phrases, and sentences in the clinic to remediate linguistic deficits. Some investigators then probed for generalization to untrained words, phrases, and sentences of the same class as those trained to see if the client produced them in natural settings. Even if successful within this approach, the clients often lacked everyday language skills—the so-called *functional language skills* that made a difference in their lives. Consequently, treatment emphasis was shifted to functional communication training or daily living skill training. Although this approach was better than remediating purely linguistic deficits, the clients were still not achieving effective and meaningful social communication and integration. In spite of improved linguistic or functional communication skills, many persons with aphasia remain socially isolated.

Therefore, several investigators have emphasized the need to approach treatment more from a social communication-integration standpoint than with an exclusive concern with grammatical accuracy and somewhat restricted functional skills (Chapey et al., 2001; Kagan & Gailey, 1993; Kagan et al., 2001; Lyon, 1997; Simmons-Mackie, 2001). These investigators have argued, collectively as well as individually, that people with aphasia need a social communication approach in which not only the client but also his or her family and caregivers are treated in such a way as to make the client an effective social-conversational partner. Within this social approach to treatment, somewhat different treatment procedures have been described (Chapey et al., 2001; Kagan & Gailey, 1993; Kagan et al., 2001; Lyon, 1997; Simmons-Mackie, 2001). Nonetheless, the varied approaches are consistent with the new World Health Organization's (2001) Classification of Function, Disability and Health (ICF), which views diseases in biological, personal, family, and social contexts. As Elman (2005) has pointed out, two patients with the same type and severity of aphasia may have vastly different outcomes. The patient with little or no support from family and social networks may perform in everyday life more poorly than the one whose family members are integrated into effective treatment programs or the one who attends group and social therapeutic activities and has a network of friends. See Appendix C for a brief description of the WHO ICF.

An important point to note is that the traditional treatment directed to improve language skills, functional language, and generalized production of quantitatively measured improvement in communication skills is not to be disregarded in using a social approach to treatment of aphasia. Going beyond, but not replacing basic and functional communication skills, is the goal of the social approach. Teaching communication skills, especially conversational skills in social settings, to improve the overall quality of life of patients with aphasia is the ultimate goal of social approach (Elman, 2005). In this light, the treatment of communication problems and social approach to aphasia are not two opposing or incompatible methods; both are more essential to a complete rehabilitation of persons with aphasia than is either of the two.

In defense of the traditional language and functional communication training, it may be said that those who advocate it do realize that adequate personal and social communication is the final goal of treatment. In criticism of this traditional approach, it may just as well be said that such a recognition has not always resulted in a broader and more effective view of aphasia treatment, viewed especially from the standpoint of people with aphasia and their families.

The main thrust of the social approach to treating aphasia, much of it from Simmons-Mackie (2001), may be summarized and expanded as follows:

- Let persons with aphasia and their family members take an active role in treatment. Research shows that people with aphasia can express their perspectives, rate services or needs, and help clinicians select treatment approaches (Kagan, 1995; Lyon, 1998).
  - Invite the person with aphasia and his or her family members to suggest the overall goals of rehabilitation and to select treatment targets. What skills are important to whom? Finalize the treatment goals and targets only after a thorough discussion with all concerned individuals, including any professional caregivers who may be involved.
- Periodically ask the person with aphasia, his or her family members, and caregivers to evaluate the progress and satisfaction with the program. Ask them to suggest changes in the program.
- Address not only communication needs but also the social needs of people with aphasia.
  - In addition to teaching language skills, implement a program in which the social isolation is reduced.
- Address the person's need to get involved in community activities (e.g., volunteering in a hospital, attending and speaking at support groups for people with strokes).
- Facilitate the rejuvenation of premorbid social behaviors (e.g., playing cards with friends or cooking in collaboration with the spouse).
- Help create new social behaviors (e.g., learning to paint with friends, tending a garden, or going to movies and talking about them).
- Treat communication skills not only in the clinic but mostly in natural settings where they are much more authentic and relevant. The traditional approach has emphasized natural training but often in a later stage of treatment.
  - Integrate natural settings from the start of treatment.

- Move treatment out of the clinic sooner and, in some cases, actually begin in the natural setting. For instance, conversational skill training may be started in many natural settings, including the client's home, a restaurant, or a shopping center.

- Target flexible, dynamic, and creative forms of communication, instead of what is *normal* according to linguistic and normative views of language (which tend to be idealized forms of language).

  - Accept communicatively effective productions even if they are linguistically truncated or incorrect. Accept sentences that communicate well even when certain grammatic elements are missing. For instance, when a person with aphasia says, "two cup," there may be little point in the naturalistic context (at the least) to insist on the plural morpheme *s*.

- Target the collaborative nature of communication. Effective communication is rarely achieved by training one person (typically and traditionally, the person with aphasia), because communication is an interdependent social behavior of two or more persons (Kagan et al., 2001; Lyon, 1997; Simmons-Mackie, 2001).

  - Train both the person with aphasia and many who interact with that person to promote natural conversation.

- Train family members, volunteers, health care workers, and any one that can be recruited in the treatment process (Kagan et al., 2001; Rayner & Marshall, 2003). As communication partners, volunteers who do not know the person with aphasia may often be more effective than family members because volunteers do not always think detrimentally how the person was premorbidly. Family members find it difficult to avoid such thoughts (Lyon, 1997).

- Train the conversational partners in strategies that support and enhance the communication skills of people with aphasia. Generally, target conversational skills in treatment sessions (Elman, 2005). Train conversational partners to (1) speak slowly and in simple sentences, (2) pause between topics, (3) introduce new topics, (4) pay attention to signs of failure to comprehend by periodically asking questions, (5) rephrase statements and be redundant when not understood, (6) avoid indirect references and make direct references (e.g., say *Tom* instead of *he*), (7) supplement verbal productions with gestures and facial expressions, (8) use props (e.g., pictures), (9) talk about the objects in the room, pictures on the wall, and (10) repeat key words (Simmons-Mackie, 2001).

- Promote adaptation of the individual with aphasia as well as those who interact with that individual. Aphasia rehabilitation, with the best possible efforts, does not eliminate all negative consequences of stroke and aphasia. Therefore, strategies of adaptation are needed. Often, unfortunately, this adaptation is a target only for the person with a disability. It should not be; those who live with a person with a disability and all those who interact with that person also need to adapt.

  - Let the conversational partners pause and give a chance to a person with aphasia who says "uh uh" before saying the right word, instead of treating this interjection as abnormal (Simmons-Mackie, 2001).

- Use all the strategies offered to train conversational partners as those strategies effectively modify the behavior of people who interact with the person who has aphasia.

Evidence in support of a social approach to treating people with aphasia is being accumulated (see Simmons-Mackie, 2001, for a summary of studies) although much needs to be done. The approach has many attractive features. It is based on sound clinical philosophy of disability and its personal as well as social consequences. Some of the methods of the social approach, however, need to be described in operational terms. The more globally described methods need to be cast in more practical methodological terms so that clinicians can readily and easily use them. Enhanced specificity in treatment procedures within this philosophical framework may be expected to facilitate increased controlled treatment experimentation and thus contribute significantly to a more complete rehabilitation of people with aphasia and their social and family milieu.

Treatment of Reading Problems

Reading skills may be more or less important to a patient with aphasia. Premorbid reading skills and current interest or need to read will dictate the extent of treatment time devoted to reading. Therefore, the first step in designing a reading treatment program is to assess the premorbid level of literacy and the current need for and interest in reading. Interviewing the client and his or her family will help obtain this information.

Functional verbal expression, not reading skills, is the primary target for clients with severe aphasia. Basic and functional reading skills may be useful treatment targets for those who are mildly or moderately aphasic (Brookshire, 2003; Rosenbek et al., 1989). Comprehension of silently read material is a more important treatment target than oral reading.

In designing and implementing a reading treatment program, the clinician should take the following steps:

- Select client-specific reading skills that may include such *survival reading skills* (Rosenbek et al., 1989) as reading letters, menus, checkbooks, bank statements, medicine labels, phone books, calendar, maps, and product labels; let the client and his or her family members suggest useful targets.

- For clients who have intact or clinically reacquired basic reading skills, consider targeting additional reading skills, including reading newspapers, books, and letters, provided the client wishes to learn them.

- Start with comprehension of printed words. Have the client read printed target words aloud on repeated trials; initially, model the words; later, prompt them. Subsequently, ask the client to silently read a word at a time and then state the meaning of the word just read.

- When the client's understanding of target words improves, construct phrases and sentences using the same words, and arrange for repeated practice of phrases and sentences. Initially, let the client read orally with the help of modeling and prompts; later, let the client read silently and answer questions to assess comprehension. Give corrective feedback and positive reinforcement.

- Use such strategies as (a) completing printed sentences that are incomplete by either saying the target word or by selecting the word among given alternatives (e.g., *Before going to the movie, we had dinner at a____*); and (b) matching sentences with pictures.

Note that reading comprehension can be improved only by having the client read more, read progressively more challenging material, and getting appropriate feedback from the clinician.

Please note that controlled data on clearly specified reading treatment techniques are extremely limited. Techniques must be used with caution. Systematic documentation of the effects is necessary to continue, modify, or abandon a technique.

Treatment of Writing Problems

Controlled research on treatment of writing problems in clients with aphasia also is limited. Available data suggest that most clients show improvement in writing with systematic treatment.

As with reading skills, writing skills may be more or less important for a given client. Therefore, the need for writing treatment should be assessed first.

The words, phrases, and kinds of continuous reading material selected for treatment should be useful to the client. Generally, oral expression problems of clients with aphasia are reflected in their writing (e.g., fluent clients write fluently and easily but communicate little through their writing, whereas nonfluent clients write less, write with great effort, but manage to communicate better with their writing).

In designing and implementing a writing treatment program, the following targets and procedures may be considered and individualized for each client:

- Target correct spelling of words and grammatically correct sentences.

- Select such functional writing skills as writing short notes, writing brief letters, signing names, making grocery lists, writing one's address, and filling out forms. Ask the client and the family or other caregivers to help make a list of useful writing skills.

- Ask the client to practice writing selected words and phrases at home; assign additional homework through spelling and writing drill books.

- Design a hierarchy of skills, such as the one Haskins (1976) suggested:
  - Say the sound a letter represents and have the client point to the correct printed letter.
  - Name an alphabet and have the patient point to the correct printed letter.
  - Say a word and have the client point to the correct printed word.
  - Have the client trace printed letters of the alphabet.
  - Have the client copy printed letters.
  - Have the client write letters and then words to dictation.
  - Have the client copy sentences.
  - Have the client write sentences to dictation.
  - Design additional steps as necessary (e.g., have the client write paragraphs, brief notes, lists of grocery items).

Group Treatment for People with Aphasia

Group formats for treating individuals with aphasia started during World War II. Veterans were treated in groups for what was then called aphasia, but was in fact the communication and behavioral consequences of traumatic brain injury. The group format was used fairly regularly until the late 1960s when it gave way to individual treatment when aphasia therapy became an established practice in speech-language pathology. Although there always have been advocates of group treatment, a lack of generalization of individually treated language skills to social settings and the cost-effectiveness of the group format forced several clinicians to rediscover the usefulness of that format in more recent years.

There are multiple group formats with varied objectives and treatment strategies (Avent, 1997; Brookshire, 2003; Elman, 1999; Helm-Estabrooks & Albert, 2004; Kearns & Elman, 2001; Marshall, 1999). Very few programs have been subjected to experimental evaluation for their effectiveness; most are based on clinical experience or case studies. Case studies lack experimental control (treatment is not compared with no treatment). Therefore, they can only claim improvement in skills but not effectiveness for the procedure (Hegde, 2003). Demonstrated improvement within case studies is important, however, because it can justifiably lead to experimental studies. Group treatment case studies that have documented improvement in communication skills of patients with aphasia include those by Aten, Caliguri, and Holland (1982) and Holland and Beeson (1999). A few controlled evaluations that have documented the effectiveness of group treatment include those by Elman and Bernstein-Ellis (1999) and Radonjic and Rakuscek (1991). Elman and Bernstein-Ellis used two groups, offering treatment to one group while the other group served as a control. When the first group's treatment was completed, the second group also received treatment. Improvement in both the groups was associated only with treatment. Therefore, the study did demonstrate the effectiveness of group therapy.

A study by Wertz et al. (1981) compared group treatment with individual treatment with no controls; the study showed that both can result in improvement in communication skills. However, whether either is better than no treatment cannot be ascertained from the results of this study.

Few aphasiologists advocate that group therapy should replace individual therapy. Most believe group therapy may be useful if it follows individual therapy (Davis, 2000; Brookshire, 2003; Helm-Estabrooks, 2004; Kearns & Elman, 2001). Simultaneous use of individual and group formats may also have some advantages, but an exclusive and initial use of the group format may overwhelm some persons with aphasia. More structured individual sessions offer better support in the initial stages of communication rehabilitation than the less structured group sessions.

Speech and language treatment groups may be formed to offer more or less direct treatment to members of the group (Davis, 1992). Groups in which communication skills are trained directly tend to be more structured than those in which the language skills are addressed globally, hence indirectly. Specific language targets may be taught with techniques used in individual therapy, including clinician-prepared stimuli, modeling, cueing, positive reinforcement for correct responses, and corrective feedback for incorrect ones. In teaching communication skills directly, the clinician takes a leading role.

The language skills targeted may include the use of specific language structures (sentence types), word retrieval skills, and description of events and stimuli. In somewhat more advanced sessions, such conversational skills as topic initiation, topic maintenance, narration of personal experiences or objective events, and turn taking may be targeted (Helm-Estabrooks, 2004). The more advanced the language skills targeted in the group format, the more likely such group treatment will follow individual therapy in which the basic skills are honed.

The groups in which speech and language skills are targeted only indirectly tend to be less structured, with the clinician playing the role of a facilitator. Group members may assume leading or relatively active roles in the indirect treatment groups. Both the target skills and the treatment procedures used in indirect treatment groups tend to be less specific. General improvement in communication skills, opportunities to practice skills learned in individual sessions, deriving and offering emotional support, learning from others about living with aphasia, and giving and receiving information may be among the main goals of the group activity.

The distinction between direct and indirect treatment groups may be one of degree. The distinction may be blurred in some cases. Some highly structured groups may target such advanced skills as conversational turn taking, topic maintenance, and narration. Similarly, some loosely structured groups may target specific language targets. Even with a considerable degree of structure in which the clinician takes an active role, more spontaneous conversational speech may be monitored and reinforced.

Intuitively and logically, group therapy should work well for practicing social communication skills learned in individual sessions. Even a small group of four to five individuals may pose an initial challenge to persons with aphasia in maintaining such social communication skills as topic initiation, topic maintenance, turn taking, and conversational repair. Nonetheless, the clinician needs to go beyond the routine clinical setup to strengthen such skills. Obviously, such skills are better practiced in groups than in isolated one-on-one clinical sessions. Therefore, group therapy in which specific skills are carefully monitored and measured may be useful in the maintenance stage of aphasia therapy.

A challenge clinicians face is the measurement of change in the communication skills of people with aphasia who participate in group therapy. The challenge is the greatest when the group structure is loose, the target skills are global or subjective, and the groups are fairly large. Observing all members accurately and recording their actions reliably can pose both methodologic and logistic problems. Although the goals are worthy, measuring the effects of such global and subjective goals as sharing information, offering and receiving emotional support, maintaining good communication, and learning from others about living with aphasia is especially troublesome. Treatment procedures directed toward such goals, too, tend to be somewhat vague. Therefore, research on group therapy should address: (a) the effectiveness of specific and replicable treatment strategies to be used in groups; (b) communication targets for which the group format is superior; (c) operational specification of skills targeted; (d) methods of measurement that will provide objective and verifiable data on the effects of treatment; (e) the relative effects of different kinds of groups themselves; and (f) experimental research that seeks to establish the effectiveness of the varied group formats.

Augmentative and Alternative Communication for Patients with Aphasia

Patients with aphasia may be candidates for augmentative and alternative communication (AAC).

Augmentative communication helps enhance, expand, or augment a person's limited verbal communication skills. **Alternative communication** provides a means of expression for persons who are extremely limited in functional verbal communication. Historically, AAC might have been considered only after attempts at verbal communication training failed in individual cases (Beukelman & Mirenda, 1989; Hux, Manasse, Weiss, & Beukelman, 2001). While AAC should definitely be considered when verbal communication training does not produce the desired effects on functional communication training, clinicians need not always wait to implement AAC until such failures are documented. In fact, functional AAC may be a target for many patients with aphasia in their early stage of assessment and treatment when verbal communication skills are lost to varying degrees; and an AAC might be helpful until verbal skills are recovered either naturally or with treatment.

All people who have aphasia to any significant extent may benefit from AAC, provided they are willing and motivated to use an external aid system. People who have mild aphasia may have less need, but their naming problems may impede full and natural verbal expression. Therefore, they, too, might benefit from an AAC system. A person with mild aphasia but significant naming problems may use a word list to scan and pick the right word; this is an example of augmentative communication (Hux et al., 2001).

When trained to use an AAC device, people with moderate aphasia may benefit to a greater degree than those with mild aphasia as they experience a greater need for it. In people with moderate aphasia, an AAC device may either supplement speech or be the sole mode of communication, depending on the situation and the complexity of the messages (Hux et al., 2001). This points out that *augmentative* and *alternative* strategies are not mutually exclusive; it is more a matter of how a device is used in a given situation by a particular individual than the classification of the device itself. While producing speech to the extent possible, patients with moderate aphasia may use gestures, point to objects or pictures, write the words (if they can still write), or draw a simple line drawing to express basic needs or express other ideas.

People with severe aphasia are, of course, excellent candidates for AAC. These patients may learn, on their own, to gesture, point to things, and write the words. Moreover, with professional training, they may be able to use more sophisticated electronic devices to communicate more extensively and effectively than without such devices. For example, a person with aphasia may use a small handheld computer and type messages that are displayed on a small screen. Another person who cannot type well may learn to display messages already stored in the computer; the person has to point at a graphic icon and click to display a stored message, which may be a word, phrase, single sentence, or group of sentences narrating an experience (Hux et al., 2001). Or, the person may use such nonelectronic (low technology) devices as a communication board on which words, messages, pictures, and symbols are posted. The client may point to words in a certain order to generate sentences that the communication partner "reads." One might also use an organized nonverbal language system, such as American Sign Language.

The patient and the listener roles may be reversed when the person with aphasia has a significant auditory comprehension problem. It is now the listener (a conversational partner) who needs to use an AAC system. Those who interact with a person with aphasia may draw, write, gesture, point to things, point to messages displayed either on a communication board or on electronic screens, type on a handheld computer, or use other electronic devices to communicate.

In selecting an appropriate mode of AAC, the clinician needs to consider the patient's and family members' preference for a particular system. Also to be considered are the literacy level, technical sophistication, manual dexterity (e.g., paralyzed right hand that may limit the use of instruments, typing, or drawing), and motivation to learn to use the left hand for writing and typing.

Various techniques have been described in the literature to help people with aphasia use forms of AAC. Space will not permit a more detailed description of them. The reader is referred to Beukelman, Yorkston, and Reichle (2000), Beukelman and Mirenda (1989), and Hux and colleagues (2001) for details. As pointed out in earlier sections of this chapter, the basic philosophical tenet of aphasia treatment is to help people with aphasia *communicate in any mode possible.* It is not the linguistic competence that aphasia treatment seeks; it seeks effective social communication that has a positive effect on the lives of individuals with aphasia and their families. Any mode of communication that serves this purpose is a useful target.

Suggested Readings

Read the following for additional information on treatment of aphasia:

Basso, A. (2003). *Aphasia and its therapy.* New York: Oxford University Press.

Beukelman, D., & Mirenda, M. (1989). *Augmentative communication: Management of children and adults with severe communication disorders* (2nd ed.). Baltimore, MD: Paul H. Brookes.

Beukelman, D. R., Yorkston, K. M., & Reichle, J. (2000). *Augmentative and alternative communication for adults with acquired neurologic disorders.* Baltimore, MD: Paul H. Brookes.

Brookshire, R. (2003). *An introduction to neurogenic communication disorders* (6th ed.). St. Louis: Mosby Year Book.

Chapey, R. (Ed.). (2001). *Language intervention strategies in adult aphasia and related neurogenic disorders* (4th ed.). Baltimore, MD: Lippincott Williams & Wilkins.

Helm-Estabrooks, N., & Albert, M. L. (2004). *A manual of aphasia therapy* (2nd ed.). Austin, TX: PRO-ED.

Hux, K., Manasse, N., Weiss, A., & Beukelman, D. R. (2001). Augmentative and alternative communication for persons with aphasia. In R. Chapey (Ed.), *Language intervention strategies in adult aphasia and related neurogenic disorders* (4th ed., pp. 675–687). Baltimore, MD: Lippincott Williams & Wilkins.

LaPointe, L. L. (Ed.). (2005). *Aphasia and related neurogenic language disorders* (3rd ed.). New York: Thieme Medical Publishers.

Marshall, R. C. (1999). *Introduction to group treatment for aphasia: Design and management.* Boston: Butterworth-Heinemann.

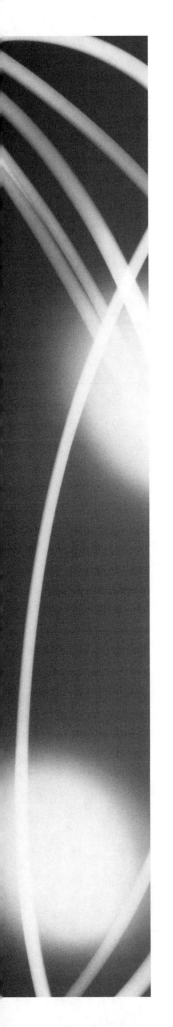

PART II

RIGHT HEMISPHERE
SYNDROME

10 RIGHT HEMISPHERE SYNDROME

Chapter Outline

- Hemispheric Asymmetry

- Right Hemisphere Functions

- Neuropathology of Right Hemisphere Damage

- Behaviors of Patients with Right Hemisphere Damage

- Deficits Associated with Right Versus Left Brain Injury

Learning Objectives

After reading this chapter, the student will:

- Describe the anatomic differences between the right and left hemisphere.

- Summarize and contrast the functions of the left and right hemispheres.

- Describe the neurological and behavioral symptoms of right hemisphere damage.

- Summarize and contrast deficits associated with right versus left brain injury.

Hemispheric Asymmetry

The two hemispheres of the brain are anatomically and functionally asymmetrical. That the right and left hemispheres of the brain tend to specialize in different functions has been well known for many decades. Historically, the left cerebral hemisphere has received much attention from clinical neurologists, speech-language pathologists, and related clinical professionals. Since Broca's investigation of aphasia associated with left hemisphere damage in 1861 and Wernicke's discovery of sensory aphasia in 1874, the research and clinical attention has largely been paid to the left hemisphere. Based on subsequent research on the relationship between brain and language, it is hypothesized that the left hemisphere is better able to handle serial, or sequential, time-related stimuli often presented to the brain by auditory mechanism. Language is thought to require serial processing, because the syllables, words, and sentences are produced serially. Tasks requiring logic and analysis of information have also been thought to be the left hemisphere function.

The two halves of the brain may look roughly the same size, but closer examination reveals structural asymmetry. Brain postmortems and such scanning techniques as magnetic resonance imaging have confirmed structural differences between the hemispheres. For instance, ultrasound scanning has shown that the diameter of the left hemisphere in male and female fetuses is slightly larger than that of their right hemispheres.

Morphological differences are the greatest in certain areas surrounding the lateral sulcus (Fissure of Sylvius). As noted in Chapter 2, the areas surrounding the lateral sulcus are important for language. The lateral sulcus in the left hemisphere is slightly longer than that in the right hemisphere; the left sulcus extends farther posteriorly than the right. One structure in the vicinity of the lateral sulcus that is especially asymmetric in the two hemispheres is the *planum temporale* on the superior surface of the temporal lobe. The planum temporale is a part of the superior surface of the superior temporal gyrus, located posterior to the primary auditory cortex. In a majority of people, the left planum temporale is larger than the right, in some cases more than five times larger. Other morphological differences include a larger *left temporal opercular region,* which is more infolded than the corresponding region in the right hemisphere. This is the region that is also known as Broca's area, the motor speech cortex. In addition, the posterior thalamus region in the left hemisphere is also larger than that in the right hemisphere (Bear, Connors, & Paradiso, 2001).

Initially, it was thought that the hemispheric difference is due to the left hemisphere's specialization in language. However, the left hemisphere is larger in fetuses (Hering-Hanit, Achiron, Lipitz, & Achiron, 2001) and apes as well. Therefore, the hypothesis that language lateralized to an existing structure is more likely to be valid than the hypothesis that language use caused the structure to enlarge. The language lateralization to the left hemisphere may partly be due to genetic factors (Nolte, 2002).

The two hemispheres are well connected. The corpus callosum (see Chapter 2) is a bundle of fibers that connect the two hemispheres. Containing more than 300 million axons, the corpus callosum, also known as *commissural fibers,* is the largest bundle of fibers found in the human brain (Nolte, 2002). Most commissural fibers connect structures that are mirror images in the two hemispheres, although many originate in one area only to connect different (not corresponding) areas.

Right Hemisphere Functions

The workings of the right hemisphere remained largely unknown until the 1950s; it was generally thought of as a silent hemisphere. The right hemisphere was thought to take over the functions of a damaged left hemisphere. During the last few decades, research on the structure and functions of the right hemisphere has increased our understanding of it. A surgical procedure designed to reduce the severity of epilepsy has taught us much about the right and left hemisphere functions. In this procedure known as *commissurotomy,* the corpus callosum is severed because these fibers help spread the sources of epileptic attacks from one hemisphere to the other. This is a last-resort treatment for intractable epilepsy. For the most part, the two hemispheres cannot communicate with each other because of lost connections. Patients who have undergone such surgery have no readily seen problems. They can lead a normal life. Their reaction to most everyday stimuli, motor coordination, and learning remain intact. Nonetheless, they show significant deficits in certain specialized tasks. Sperry (1964) conducted some of the original experiments designed to find deficits due to commissurotomy done in animals. Clinical neurological and behavioral research evidence accumulated since then has shed much light on the functions of the right hemisphere.

In individuals with an intact right hemisphere and normal hemispheric connections, the right brain seems to handle:

- *Arousal, orientation, and attention.* The right hemisphere is mostly responsible for these functions although there is a competing hypothesis that the left hemisphere is dominant. The right-dominant hypothesis has received significant evidential support. In the right-handed individuals, the right hemisphere is dominant for:
  - Arousal, which is a general readiness to respond to external stimuli
  - Orienting, which is directing one's attention to a specific stimulus, event, or location
  - Vigilance, which is sustained attention to detect changes in stimuli
  - Selective attention, which is ignoring some while paying attention to certain specific stimuli
  - Sustained attention, which involves prolonged periods of attention to stimuli or tasks (not necessarily involving changing stimuli as in vigilance)
- *Visual perception.* The right hemisphere is dominant for visual perception, which requires attention and its various components. Specifically, the right hemisphere appears to process:
  - *Holistic, gestalt-like stimuli.* The right brain is especially efficient in grasping the meaning of a total stimulus (e.g., a picture), with little time spent analyzing its component.
  - *Geometric and spatial information.* The right hemisphere seems to be significantly

involved in understanding and recognizing stimuli that include spatially organized shapes and figures. For example, the right brain is adept at recognizing handwriting of a known person.

- *Facial recognition.* The right hemisphere is largely responsible for recognizing familiar faces. Even 4- to 10-month-old infants show a right hemisphere advantage for recognizing their mother's face.

- *Body image.* The right hemisphere is especially proficient in maintaining a proper body image. As we shall see in the next section, people with right brain injury neglect their left side.

- *Emotional experience and expressions.* Generally, the right hemisphere seems to be dominant for emotional experiences. Specifically:

  - The right hemisphere seems to be dominant for expressing angry and happy emotions evoked by environmental stimuli (e.g., pictures of human faces expressing such emotions).

  - The posterior region of the right hemisphere is more active than the left hemisphere when individuals experience emotions.

  - Some controversial evidence indicates that negative emotional experiences (e.g., anger and fear) are lateralized to the right hemisphere (whereas such positive emotional experiences as happiness are lateralized to the left hemisphere).

  - Deaf children who have not had experience with oral language may not show right lateralization for recognition of emotional experience shown in pictures. In such children recognition of emotional expressions may be processed in both hemispheres.

- *Perception of temporal order.* The right hemisphere is dominant for perceiving the temporal order or sequence of events.

- *Perception of musical harmony.* The right hemisphere may be dominant for perception of musical harmony.

- *Certain aspects of communication.* Although language is left lateralized in most people, the right hemisphere is involved in certain aspects of communication. For example:

- To some extent, the right hemisphere may process discourse comprehension and production. There is some evidence that both the hemispheres are involved in discourse comprehension and production.

- Some evidence suggests that the right hemisphere may be less efficient in understanding *verbs* than *nouns.*

- The right hemisphere may help make complex inferences implied in verbal exchanges.

- Communicative efficiency and specificity may be lateralized to the right hemisphere.

- Understanding alternative and ambiguous meanings may require the participation of the right hemisphere.

- Understanding or expressing emotional tone of verbal expressions is largely a right hemisphere function.

- Understanding or expressing prosodic aspects of speech also is largely a right hemisphere activity. The right inferior frontal gyrus participates in the *production* of prosody, and the right posterior temporoparietal region participates in *understanding* prosodic features of speech.

- Understanding contextual information of verbal expression is largely a right hemisphere function.

- Managing pragmatic communication skills may be a right hemisphere activity. Such skills as turn taking, topic maintenance, social appropriateness of communication, and eye contact may be better managed by the right hemisphere than the left.

Studies of individuals who have undergone commissurotomy (split-brain) have revealed some interesting findings about the workings of the right and left hemispheres and their interactions. Such studies also have revealed the nature of interaction between verbal and nonverbal behaviors. Investigators have used a technique in which a visual stimulus is presented to only one eye for a brief duration; the patient's verbal or nonverbal response is then measured. The patient may be asked to perform a task with either the left or right hand (with and without seeing the action being performed) to assess perception or understanding of what is being done. Such studies have shown that right-handed individuals with split brains:

- Can describe numbers, words, and pictures presented only to the right visual field because the information from the right field is processed in the left hemisphere, which has language.
- Cannot describe similar stimuli presented to the left visual field because the right hemisphere that receives the stimuli cannot speak. Nonetheless, the right hemisphere can understand those stimuli if the patient is asked not to describe them but to match them by selecting an appropriate object by touch. For instance, the patient who cannot see the word *ball* presented to the left visual field will select a ball by touching it to match the word. Persons with split brain cannot do this with more complex words or sentences.
- Can create a block design with their left hand, directed by the right hemisphere, but not with their right hand, directed by the left hemisphere.
- Can copy figures using their left hand, which is directed by the right hemisphere, but do poorly with their right hand, directed by the left hemisphere.
- Can verbally describe an object placed in their right hand (which is blocked from their sight). This is because the left hemisphere receives the sensory information and has language to describe it.
- Cannot describe the same object held out of sight in their left hand because the right hemisphere that receives the sensory information from the left hand has no language to describe it. The patients may say there is nothing in their left hand.

Descriptions of right brain functions should be taken with caution. Most studies have shown individual differences that do not conform to generalized statements. Conclusions based on most studies apply only to group performances, not to individual patients who may present unique or unexpected findings. For example, in most people, the left hemisphere may control speaking and writing, but a woman who had commissurotomy could say the words flashed to her left hemisphere, but she could not write them. The same woman could write but not speak the words flashed to her right hemisphere. Individual differences in hemispheric specializations and localization of brain functions limit generality of research findings.

The difference between right brain injury and commissurotomy should be clear as well. Right brain injury in individuals may present a complex clinical picture because such injuries do not exactly resemble surgically induced disconnection between the two hemispheres. Obviously, effects that pathological factors create are different from those of commissurotomy. We will consider such pathological factors before describing the symptoms of right hemisphere injury.

Neuropathology of Right Hemisphere Damage

The same neuropathological factors that affect the left hemisphere also affect the right hemisphere (see Chapter 3 for details). Factors that cause right hemisphere damage (RHD) include:

- *Cerebrovascular accidents.* Ischemic and hemorrhagic strokes are the most common cause of right hemisphere damage.
- *Tumors.* Various kinds of brain tumors in the right hemisphere tend to cause more focal symptoms than the cerebrovascular accidents.
- *Head trauma.* This factor also tends to produce more focal symptoms than cerebrovascular accidents.
- *Various neurological diseases.* For example, Alzheimer's disease also may affect the functioning of the right hemisphere. The clinical picture, however, will be much more complex than what is found in patients with straightforward right hemisphere damage.

Typically, patients who sustain RHD because of posterior lesions do not have motor disabilities (hemiparesis or hemiplegia). On the other hand, those who sustain RHD because of frontal lobe injury do have motor disabilities. Possibly, a disproportionate number of patients with right hemisphere frontal lobe lesions has been included in group studies because these patients tend to be hospitalized longer and therefore are available for research studies.

Behaviors of Patients with Right Hemisphere Damage

As in patients with left hemisphere damage, those with RHD show varying degrees of functional involvement, depending on the site, nature, and extent of damage. With the same site, nature, and extent of damage, individual differences may exist.

The varied symptoms patients with RHD exhibit may be grouped under the following three categories:

- Perceptual and attentional deficits
- Affective (emotional) deficits
- Communication deficits

Perceptual and Attentional Deficits

Several categories of deficits have been described as *perceptual* and *attentional* in nature. Such deficits may cause some of the problems patients exhibit in communication. Perceptual and attentional deficits include left-neglect, visuospatial impairments, and forms of disorientation.

Left-neglect. Generally, **neglect** is reduced sensitivity to stimuli, reduced awareness of space, or absence of previously learned responses to stimuli in certain visual fields. Damage to any lobe in any hemisphere may produce neglect. Therefore, neglect can be right- or left-dominant. Left hemisphere damage can produce right-neglect, but only in 2 to 15 percent of patients. Right parietal lobe damage produces left-neglect in 31 to 90 percent of patients. Left-neglect, also known as *left hemispatial neglect,* tends to be more severe and consistent, almost incredibly so, than right-neglect.

It is thought that the right hemisphere is dominant for spatial attention. Therefore, it can compensate for spatial attentional impairment due to left hemisphere damage. However, when the right hemisphere is damaged, the nondominant left (for spatial attention) cannot compensate for the deficit. Lesions in the right hemisphere's posterior parietal cortex are the most common cause of left-neglect. Less commonly, lesions in the prefrontal cortex of the right hemisphere also may cause left-neglect.

Left-neglect is characterized by greatly reduced responsiveness to stimulation on the left side of the body and impaired awareness of left-sided space. Visual, auditory, and tactile modalities may all be involved in left-neglect, although visual neglect has been the most frequently tested. Patients with visual neglect also may have left visual field blindness, but this form of neglect may be found in patients with an intact visual field. Within a few weeks or months postonset, patients recover from neglect either partially or completely.

With varying degrees of severity across patients, the following characterize left-neglect (Myers, 1999; Tompkins, 1995):

- *A right focus.* There is a strong tendency for the stimuli on the right side to capture and hold the patient's attention.
- *Difficulty shifting attention from right to left.* Patients exhibit a generalized difficulty in shifting attention from the stimuli on the right side to those on the left side.
- *Failure to perceive left-sided tactile or perceptual stimuli.* For example, patients may have difficulty in perceiving touch or pinprick stimuli applied to the left side of the body. When both the left and right side of the body are simultaneously touched (or otherwise stimulated) in a test called *extinction,* the patient may report sensation only on the right side. Some mildly impaired patients can report left tactile stimuli only when the left side is stimulated but not when both the sides are simultaneously stimulated.
- *Failure to copy the left side of a picture or a geometric design.* For example, the patient may copy only the right side of a clock; he or

she may crowd all the numbers into the right half of the circle.

- *Painting only the right half of faces or other images.* For example, in creating a self-portrait, a painter may paint only the right side of his or her own face.

- *Paying extreme right-centered attention in an array of stimuli.* For example, a patient may point to only the objects or pictures found at the extreme right, when several are placed to the *right* of the patient. This implies that what is *right* is relative.

- *Paying attention only to the right side of a space while describing it from memory.* For example, while describing houses on his or her street, the patient may describe only those on the right side of the street. However, depending on whether the patient is imagining going in one or the other direction, he or she is capable of describing houses on either side, suggesting again that *right* is relative to the patient's real or imagined location.

- *Bumping into things or persons on the left side.* A patient in a wheelchair may keep hitting objects on the left side. Patients may not notice objects or structures that trap their left side. For example, a patient may not realize that his or her left shirt sleeve is stuck in a door knob.

- *Using only the right-sided objects.* For example, the patient may use only the right-sided pockets or drawers.

- *Disownership of left body parts or their belongings.* The patient may deny the existence of his or her own left hand or leg or may not recognize the ring or watch worn on the left hand. When the ring and watch are worn on the right hand, or when held by someone else, the patient may recognize them as his or her own.

- *Denying illness (anosagnosia).* The patient may deny the existence of a paralyzed left arm or leg or may say that paralyzed body parts belong to someone else. Some patients who admit to their problems may underestimate the extent or effects of such problems; others may be indifferent to admitted problems or their consequences.

- *Auditory neglect.* Although less common than visual neglect, some patients may neglect sound from the left side. For example, they may not answer a telephone ringing on the left side or may not respond to people talking on their left side. In addition, posterior lesions can cause sound localization problems independent of auditory neglect.

- *Motor neglect.* The patient behaves as though the left side is paralyzed, although in fact it is neurophysiologically normal. The patient's left leg or arm may drag while the patient moves, or he or she may fail to withdraw the left limb from painful stimuli. The patient may lose balance because of poor posture caused by left motor neglect. Movements of the left limb may be slow, sluggish, and weak.

- *Left-neglect in reading.* The patient may read aloud only the right portion of the text. While reading only the right half of each line, the patient may complain that what is read is meaningless. The patient also may omit the left-most letters in words (e.g., read *pastime* as *time*).

- *Left-neglect in writing.* Failure to give the left margin in writing is a common symptom. Other writing errors include inconsistent left margin, extra space between letters, split words, and letter repetitions or omissions. Frontal lesions tend to cause letter repetitions, and postrolandic lesions tend to cause left margin and other spatial errors in writing.

Facial recognition deficits. Also known as *prosopagnosia,* facial recognition deficits are a part of the perceptual and attentional deficits evident in some patients with RHD. These deficits are seen in patients with posterior right hemisphere damage. Bilateral damage may produce more persistent deficits.

Prosopagnosia involves:

- *Difficulty recognizing familiar faces.* This is most apparent when the patient is shown line drawings or photographs of familiar faces, but the difficulty may extend to pictures or actual faces of familiar animals, distinguishing faces of older and younger persons and male and female individuals. The difficulty may be limited to faces only. Patients with

RHD usually can recognize a face as soon as the person speaks, moves, and does something. Such physical characteristics as body size, hair color and style, and gait also may prompt correct facial recognition.

- *Difficulty choosing pictures of faces just shown.* Patients may find it difficult to choose the picture of a face they were just shown from a collection of pictured faces that includes those not shown.

- *Problems naming the pictures of faces of famous persons.* The patients may find it difficult to name pictures of persons they normally would know.

A rare and an extreme consequence of prosopagnosia is known as *Capgras syndrome.* Patients who have this syndrome entertain a delusional belief that their friends and family members are not their real selves but imposters or doubles.

Constructional impairment. Parietal or parietooccipital damage is most often associated with **constructional impairment,** a form of visuospatial (perceptual) impairment characterized by:

- *Problems constructing block designs.* Patients may find it difficult to construct block designs by looking at printed designs.

- *Difficulty reproducing two-dimensional stick figures.* Patients are likely to find it difficult to construct a copy of shown models.

- *Errors in drawing or copying geometric shapes.* The patient may make numerous errors in drawing or copying actual or printed geometric shapes.

Constructional impairment often is seen in patients with all kinds of brain damage, although it is most prominent in patients with RHD. Generally, the kinds of constructional errors the patients with left hemisphere damage make can be distinguished from those made by the patients with RHD.

The patients with left hemisphere involvement draw with difficulty but make fewer mistakes; their drawings bear greater resemblance to models; their drawings are better with models than without.

On the other hand, patients with RHD draw hastily, make many mistakes, add unnecessary lines to correct mistakes, turn three-dimensional figures into two-dimensional, and do not show improvement when provided with models.

Attentional deficits. Injury to the right or the left hemisphere tends to impair attention. Patients with RHD are likely to show various forms of attentional deficits that create problems in communication as well. The specific problems include:

- *Reduced state of arousal.* As noted, arousal is physiological and behavioral readiness to respond to stimuli. Patients with RHD are described as hypoaroused: reduced arousal reduces attention to stimuli.

- *Difficulty in sustaining attention.* The patient's attention may wander from task to task or from stimulus to stimulus. This can pose problems in treatment, with the patient unable to maintain attention on treatment activities.

- *Difficulty in paying selective attention.* The patient may find it difficult to pay attention to a particular stimulus embedded in an array of stimuli. Because of this problem, patients with RHD are easily distracted by unimportant or irrelevant stimuli.

Because of these attentional deficits, patients with RHD find it difficult to respond promptly, sustain their conversation, sustain conversational topics, and maintain attention to a speaker's messages. Their speech may be incoherent at times because of their lack of attention to what others say.

Disorientation. Patients with RHD may show a variety of problems involving orientation. Their orientation problems may be due to impaired visual attention to environmental cues. Some of the specific problems of orientation include:

- *Topographic disorientation.* Also known as *topographic impairment,* topographic disorientation is confusion about space. Patients have difficulty finding their way in familiar surroundings (e.g., one's own room in a house), understanding maps, and giving directions.

- *Geographic disorientation.* This is patients' confusion about their geographic location.

Few patients show this form of disorientation, but those who do may believe that their hospital or house is located in a state or country different from the actual location.

- *Reduplicative paramnesia.* Also a rare condition, it involves a belief in the existence of multiple and identical persons, places, and body parts. Brookshire's (2003) examples include a patient who believed in the existence of two identical hospitals in the same city; another believed he had two left legs, and another woman thought she had two identical husbands at home.

Patients with RHD who show disorientation of the kind specified can be distinguished from other patients (e.g., those with dementia) who also are disoriented. Patients with RHD may not be disoriented to time, space, and persons in general; they are confused about themselves, as patients with dementia may be. Patients with RHD who are lost in their familiar surrounding can usually find their way back. Patients with dementia who are disoriented and confused usually cannot accomplish this.

Visuoperceptual deficits. Patients with RHD may have visuoperceptual deficits that are typically limited to:

- Difficulty recognizing line-drawn pictures or incomplete drawings
- Drawings that distort the representation by showing unusual size, dimension, or orientation
- Drawings that are superimposed on other drawings

It should be noted that patients with RHD do not have difficulty recognizing real objects or objects depicted fully and naturally.

Affective Deficits

While emotions are felt internal bodily states, affects are behavioral expressions of those emotional states or experiences. Normally, the limbic system mediates most biological functions, including emotions, affect, thirst, hunger, and sexual arousal. A system of marginal ("limbic") structures of the frontal, parietal, and temporal lobes, the limbic system is a horseshoe-shaped structure that forms a circle over the brainstem. A major portion of the limbic system, called the *cingulated gyrus,* sits on top of the corpus callosum, mostly encircling it. The medial surface of the temporal lobe, including the hippocampus, also is a part of the limbic system. Paul Broca, who discovered it, called it the *limbic lobe* and thought it was responsible for olfaction (smell), a view not currently held.

Although the limbic system is responsible for the actual experience of emotions, the right hemisphere is largely responsible for mediating the *expression* of emotions and *appreciation* of emotions other people express. Electroencephalographic (EEG) studies have shown increased right hemisphere activity when patients experience strong emotions or recall emotionally charged experiences. When experiencing failure to complete difficult and stressful tasks, patients with left hemisphere damage tend to react emotionally (known as *catastrophic reaction* and includes crying and cursing). In a similar situation, patients with RHD tend to be emotionally indifferent. Unless the limbic system also is involved, the patient with RHD can *experience* emotions normally but may have *difficulty expressing* them.

Patients with right hemisphere damage may exhibit:

- *Difficulty understanding emotions.* The patients may not understand emotions other people express through their facial expressions. The data are mostly based on patients' judgment of static pictures that depict emotional expressions, however.

- *Difficulty stating the emotions depicted in pictured story scenes.* Patients may miss emotional expressions shown in pictures that tell stories.

- *Problem recognizing emotions expressed in isolated spoken sentences.* This finding is controversial, as it is observed only in some patients.

- *Problems understanding emotional tone of voice.* Patients may find it difficult to appreciate emotions speakers express through such cues as tone of voice and prosody of spoken speech (more about this in the next section).

- *Difficulty in emotional expressions.* Patients may have problems in expressing their own emotions correctly.

Communication Deficits

Communicative problems are found in about 50 percent of individuals who have right hemisphere damage. Communicative problems are more common in individuals who are left-handed and then sustain right cortical injury, presumably because of the right hemisphere dominance for language in these individuals. However, not all left-handed individuals who sustain right hemisphere damage exhibit predominant language problems. This is because the left hemisphere is still dominant for language in many left-handed individuals.

Communicative deficits associated with RHD are unlike those associated with left hemisphere damage. Also, it is important to note that certain language skills are relatively preserved in patients with RHD. Generally, patients with RHD do not experience word-finding problems. The patients can define words or name objects described to them. If there is any difficulty in individual cases, it is likely to be mild and more pronounced in naming categories or collective nouns (e.g., the patient may name such individual elements of a category as *roses, petunias,* and *marigolds,* but may not readily name *flowers*).

Consequently, paraphasias and circumlocution due to word-finding problems are also not significant in patients with RHD. Any circumlocution they may exhibit is due to their attentional and cognitive problems that make it difficult for them to be precise and direct in their communication. On the other hand, the patients with LHD do not have such attentional and cognitive problems; their circumlocution is due to word-finding problems. For these and other reasons, patients with RHD are not described as aphasic.

For the most part, patients with RHD speak in grammatically accurate sentences. They may have difficulty with abstract or metaphoric meaning but not literal meaning of language they hear. Although the right hemisphere may be involved in processing single words and sentences (Meyers, 1999), most patients with RHD understand the main meaning of single words spoken to them. On tests of aphasia, patients with RHD exhibit normal comprehension of sentences, especially of simple sentences. The patients' attentional deficits may account for any difficulty they show in understanding complex sentences.

A summary of the most notable communicative deficits of patients with RHD follows.

Prosodic deficits. *Prosody* of speech refers to the stress patterns, intonation, rhythm, and melodious qualities of speech that convey meaning. Prosodic features sometimes convey meanings not conveyed by the words and phrases; sometimes such features may convey the opposite of what the words mean. For example, "Sure, you are invited to my party" may be said with such prosodic features to mean *please stay away.* Speech with adequate prosodic features is variable in intensity, pitch, stress, vocal quality, and duration of syllables. When prosodic features are diminished, the speech may sound monotonous and fail to provoke interest. Lacking in variation, speech with limited prosody fails to convey subtle but important extralinguistic meanings, connotations, and emotional tone of experiences being expressed.

The right hemisphere damage may impair both production of normal prosodic features and comprehension of meanings others express through prosodic variations. Although the speech of depressed people shows reduced prosodic features, prosodic deficit of patients with RHD is not due to depression. Similarly, although patients with dysarthria (motor speech disorder) may show prosodic deficits, such deficits in patients with RHD may not be due to motor disturbances. Finally, prosodic deficits of patients with RHD are not attributable to a language disorder as the patients generally have intact language skills. Although such terms as *aprosodia, auditory affective agnosia,* and *dysprosodia* have been suggested to describe the prosodic problems of patients with RHD, the terms *prosodic deficits* or *prosodic impairments* are better suited to describe such problems (Myers, 1999).

Prosodic deficits may be severe in a few cases but are mild in most. The speech of the patients with RHD may be:

- *Monotonous.* The speech may lack prosodic variations; the speech may fail to indicate different kinds of sentences by intonational variations (e.g., patients may fail to show a rising intonation to suggest a yes/no question). A limited fundamental frequency of voice is a part of this monotonous speech.

- *Impaired in stress patterns.* Instead of changing pitch to stress words, the patients may change amplitude (loudness).

- *Reduced in rate.* A slow rate may also contribute to the monotonous quality of speech.

- *Devoid of emotions.* The speech may fail to convey emotional tones and meanings.

- *Impaired in prosodic comprehension.* The patients may have marked difficulty understanding the emotional tone of speech they hear.

Patients with RHD may be aware of their prosodic deficits (Brookshire, 2003). Some patients, surmising that their emotional tone is not clear to the listener, may then resort to direct verbal expression of their emotion (e.g., a patient might say, "If it is not clear to you, I am very angry").

Impaired discourse. *Discourse* is a set of social communication skills. Discourse may involve description of events (narration), objects, and performance (procedures); it also may involve extended talk on a given topic (expository discourse). Finally, discourse involves conversation between two or more participants.

Many patients with RHD have their discourse skills impaired to a greater extent than those with LHD. Such an impairment may be the most significant aspect of communicative deficits of patients with RHD (Myers, 1999). They have difficulty narrating events, pictures, or personal experiences in a coherent, well-organized, and precise manner. This skill often is tested through description of story pictures. Such descriptions tend to show:

- Problems in distinguishing significant from irrelevant information; the patient tends to focus on irrelevant, tangential, or inconsequential aspects of pictures shown. In conversational speech, too, the patient tends to focus on irrelevant elements or tangential topics.

- Difficulty understanding implied meanings, abstract words, metaphors, irony, and humor expressed in conversational speech (please see the next section).

- Premature and incorrect inferences made during discourse; because of such inferences, the patient may give incorrect or puzzling responses during conversation.

- Confabulation and excessive speech; by inferring too much from stimulus events and by paying too much attention to irrelevant details, many patients say too much that borders on confabulation. Even though they say too much, they produce less meaningful speech because of their rambling; occasionally, the speech may be inappropriate as well.

- Unelaborated narratives; a few patients may give excessively restricted and limited description of pictures or events.

It should be noted that many patients who show difficulty understanding abstract meanings or humor or in interpreting stimuli in test situations may behave appropriately or nearly appropriately in actual situations that provide more contextual information. This suggests that natural observations of patients' skills are more valid than standardized linguistic tests.

Semantic problems. The left hemisphere seems to be active in promptly and quickly understanding concrete meaning of words. On the other hand, the right hemisphere may be involved in understanding or producing words with complex, abstract, metaphoric, and multiple meanings. While the left hemisphere seems to react more quickly in understanding direct and concrete meaning of words, the right hemisphere may react more slowly in understanding alternate, abstract, metaphoric, or multiple meanings of words (Myers, 1999). For instance, normally the left hemisphere may quickly grasp the concrete meaning of the phrase *open book,* while the right hemisphere may take a bit more time to grasp its metaphoric, abstract, or alternative meanings (e.g., something transparent).

Patients with RHD tend to exhibit the following kinds of semantic problems:

- Difficulty understanding implied, alternative, or abstract meanings. Patients with

RHD have difficulty going beyond the literal meaning of situations or verbal expressions to deduce the abstract, alternative, or implied meanings of utterances.

- Failure to grasp the overall meaning of situations, events, stories, or story pictures. They may miss the central message of a communication or the theme of a story. Their description of story pictures may include naming individual elements with no understanding of the inherent theme or story, showing lack of integration of individual elements.

- Failure to understand the meaning of proverbs, idioms, and metaphors. The patients may impose literal interpretations on such complex and abstract expressions.

- Problems in naming abstract categories in contrast to the names of individual items within categories. For example, patients may name individual items in a category (e.g., *carrots, beans, spinach*) but may not name the category (*vegetables*).

- Difficulty understanding irony, humor, and sarcasm. The patients may not understand such relatively abstract expressions.

- Problems in understanding logical errors in sentences. Detection of logical errors also requires abstract reasoning, which may be difficult for patients with RHD.

It must be noted that patients with RHD may perform better in understanding multiple or alternative meanings in real-life contexts than in clinical assessment situations. Larger and real contexts of communication may help them deduce such meanings.

Pragmatic deficits. Many, but not all, patients with RHD tend to show pragmatic language problems. Some of the more commonly observed pragmatic deficits include:

- *Difficulty in conversational turn taking.* The patients' tendency to ramble and to get distracted may make them especially vulnerable to this problem. Those who do exhibit this problem may fail to yield to their conversational partners.

- *Difficulty in topic maintenance.* The patients' attentional deficits may be responsible for frequent and irrelevant topic changes during conversations.

- *Difficulty in maintaining eye contact.* While talking excessively or rambling, the patients with RHD may fail to maintain eye contact with their conversational partners.

- *Insensitivity to communicative contexts.* The patients may assume too much about what their listeners know about the topic of conversation (e.g., patients may talk about their friends or colleagues as though the clinician knows them). The patients also may introduce new topics when their partners indicate a closure to discourse.

Significant individual differences in pragmatic skills of patients with RHD have been noted. Some may have essentially normal skills while others have severe impairments. Therefore, careful assessment of intact and impaired skills is necessary to design client-specific management programs for patients with RHD. Assessment and management procedures and issues are addressed in Chapter 11.

Deficits Associated with Right Versus Left Brain Injury

A brief comparison of patterns of deficit found in patients with RHD versus those with LHD will help understand the unique characteristics of patients in these two groups. The major similarities and differences include the following:

- The patients with LHD and RHD are similar in the sense that they all have communicative deficits that are a result of neural pathology. But the site of that pathology produces distinct patterns of deficits.

- LHD generally produces a more focal pattern of deficits than RHD. RHD produces a more diffuse pattern of deficits.

- The more diffuse deficits patterns of RHD are less concrete and more abstract than the focal and more concrete deficits of LHD. Consequently, the deficits of RHD are somewhat harder to quantify than those of LHD. For instance, patients with LHD have such specific and relatively easily quantifiable communication deficits as naming problems and grammatical deficiencies. In contrast, patients with RHD have such abstract and somewhat more complex deficits as difficulty understanding or conveying emotional tone of verbal expressions, difficulty understanding metaphoric use of language, and social appropriateness of communication.

- The communication deficits of patients with RHD may be partly be due to other deficits, whereas those of LHD may be a more direct result of their brain injury. For instance, the naming and grammatical difficulties of patients with LHD are a more direct result of the specific lesions whereas some of the communication problems of patients with RHD may be due to their attentional deficits.

- The communication deficits of patients with RHD are further complicated by their denial of illness, indifference to their impairments, confabulation, left-neglect, impulsive behavior, reduced attention and increased distractibility, and deficits in reasoning skills. The communication deficits of patients with LHD are not so complicated with related behavioral deficits. Furthermore, patients with LHD may be generally less motivated for therapy than those with RHD.

The major differences between these two sets of patients have important assessment and treatment considerations to be described in the next chapter.

Suggested Readings

Read the following for additional information on right hemisphere syndrome:

Myers, P. S. (1999). *Right hemisphere damage.* Albany, NY: Thomson Learning.

Tompkins, C. A. (1995). *Right hemisphere communication disorders: Theory and practice.* Clifton Park, NY: Thomson Delmar Learning.

11

ASSESSMENT AND TREATMENT OF RIGHT HEMISPHERE SYNDROME

Chapter Outline

- Assessment of Patients with Right Hemisphere Damage
- Treatment of Patients with Right Hemisphere Damage

Learning Objectives

After reading this chapter, the student will:

- Describe the bedside screening of clients with right hemisphere syndrome.

- Give an overview of standardized assessment tools for clients with right hemisphere syndrome.

- Describe procedures to assess visual neglect and visuospatial skills.

- Describe and evaluate procedures designed to treat the various deficits in clients with right hemisphere syndrome.

Assessment of Patients with Right Hemisphere Damage

Assessment of patients with right hemisphere damage (RHD) requires an analysis of affective, attentional, perceptual, and communicative behaviors. Rehabilitation of patients with RHD has received attention only in recent years. Therefore, research on assessment and treatment of such patients is limited.

The standard aspects of assessment apply, including case history, hearing screening, interview of the patient and family members, orofacial examination, language sampling, and administration of standardized and client-specific procedures.

The case history should concentrate on the circumstances of hospitalization. More often a stroke and in some cases traumatic brain injury or such neuropathology as a brain tumor may bring the patient to the hospital. Information on the premorbid intellectual and communicative skills of the patient will be helpful in assessing the current deficits. In many cases, this information may have to be obtained in subsequent contacts with family members.

A few special considerations are important in assessing patients with RHD. For instance, denial of illness may make it difficult to assess some of the problems strictly through client reports. Nonetheless, asking the patient to describe his or her problem may be helpful in assessing insight (the patient's awareness of his or her problems). Interview of family members and other caregivers will provide additional information that may reveal specific deficits the patient is not aware of or is unwilling to admit to the clinician in initial sessions.

Some family members may not appreciate the subtle communicative problems of the person with RHD, while others may be keenly aware of them. Therefore, to get a more complete view of the deficits, it may be necessary to interview multiple members of the patient's family.

Family members may think the patient is confused. The patient's lack of facial recognition and neglect may prompt this idea. Giving family members brief background information on RHD might be helpful. Interviews of the family members should include questions about the patient's orientation, memory, and attention.

Initial Screening of Patients

An initial screening of major deficits of patients with RHD will help plan a detailed assessment. The clinician may first see patients with RHD soon after hospitalization. Such patients are not ready for the demanding and time-consuming assessment ordeal. Therefore, the initial screening may be done at the bedside to identify major deficits that need to be assessed further. Family members may have been interviewed prior to screening or may be interviewed soon thereafter.

As a part of the screening, the patient is interviewed. The clinician will ask why the patient thinks he or she is in the hospital and ask the patient to describe the events leading to hospitalization. The clinician will also ask the patient about his or her family, work, hobby, daily activities, personal problems the patient experiences, and so forth. It may be noted that patients with RHD may often ramble when asked such simple questions as "Why are you in the hospital?" While most patients may give a direct answer (e.g., "I think had a stroke" or "I fell down and hurt myself"), the patient with RHD may begin to describe irrelevant events or trivial problems (Myers, 1999).

An extended interview, conducted with short breaks if necessary, will help gain an initial impression of the patient's communicative and cognitive deficits that need to be assessed further. The clinician may find that the patient not only rambles but does not maintain eye contact, does not stay on a topic of conversation, does not use gestures appropriately, speaks in an emotionally flat tone, and shows signs of left neglect.

As a part of screening, the clinician should sample the patient's *narrative skills.* Clinicians have found the "Cookie Theft Picture," which is a part of the Boston Diagnostic Aphasia Examination (see Chapter 8), helpful in evoking narrative descriptions that may reveal various kinds of discourse problems (Myers, 1999). Asked to "tell what is happening in the picture," the patient may give descriptions that are incomplete, inaccurate, or both. The patient may fail to make correct inferences about the events that led to the current scene and the events that are likely to follow.

Screening the patient for *neglect* is an important task. Neglect may be initially screened with a few simple tests. For instance, brief tests of *cancellation* may be useful in screening neglect. Most paper-and-pencil cancellation tests contain a page on which short lines, small squares, or a combination of two kinds of stimuli (e.g., flowers and snowflakes) are drawn. The patient is asked to cross out or draw a line through all stimuli or a specific kind of stimuli (e.g., only the flowers that are mixed with snowflakes). On most such tests, patients may fail to cancel out the targets on their left side.

Other tests of neglect include copying line drawings, freehand drawing, and line bisection. When patients are asked to copy simple line drawings shown to them, they may fail to copy parts of the picture displayed to their left. They may make similar mistakes when asked to draw freehand. The patient's drawing of a flower or a man may have missing parts to the left. Line bisection involves making a mark in the middle of a printed line that is at least 20 cm long. The patients with RHD tend to make the mark more toward their right, thus missing the midline because of left-neglect. Details of such tasks and descriptions of specific standardized tests of neglect are given in the next section.

Ethnocultural Considerations in Assessment

There is little or no research on ethnocultural issues in the assessment of patients with RHD. However, the issues are similar to those raised in the assessment of aphasia. Therefore, suggestions offered in the assessment of aphasia in ethnoculturally diverse clients are applicable to patients with RHD. See Chapter 8 for details.

Standardized and Nonstandardized Assessment Tools

Although there are many standardized tests for aphasia, only a few are available to assess patients with RHD. These few standardized and nonstandardized assessment tools help evaluate the varied symptoms of patients with RHD. Some assessment protocols contain more items to evaluate communication than other kinds of skills; similarly, other protocols contain more items to test nonlinguistic skills than linguistic skills.

The Mini Inventory of Right Brain Injury (Pimental & Kingsbury, 1989) is a standardized test that evaluates 10 categories of skills: visual scanning, integrity of gnosis (finger identification, tactile perception, two-point tactile discrimination), integrity of body image, reading and writing, serial 7s (e.g., subtracting 7 from 100 and subtracting 7 from the remainder), drawing, affective language, abstract language (e.g., absurdities, similarities), affect and general behavior, and appreciation of humor. The test was originally developed to distinguish right hemisphere damage from left hemisphere damage. The test was standardized on 30 patients with RHD, 13 patients with left hemisphere injury, and 30 with no brain injury. Because each skill is sampled only with a few items, it is probably best used as a screening device.

The Right Hemisphere Language Battery (2nd ed.) (Bryan, 1995) is a standardized test that helps assess such skills as: comprehension of spoken and printed metaphors, comprehension of inferred meanings, appreciation of humor, discourse analysis (including such pragmatic skills as turn taking, formality of language and behavior, greetings, complaining, demanding, and criticizing), and matching spoken words with printed words (lexical semantic recognition), and emphatic stress production (prosody). This test was standardized on 30 persons with no brain injury, 40 with RHD, and 40 with LHD (aphasia). The test's reliability and validity measures have been questioned, however (Tompkins, 1995).

Standardization of *The Burns Brief Inventory of Communication and Cognition* (Burns, 1997) included only the patients with RHD. The test includes tasks to evaluate scanning and tracking (e.g., single word tracking), visuospatial skills (e.g., recognition of familiar faces, visuospatial construction, and spatial distribution of attention), expressive and receptive prosody, inferences, and metaphoric use of language. The test allows a comparison of RHD patients' performance with that of LHD patients and patients with other neuropathological conditions.

A comprehensive and standardized evaluative tool is the *Rehabilitation Institute of Chicago Clinical Management of Right Hemisphere Dysfunction*

(Halper, Cherney, & Burns, 1996). In addition to allowing for an evaluation of the typical skills of interest (e.g., visual scanning and tracking, awareness of illness, attention, orientation, facial expression, intonation, storytelling task, written expression, and pragmatic language skills), the protocol includes an interview schedule to be used with the patient and observation of the patient as he or she interacts with family and caregivers. Pragmatic language skills assessed in the test include nonverbal communication (e.g., intonation, eye contact, facial expression, topic maintenance, and narrative skills). The test was standardized on 40 patients with RHD and 36 persons with no brain injury.

A nonstandardized assessment protocol is that of Gordon and associates (1984). This protocol provides a framework for assessing most skills of interest, including visual scanning and inattention (including neglect), activities of daily living (including arithmetic, reading, and copying), sensorimotor integration (including tactile perception, estimation of body midline, and manual dexterity), visual integration (including facial recognition and copying geometric forms), linguistic and cognitive flexibility (including analogies, auditory comprehension, and generative naming), higher cognitive performance (as evaluated by verbal and performance subtests of the Wechsler Adult Intelligence Scale), and affective state (including comprehension of affect and examiner's rating of mood). The authors provide extensive information on the performance of 385 patients with RHD.

Other Means of Evaluating Aspects of Communication Deficits

Several other measures may be useful in evaluating communicative deficits—especially the pragmatic deficits—of patients with RHD. For instance, the *Pragmatic Protocol* (Prutting & Kircher, 1987) helps assess a variety of pragmatic language skills, including turn taking, topic maintenance, vocal intensity and quality, prosody, fluency, posture, and eye contact.

Some tests that were intended to assess communication deficits in patients with aphasia also may be used with patients who have right hemisphere injury. For instance, the *Communicative Effectiveness*

Index (Lomas & Associates, 1989) and the *Communication Activities in Daily Living* (Holland, Frattali, & Fromm, 1998) were designed to helps assess functional communication skills in patients with aphasia. Both tests may be useful in assessing functional communication skills in patients with RHD. Similarly, the *Discourse Abilities Profile* (Terrell & Ripich, 1989) is a test that is primarily concerned with discourse skills of patients with aphasia, but it may be useful in evaluating such skills in patients with RHD.

Myers (1999) provides an informal protocol to assess prosodic performance of patients with RHD. Her protocol includes such skills as *comprehension* of the emotional tone of spoken sentences (e.g., happy or sad); identifying emphatic stress in spoken words, phrases, and sentences; and distinguishing spoken interrogative versus declarative sentences. The protocol also includes *production* of emotional sentences, emphatic stress in sentences, and the use of prosody to indicate differences in intonation.

Tests of Visual Neglect and Visuospatial Skills

As noted previously, several measures are available for visual neglect. It is usually necessary to give more than one test because only multiple measures can correctly identify neglect in most patients.

The Test of Visual Neglect (Albert, 1973) is a paper-and-pencil test. It contains a printed page on which short lines are printed randomly. The patient is asked to cross out the lines. Patients with RHD tend to cross out lines only on the right side of the page.

The Bells Test (Gauthier, Dehaut, & Joanette, 1989) requires selective attention because it contains both target and nontarget drawings. The printed page contains the drawings of bells and other objects scattered across a page. The patient is asked to circle only the bells. The patient may neglect to cross out the bells on the left side.

The Behavioral Inattention Test (Wilson, Cockburn, & Halligan, 1987) is a battery of standardized tests for assessing neglect. The test includes such paper-and-pencil tests as cancellation task, figure and shape copying, line bisection, representational drawing, picture scanning, and card sorting. In addition, the battery also includes techniques to assess neglect in such functional tasks as reading maps, menus, and newspapers; using a telephone; and sorting coins. Therefore, the test is especially useful in assessing neglect in daily functional activities.

The Test of Visual Field Attention (CoolSpring Software, n.d.) allows for computer presentation of and scoring of stimuli. Visual stimuli randomly appear in one of four quadrants on the computer monitor. The patient is asked to press the mouse button in response to target stimuli. Errors and reaction time for each quadrant are calculated to assess left-neglect.

Clinicians may generate various *copying and drawing stimuli* to assess neglect. Stimuli selected for drawing should be symmetrical, with the same kind of elements to be drawn on the left and the right side of the picture midline. Drawings of human or animal faces, clocks, and flowers have frequently been used. The patient may be asked to draw objects or scenes from memory. The patient with left-neglect will omit details on the left side of the copied or drawn picture.

Scanning tests allow the clinician to assess neglect by asking patients to cross out or circle a target item (e.g., the letter T or the number 7) in an array of letters or numbers printed horizontally.

Visuospatial or visual organization skills are often a target of assessment in patients with RHD. Most assessment tools include such tasks as naming an incompletely drawn picture (e.g., a human face drawn in dotted lines) or naming a picture that shows parts of a larger picture separated and randomly arranged (e.g., pictures of parts of the human body).

Treatment of Patients with Right Hemisphere Damage

Compared to treatment of aphasia, treatment of patients with RHD is new. Treatment efficacy studies involving patients with RHD are extremely limited. Consequently, the advocated techniques are based largely on clinical experience, untested theories, expert opinion, or positive outcomes in treating such other disorders as aphasia. Although there are strong recommendations about treatment targets or strategies, controlled experimental research to support such recommendations is lacking.

There is disagreement about treatment targets themselves. Some clinicians prefer to design treatments for specific skills (e.g., eye contact or conversational turn taking) while others prefer to address the hypothesized underlying processes (e.g., attention) of observed behavioral deficits. Myers (1997) describes treating specific skills as *task-oriented therapy* and treating underlying processes as *process-oriented therapy*. Process-oriented therapy is mostly theory-driven; theories themselves are mostly a collection of untested hypotheses. Furthermore, there is no convincing controlled experimental evidence to show that treating underlying processes is more effective or results in more generalized learning of related skills than direct skill training. Until evidence shows that process training is better than direct skill training, the latter is both clinically practical and theoretically parsimonious.

Ethnocultural Considerations in Treatment

There is little or no empirical data on treating ethnoculturally varied clients who have RHD. In the absence of specific data, the clinician can follow general guidelines considered appropriate for treating communicative disorders in ethnoculturally varied clients. Only with caution can treatment procedures that have not been applied to a particular ethnocultural group be used to treat a member of that group. Careful documentation of improvement or its absence will help assess its usefulness to other patients belonging to that group. Such documentation also will help design experimental studies on treatment effectiveness.

Guidelines on treating ethnoculturally varied patients with aphasia are applicable to those with RHD. Please see Chapter 8 for details.

Treatment Targets and Strategies

Major treatment targets for patients with RHD include (a) denial and indifference, (b) impaired attention, (c) visual neglect, (d) impulsive behavior, (e) pragmatic language skills, (f) impaired recognition of absurdities, and (g) impaired comprehension of metaphors and proverbs. Our treatment description will emphasize communication deficits that include prosodic, pragmatic, affective, and discourse aspects. Other skills addressed in this section are those that directly affect communication.

Denial and Indifference

Most clinicians believe that denial of illness and indifference to one's own deficits are the most difficult problems to treat. Also, the patient who denies disabilities is least motivated to work during treatment sessions, complete home treatment assignments, and accept suggestions or help from family members. Even those who participate in treatment sessions without much complaint may do so only halfheartedly and offer confabulated reasons for their failure to cooperate fully (Brookshire, 2003). In some cases, treatment may be delayed until a time when the severity of denial and indifference is reduced (Tompkins, 1995). Improved neurologic status usually results in improved insight into one's own health and behavioral status. Such patients are then likely to meet the demands of treatment.

Increasing a patient's awareness of his or her problems may be the key to reducing denial and indifference. Behavioral awareness is typically a function of response-contingent feedback. Therefore, to increase such awareness, the clinician should give immediate, systematic, and response-contingent corrective feedback on errors the patient makes. Speech-language pathologists should give such feedback during all communication treatment activities. Brookshire (2003) recommends videotaping treatment sessions in which the patient shows little or no appreciation of errors and reviewing tapes with the patient to give response-contingent feedback. Other professionals who work or regularly interact with the patient should be trained to give response-contingent corrective feedback on errors or deficient behaviors.

Positive reinforcement for appropriate behaviors—equally systematic and response-contingent—should accompany corrective feedback on the patient's errors and deficient behaviors. Appropriate behaviors may include acceptance of feedback on errors, verbal statements that acknowledge one's own errors, willingness to imitate a modeled correct response, self-correction of errors, and seeking help to perform better. All such behaviors should be promptly acknowledged with verbal praise and requested help.

To encourage self-correction that follows an awareness of one's own errors, the clinician should teach self-monitoring skills. As the clinician gives feedback on errors, the patient may be asked to chart or simply count his or her errors. An error the patient misses may be pointed out to improve self-monitoring skills.

Brookshire (2003) cautions that unless a carefully programmed maintenance program is implemented, the patient's lack of awareness or denial may continue in the natural environment. To promote maintenance, the clinician should work closely with family members or professional caregivers. They, too, should learn to give corrective and positive feedback to the patient in his or her everyday activities.

Impaired Attention

Impaired attention is an impediment to effective communication. Such an impairment also affects other skills and behaviors. Clinically, attention may be treated as an exclusive or independent target or as a target integrated with such other treatment targets as communication skills or nonverbal behaviors. When attention is treated as an exclusive target, clinicians may use paper-and-pencil tasks (e.g., cancellation of a target letter printed among nontarget letters). On computerized tasks, the patient may be asked to press a key when dots appear or disappear against a background of dots. On repeated trials, the clinician may give corrective feedback for missing specified targets and positive reinforcement for canceling the targets or reacting in some way to the specified stimuli (such as pressing a key on a computer keyboard). Eventually, the patient will be more proficient in reacting to the target stimuli.

There is an expectation that improved attention on such nonfunctional tasks as letter cancellation or dot detection will improve attention paid to functional tasks in everyday living. Unfortunately, there is no compelling evidence that attention treated as an exclusive target helps improve functional skills in the natural environment. In other words, patients who become proficient at canceling letters printed among geometric shapes on a piece of paper or in detecting appearing and disappearing dots on a computer monitor may still be inattentive during communication exchanges or in performing such nonverbal tasks as dressing or eating at a dinner table. Attention paid to performing daily activities may have to be treated in the context of such activities. Therefore, it may be most effective to reinforce attending behaviors during communication and nonverbal skill training.

Clinicians who treat attention in the context of communication training use such strategies as frequently drawing attention to treatment stimuli, giving specific directions to follow, repeating such directions throughout treatment, and reinforcing attention during discourse training. For example, the clinician might make attention a part of treatment contingency while training such pragmatic skills as:

- *Attention to maintaining topics of conversation.* The patient may be stopped when he or she begins to wander away from the selected topic of conversation. He or she then may be prompted to get back on track. The patient may be reinforced for picking up the interrupted topic and for paying attention to the same topic for progressively longer durations. The reinforcement may be continuous in the beginning and intermittent as the patient makes progress in sustained attention. To promote maintenance in natural settings, interactions between family members and the patient may be targeted for treatment. Initially, family members may be asked to watch the clinician's treatment procedures. Subsequently, family members may be trained to give corrective and positive feedback for inattentive and attentive behaviors, respectively.
- *Attention as a part of eye contact.* To encourage eye contact, the clinician might use the same strategy used in strengthening topic maintenance skills. The clinician will reinforce the patient for maintaining eye contact

and stop inattentive behaviors that may result in loss of eye contact.

- *Attention to giving appropriate responses to questions.* To decrease inappropriate responses to questions asked of the patient (possibly because of lack of attention), the clinician may first draw the attention of the patient before asking a question. For example, before asking a question, the clinician may say, "I am about to ask you a question. Please listen carefully."

- *Attention to treatment stimuli.* To decrease inappropriate responses to treatment stimuli, the clinician might say, "I am about to show you a picture and ask some questions. Please look at the picture carefully before you say something."

In each of the tasks described, the clinician may reinforce progressively longer durations of sustained attention. By systematically training family members and professional caregivers, the clinician may help promote better attentional skills in everyday situations. Furthermore, as the patient becomes more proficient in paying attention and staying on target, progressively more complex tasks may be introduced. For instance, the patient may be reinforced for appropriately shifting attention from one topic to another. Or, the patient may be reinforced for paying sustained attention to the same topic when such distractions as extraneous comments, background conversations, and noise are present.

Visual Neglect

Occupational therapists are likely to treat visual neglect through daily activities. Patients with moderate to severe left-neglect need treatment to accomplish such tasks as dressing, grooming, eating, and walking without the negative consequences of their neglect. Speech-language pathologists treat this problem as well because left-neglect negatively affects reading and comprehension of read material. Left spatial neglect may also reduce communicative effectiveness in group interactions because the patient fails to attend to people talking on the left side. The patients who are talking about events and objects in front of them may give incomplete descriptions because of their left-neglect. Therefore, left-neglect is a communication treatment target.

Most of the available treatment procedures are designed to reduce neglect in reading. As with the treatment procedures designed to improve attentional skills, some of the techniques include such indirect skills as tracking moving objects, responding to lights that flash across a computer monitor, and letter or other kinds of stimulus cancellation. Once again, in the absence of controlled evidence that indirect target training improves reading and reading comprehension, it may be best to spend treatment time and energy on treating visual neglect in the context of reading skills themselves.

Forcing a patient's attention to the left side of the visual field and then positively reinforcing that behavior are the two essential elements of treating neglect. Various procedures are available to force a patient's attention to the left visual field. For instance, in treating reading errors due to left-neglect, the clinician may use:

- *Discriminative stimuli on the left margin.* Special stimuli that draw attention to the beginning of each printed line of text may be drawn on the left margin. For example, thick and brightly colored vertical lines may be drawn on the left margin. Colored dots may be placed on the left margin, at the beginning of each sentence. Such special stimuli help draw attention to the left side of each page.

- *Verbal prompts.* Frequently given verbal prompts to "look to the left" and "go to the beginning of the line" as the patient reads aloud may be effective in themselves or when combined with other discriminative stimuli (e.g., colored vertical lines or dots in the left margin). Verbal prompts may also draw attention to the specific stimuli in the margin. For instance, the patient may be asked to "notice the line (or the dot) to your left."

- *Finger on the left margin.* The patient may be asked to keep a finger on the left margin as a reminder to go to the beginning of each line. This strategy, too, may be combined with verbal prompts to go back to the beginning of the line.

- *Pointing to the beginning of each line.* With a pencil, the clinician may point to the beginning of each line as the patient comes to the right end of each line.

- *Manipulation of printed text.* The size of the printed text may be manipulated to draw attention to the entire sentence. For instance, in one treatment program, patients read sentences printed with large letters and increased space between words (Stanton & Associates, 1981). Gradually, the letter size and spaces are reduced to normal size.

- *Use of words and sentences that encourage leftward search.* Some words and sentences encourage leftward search whereas others do not. Myers (1999) recommends the use of verbal material that encourages leftward search. Compound words like the following do not encourage leftward search because the patient may ignore the letters to the left and still read something that makes sense.

    steamship
    butterball

On the other hand, the following words when read only partially do not make sense and may force attention to the left side.

    school
    stick

Similarly, sentences like the following encourage leftward attention:

    Our hats were off to them.

Whereas sentences like the following do not encourage leftward search:

    She found that Tom was nice.

- *Positive reinforcement for left-attention.* In each procedure, the clinician should positively reinforce either requested, special stimulus-driven (e.g., colored margins), or spontaneously exhibited left-attention.

- *Corrective feedback for left-neglect.* Patients should be stopped every time they miss words on the left side. Prompts to look to the left side should then be repeated.

- *Fading the special discriminative stimuli.* All discriminative stimuli (colored vertical lines, dots, the finger on the left margin, verbal prompts, and manipulation of printed texts) should be faded to promote maintenance of left-attention in natural settings.

It should be noted that research on the efficacy of procedures described in reducing visual neglect is extremely limited. Clinicians should watch for treatment efficacy studies and use techniques that gain experimental support.

Impulsive Behavior

Patients with RHD often give hasty and impulsive responses to stimuli and questions, leading to wrong responses. To reduce such errors, the clinician needs to teach more thoughtful responses. Patients who take their time to respond may give more accurate responses. Therefore, to reduce impulsive and hasty responses, the clinician might use several nonverbal and verbal techniques:

- *Nonverbal signals.* The clinician may give such nonverbal signals as a hand gesture or a tone that signals the patient to wait a few seconds before giving a response.
- *Verbal signals.* The clinician also may give verbal signals that encourage a more thoughtful response. For example, the clinician might say, "wait for a few seconds and then respond." Such other verbal instructions as "wait until I am finished" may also help reduce interruptions in conversation.

Pragmatic Language Skills

Treatment of pragmatic language skills is an important part of speech-language pathologists' work with patients who have RHD. Treatment may target such common pragmatic language skills as eye contact, topic maintenance, and turn taking.

Brookshire (2003) recommends a videotaped baseline measure of a patient's conversational skills before treatment is started. Conversation between the patient and the clinician or between the patient and another person (e.g., a family member or a professional caregiver) may be videotaped. Brookshire also recommends the use of videotaped conversations between other persons that show appropriate and inappropriate pragmatic behaviors to draw the patient's attention to such behaviors. These videotapes may be used to enhance the patient's awareness of appropriate and inappropriate pragmatic language skills and to assess improvement during treatment sessions. Specific pragmatic skills may then be treated as follows:

- *Eye contact.* Some clients may need frequent verbal reminders to maintain eye contact during conversation (e.g., "look at me"). Other patients may need a shaping procedure in which the duration of eye contact is progressively increased. Initially, the duration might be brief; in gradual steps, the duration for which the eye contact is maintained may be increased. Positive reinforcement in the form of verbal praise for maintaining eye contact may be provided. The reinforcement should be initially continuous and subsequently intermittent.

- *Topic maintenance.* In teaching topic maintenance, the clinician may start with simple topics and move to more complex topics. Viewing previously recorded videotapes may help increase the patient's difficulties in maintaining a topic of discourse. Initially, the clinician may set a brief duration during which the patient is asked to maintain discourse on a simple topic. As the patient becomes more proficient in maintaining simpler topics of discourse for specified periods of time, both the duration and the complexity of the topics may be increased. At each stage of treatment, the clinician should reinforce the patient for staying on the topic of discourse. The clinician should stop the client at the earliest sign of departure from the topic. The clinician may then give such verbal prompts as "You were saying that . . ." to help the patient get back on the topic of discourse. Reinforcement and verbal prompts should be reduced in frequency to encourage topic maintenance in the absence of such explicit behavioral contingency.

- *Turn taking.* Reviewing videotaped interactions might help identify the patients' deficiencies as well as appropriate turn taking behaviors during conversations. To teach turn-taking, the clinician and the client may role-play. Selecting simple discourse topics, the clinician and the client may engage in a highly structured conversation. Each partner may say only a few words and yield the floor to the other. Such verbal instructions as "it is my turn" or "it is your turn" may help regulate smooth turn taking in conversation.

- *Left-neglect in group interactions.* In group interactions, the patient may neglect conversational partners on his or her left side. To reduce or eliminate this problem, the clinician may arrange group discussion sessions, preferably involving family members, in which the patient is prompted to pay attention to conversational partners on the left side. The partners also may be taught to draw attention to themselves before speaking. For instance, the partners who are in the patient's left visual field may say "Look at me, here. I want to tell you something . . ." to draw the patient's attention to themselves. Both the clinician and the conversational partners will verbally reinforce the patient for paying attention to those on the left side.

- *Training family members and other caregivers.* To sustain the clinically reestablished pragmatic skills of language, those who frequently interact with the patient should be trained in maintenance strategies. Professional caregivers may be offered suggestions on stopping the client for violating any of the pragmatic language rules and reinforcing appropriate behaviors. Family members may be asked to initially observe treatment sessions and subsequently be trained in providing corrective and positive feedback to the patient.

Impaired Inference

The patient who cannot make correct inferences from limited but available information during discourse may not respond appropriately. Similarly, difficulty making inferences while reading or while looking at pictures will make it difficult for the patient to understand stories or individual stimulus items. Therefore, impaired inference is a treatment target for patients with RHD. To treat impaired inference, the clinician may use several strategies that Myers (1999) suggests.

- *Pictures.* Pictures that depict situations (e.g., those by Norman Rockwell) may be used to encourage the patient to make correct inferences about the depicted scenes. Myers (1999) recommends the use of line drawings or colored photographs. The patient who makes correct interpretation of pictured scenes is credited with correct inferences. For example, the clinician may show a picture of a dog shaking on a beach and ask what the dog had been doing. The correct inference in this case is that the dog had been *swimming*. Pictures that depict sad or happy scenes may be used to prompt correct inference of feelings expressed on the faces of pictured individuals. The patient who fails to make correct inferences may be prompted to pay attention to the relevant aspects of the picture and the antecedents and consequences of depictions. This may prompt correct inferences.

- *Brief stories.* The clinician may tell brief stories and then ask questions to evoke implied information. Simple inferences may be provoked by such brief stories as the following:

  > *While eating in a restaurant, a man noticed that all waiters and waitresses handed a flower to every woman as soon as she was seated. He then suddenly realized that it was a special day and that he forgot to call someone in his life.*

  The clinician can then ask the patient questions such as "What was the special day?" or "Whom do you think he was going to call?" Necessary prompts may help make the correct inference (*Mother's Day*).

Impaired Recognition of Absurdities

Patients who have difficulty recognizing absurdities will misinterpret situations, leading to ineffective communication. Therefore, procedures designed to help patients recognize absurdities are a part of treating patients with RHD. To promote this recognition, the clinician may use several strategies.

- *Logical and absurd statements.* The clinician may present a list containing both absurd and logical statements and ask the patient to pick the absurd ones. The clinician can generate statements such as the following: *(a) On my way home from work yesterday, I felt so hungry that I stopped by a movie theater and watched a movie; (b) On my way home from work yesterday, I felt so hungry that I stopped at a restaurant and ate dinner before reaching home.*

- *Explanation of absurd statements.* The clinician may present only absurd statements and ask the patient to explain recognized absurdities. A statement such as (a) in the previous example may be presented with a request to explain its absurdity.

- *Pictures that represent logical and absurd situations.* The clinician may present pictures that represent absurd situations (e.g., a bird chasing a dog) along with those that represent logical situations (a dog chasing a man). The clinician then may ask the patient to alternately point to the absurd ones and logical ones.

- *Explanation of absurd pictures.* The clinician may present only those pictures that represent absurd situations and ask the patient to state the absurdities and explain them.

Impaired Comprehension of Metaphors and Proverbs

A metaphor is an expression that suggests an implicit (not a literal) comparison. Such statements as *quiet as a mouse* or *a tower of strength* suggest implied comparisons. Proverbs are popular sayings that capture some truth or wisdom; they too, suggest implied, not literal, meanings. Such sayings as *a stitch in time saves nine* and *slow and steady wins the race* are proverbs. Neither metaphors nor proverbs should be interpreted literally. Patients who cannot understand metaphors and proverbs miss the implied meanings because they tend to interpret such statements literally. To treat this problem, the clinician should select metaphors and proverbs that are appropriate for the patient's educational level. The clinician may state metaphors and proverbs and ask the client to select printed or verbal statements that give literal or correct (metaphoric or implied) meanings. The clinician should start with more common metaphors and proverbs and proceed to more complex ones. Prompting correct responses and positive reinforcement for correct interpretations may be needed at all stages of treatment.

As noted earlier, much treatment research is needed to establish the efficacy of suggested procedures. Clinicians should watch for treatment research that supports or refutes procedures described in the literature. In addition, clinicians should collect systematic baseline and treatment session data to document improvement under applied procedures.

Suggested Readings

Read the following for additional information on treating clients with right hemisphere syndrome:

Myers, P. S. (1999). *Right hemisphere damage.* Albany, NY: Thomson Learning.

Tompkins, C. A. (1995). *Right hemisphere communication disorders: Theory and practice.* Clifton Park, NY: Thomson Delmar Learning.

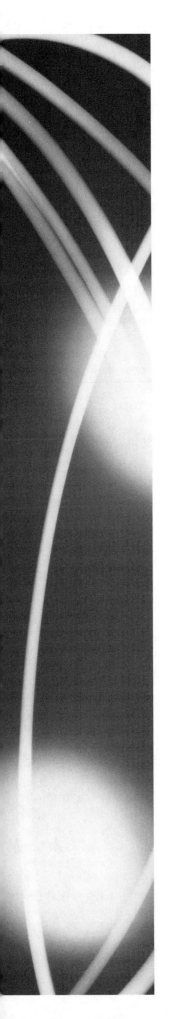

PART III

TRAUMATIC BRAIN INJURY

TRAUMATIC BRAIN INJURY: CAUSES AND CONSEQUENCES

Chapter Outline

- Defining Traumatic Brain Injury (TBI)
- Incidence and Prevalence of TBI
- Common Causes of TBI
- Types of Brain Injuries
- Biomechanics of Nonpenetrating Brain Injuries
- Primary Effects of TBI
- Secondary Effects of TBI
- Variables Related to Recovery
- Neurobehavioral Effects of TBI
- Communicative Disorders Associated with TBI

Learning Objectives

After reading this chapter, the student will:

- Define TBI and describe its prevalence and incidence.
- Specify the causes of TBI and the kinds of damage or injury produced.
- Distinguish the causes and consequences of penetrating and nonpenetrating TBI.
- Describe factors that affect recovery from TBI.
- Distinguish and describe the various neurobehavioral and communicative deficits associated with TBI.

Defining Traumatic Brain Injury

Traumatic brain injury (TBI), also known as *craniocerebral trauma,* is a frequently encountered medical emergency. The young people in all societies are especially prone to TBI. TBI is the most common cause of death and disability in younger populations throughout the world. TBI is an expensive social, medical, and personal problem. The high cost of caring for persons with TBI is escalating; estimates go as high as $25 billion a year (Adamovich, 1997; Bigler, 1990). Initial hospitalization and subsequent rehabilitation costs, along with lost wages or permanently decreased earning power, may all add up to nearly $5 million for each individual who sustains TBI (Hartley, 1995).

In the case of TBI, the immediate concern is medical treatment and the long-term concern is rehabilitation of the patient. Rehabilitation includes assessment and treatment of communicative deficits. Therefore, speech-language pathologists are involved in the rehabilitation of individuals with TBI.

The term *traumatic brain injury* excludes cerebral damage from strokes, tumors, infection, progressive neurological diseases, metabolic disturbances, toxic agents, and inherited or congenital conditions. **Traumatic brain injury** is injury to the brain sustained by physical trauma or external force. It is brain injury that impairs various skills and general behavior, requiring extensive and often prolonged rehabilitation services.

Head trauma and traumatic brain injury are not the same, although the former is involved in the latter. When a person sustains head trauma, the brain may or may not be injured and facial structures may be damaged. Only when the brain is injured does a long-term concern of multidisciplinary rehabilitation arise. Therefore, this chapter is about persons who have sustained brain injury.

Incidence and Prevalence of TBI

Results of the studies on the incidence of TBI vary by wide margins. Such variations are due to methodological problems of epidemiological studies on TBI. For example, some investigators include patients with any kind of head injury (even without brain injury) whereas other investigators include only patients who have sustained brain injury. Some investigators may exclude cases of mild injury or those who did not survive their injuries whereas others may include all such cases (Kraus & McArthur, 2000).

Several sources suggest an incidence of about 150 to 200 TBI cases per 100,000 persons in the U.S. general population, although some reports suggest as high an incidence of 367 per 100,000 persons. Based on the 1998 U.S. population and TBI incidence of a conservative estimate of 150 cases per 100,000, more than 400,000 people suffer brain injury annually; approximately 54,000 persons die of brain injuries before they reach a hospital. At least 350,000 people are hospitalized and need medical care for varied durations after their discharge (Kraus & McArthur, 2000). More than 70,000 people with moderate to severe injuries may have some degree of permanent disability.

Prevalence rates and age are significantly correlated. Prevalence of TBI is the highest in the 15 to 24 age group, concentrated especially among young people 15 to 19 years old (400 to 700 per 100,000, depending on the study). The prevalence picks up again for those who are 75 and older (300 per 100,000). TBI poses a high risk of additional injuries.

Prevalence rates and gender also are significantly correlated. For every female with TBI, there are three to five males with the same condition. Males are more likely than females to die from TBI. Toddlers and young children are prone to TBI, but much less than adolescents and young adults. A higher incidence of TBI among people living in urban areas of high population density and low socioeconomic status has been reported (Hartley, 1995).

Data on TBI in different ethnic groups are extremely limited. In various hospital records, several groups were not at all represented or are included under the "other" ethnic category. Limited data suggest that TBI is more common in African Americans and Hispanics than in whites. Head injury due to assault, gunshot wounds, and other forms of violence may be higher in ethnic minorities living in poor inner cities. Poor elderly people who live in inner cities may be more frequent targets of criminal attacks resulting in TBI than affluent elderly people living in safer suburbs (Payne, 1997).

Common Causes of TBI

Most reports on TBI do not adequately document the cause or the causes; therefore, most reported figures are estimates. Automobile accidents account for 30 to 50 percent of all cases of TBI. In fact, about 70 percent of injuries sustained in automobile accidents are TBIs. Occupants of cars and trucks sustain most transport-related TBIs. Numerous studies have shown that severe or fatal injuries due to automobile accidents may be reduced by 22 to 54 percent by wearing seat belts.

Pedestrians face a significant risk; up to 15 percent of pedestrians involved in traffic accidents may sustain TBIs. In countries where foot traffic on roads is high, a high proportion of pedestrians may sustain TBIs (Kraus & McArthur, 2000). As pedestrians, older children are especially likely to sustain TBI.

Motorcycle riders face a disproportionately high incidence of TBI and death due to TBI. Their death rate due to accidents is about 15 percent higher than the rate for occupants of passenger cars. Head injury is associated with more than 50 percent of all those who die of motorcycle accidents. In states with helmet laws, the death rate due to motorcycle accidents is 30 percent lower than in states without such laws. Bicycle riders also face the risk of TBI; in 1998, 169,000 people were treated in emergency rooms for bicycle-related injuries. More than 35,000 of them sustained some form of head injury, and 26 percent required hospitalization.

Falls are the second major cause of TBI in the general population. Among children, falls, along with abuse, are the major cause of TBI. Among elderly people (aged 75 years and older), falls are also the major cause of TBI (Murdoch & Theodoros, 2001).

Interpersonal violence accounts for about 7 percent of TBIs sustained in rural areas and 40 percent in urban areas. In large inner cities with a high density of population, TBI related to assault and firearms may exceed that of TBI due to transportation accidents (Kraus & McArthur, 2000).

Injuries related to sports and recreational activities are another cause of TBI. Such injuries may be more common in children.

Additional factors that contribute to varying and undetermined extents include abuse of alcohol and other drugs, serious and preexisting learning disorders, psychiatric disturbances, and a prior history of TBI (Hartley, 1995). Alcohol is a significant factor in motor vehicle accidents that cause TBI. Nearly a third of all people suffering TBIs in vehicular accidents may be intoxicated at the time of the accident. Alcohol-related accidents tend to be single vehicle accidents, often occurring at night and causing severe injuries (Kraus & McArthur, 2000).

The monthly trend in the incidence of TBI varies. It is the highest from May through October. Outdoor activities that predispose people to TBI probably account for the increase in the frequency of TBI during these months.

Types of Brain Injuries

There is a varied classification of brain injuries. A common classification of brain injuries includes two types: *penetrating injuries* (also called *open head injuries*) and nonpenetrating injuries (also called *closed head injuries*). Nonpenetrating brain injuries cause the most long-lasting effects that require extensive rehabilitation efforts. Therefore, we will briefly review penetrating brain injuries and then consider nonpenetrating injuries in detail.

Penetrating Brain Injuries

Penetrating brain injuries involve an open wound in the head (hence, *open head injuries*) due to some crushing or penetrating agent, resulting in fractured or perforated skull, torn brain coverings (meninges), and various degrees of brain tissue damage. Either the penetrating object or the fragments of fractured skull may damage the brain tissue. Penetrating objects such as bullets, nail guns, lawn darts, knives, and crossbows are described as *missiles* because they travel through air and strike the head.

Causes of Penetrating Brain Injuries

The basic cause of penetrating brain injuries is the piercing of the skull by an external object. The piercing object may also pass through the head. Depending on the speed with which a penetrating object strikes the head, the injury may be of high velocity (impact) or low velocity.

Generally, such agents as an arrow, nail gun, knife, and other projectile produce **low-velocity injuries.** Civilian handguns, blows to the head, and automobile accidents also produce low-velocity injuries. In the United States, bullets shot from handguns cause most of the low-velocity penetrating brain injuries. The incidence of gunshot head injury is higher among adolescents and young adults than it is among children or older people. Penetrating gunshot wounds also tend to cause the highest mortality rate, as high as 60 percent in some studies (Harrington & Apostolides, 2000).

Military weapons, rifles, and other automatic assault weapons produce **high-velocity injuries.** Clinicians who work with military personnel, especially in battlefields and beyond, deal with high-velocity injuries. Clinicians in most civilian facilities work with patients who have suffered low-velocity injuries.

Effects of Penetrating Brain Injuries

The effects of penetrating brain injury depend on several factors, including the following:

- *The projectile's entrance velocity.* The higher the speed with which the object penetrates the skull, the greater is the extent of injury.
- *The size of the missile (object) penetrating the skull.* The larger the object, the greater is the injury to the brain.
- *The degree of the projectile's yaw. Yaw* is the tendency of moving objects to change their course. An object that enters the skull and moves in a straight line produces less damage than the one that follows a zigzag path within the brain.
- *The amount of missile fragmentation.* The bullet or any other object that shatters within

the brain causes greater damage than the one that stays intact as it moves within the brain.

- *The number of wounds.* Objects that cause multiple wounds cause more damage than the ones that cause a single wound.

Of these variables, the velocity at entrance is the most critical factor that determines the extent of penetrating brain injuries (Harrington & Apostolides, 2000). Among the different kinds of bullets, those that are steel-jacketed (military issue) tend not to fragment in the brain. Hollow-point ammunitions tend to fragment and cause extensive damage.

Depending on the factors just described, the effects of penetrating brain injuries vary but may include the following:

- *Increase in intracranial pressure.* There is an instant increase in intracranial pressure when impact occurs. The pressure waves tend to spread to all areas of the brain and the spinal cord. There also is a subsequent and second increase in intracranial pressure. This increase takes place within 2 to 5 minutes of impact.
- *Death.* Death may occur immediately after the TBI, soon thereafter, or sometime later. Penetrating brain injury is survivable, although the death rate is high. The likelihood of immediate death is related to increased intracranial pressure. Seventy percent of those who suffer gunshot wounds die immediately or soon thereafter. Death sometime later is a likely result of respiratory and cardiac failures. Severe injury to the brainstem increases this possibility. Generally, mortality rate for low-velocity injury is lower (about 25 percent) compared to high-velocity injury (about 47 percent).
- *Fluctuating blood pressure.* Blood pressure drops immediately after the impact, rises and exceeds normal after 5 to 10 minutes, and then falls again.
- *Reduced cerebral blood flow.* Blood flow to the brain may remain depressed for up to 12 hours because the cerebral metabolic rate and oxygen consumption also remain depressed.

- *Destruction of brain tissue.* Evident on the projectile tract, the amount of destruction will depend on the previously listed variables (e.g., the velocity and mass of the missile).
- *Further destruction of brain tissue and infection.* Subsequently, penetrating bone fragments, hair, skin, glass, metal, and other particles may lead to these additional consequences.
- *Bleeding, infection, swelling, and hydrocephalus.* These consequences that soon follow the TBI complicate the recovery process.
- *Physical, cognitive, and language deficits.* These are typically long-term effects, requiring extensive rehabilitative efforts. See subsequent sections for a description of such long-term effects and required rehabilitation efforts.

Nonpenetrating Brain Injuries

The skull may be fractured in nonpenetrating (closed head) injuries; however, if the meninges remain intact, it is considered a **nonpenetrating injury.** Suffering indirect impact, the brain is damaged with or without skull fractures. No foreign substance enters the brain, however.

Nonpenetrating injuries induce more complex symptoms than penetrating injuries. Nonpenetrating injuries also produce long-lasting symptoms, requiring extensive rehabilitation programs. Most research, writing, and rehabilitation efforts have been directed toward patients who sustain nonpenetrating injuries.

Causes of Nonpenetrating Brain Injuries

Two kinds of forces cause nonpenetrating brain injuries. In the first kind, an external object strikes a stationary head with a certain degree of force, although there is no penetration. In the second, the head moves back and forth because of a force acting elsewhere on the body. Some specific causes that produce these forces include:

- *Various kinds of accidents.* Industrial, domestic, or sports-related accidents in which force is applied to a stationary head are a frequent cause of nonpenetrating brain injury. The collapse of an automobile on the head of a mechanic working under it (while lying on his back) is an example of force applied to a stationary head.

- *Falls.* When a person sustains a fall, the head may hit a stationary object (e.g., the floor or furniture). As noted previously, this is a common cause of TBI among the very young and the old.

- *Blunt blow to the head.* Often a result of personal violence, a blow to the head with a blunt object or instrument is a common cause of nonpenetrating brain injuries. In this case, the head may move, causing additional damage to the brain.

- *Automobile accidents.* Two kinds of forces may operate in automobile accidents. In the first kind, the force is applied directly to the movable head, which results in rapid back-and-forth movement of the brain in the skull. In the second kind, the force is applied elsewhere in the body (as in whiplash injuries in accidents); and, as a result, the head and the brain move back and forth, causing internal brain injury.

- *Abuse and interpersonal violence.* Various kinds of interpersonal violence (including domestic violence) and abuse also are causes of nonpenetrating brain injuries. A Canadian study has reported that shaken baby syndrome is a significant cause of brain injury in children under 5 years of age. Most of the children subjected to shaking had intracranial, intraocular, and cervical spinal injuries, and 19 percent of them died due to such injuries (King, McKay, & Sirnick, 2003).

Biomechanics of Nonpenetrating Brain Injuries

Experimentally induced models of brain injuries in animals have produced extensive information about the mechanisms of such injuries. Nonpenetrating brain injuries may be of two kinds: acceleration/deceleration injuries and nonacceleration injuries. These injuries are a function of biomechanical forces acting on the skull and the brain inside. To fully appreciate how the brain gets damaged when the head accelerates and then decelerates, it is necessary to understand that movement of the head and movement of the brain inside are related but separate events. When the head begins to move, the brain does not; and when the head stops moving, the brain inside the skull may keep moving. The difference in the movements of these two structures causes varied injuries to the brain.

To understand the nature of varied brain injuries, it is necessary to understand the biomechanics of forces that cause such injuries.

Acceleration. Accelerating and then decelerating movement of the head and the brain inside it are important biomechanical events that cause injuries collectively known as **acceleration/deceleration injuries.** These injuries occur when (a) a moving object strikes an unrestrained head and thus propels the head, or (b) physical forces set the head itself into motion, which then strikes a stationary object. The head may accelerate even when nothing strikes it. This happens, for example, when the chest hits a steering wheel in an automobile accident and sets the head into rapid, forward motion. Rapid acceleration of the head results in brain injury even if the head does not strike anything. Acceleration/deceleration injuries are up to 20 percent more severe than nonacceleration injuries. The type and severity of injuries that result from acceleration depend on whether it is linear or angular.

Linear acceleration. A force striking the head midline causes linear acceleration of the head. The force that is applied to the midline of the head will cause the head to move back in a straight line (linear). Linear acceleration sets off a chain of events as follows:

- The head suddenly begins to move linearly. The brain, however, remains still for a few milliseconds because of its inertia.
- At the point of impact trauma, the brain is injured because of the compression of the

skull; this injury is called **coup injury** (pronounced *coo*, which is "blow" or "impact" in French).

- When its inertia is overcome, the brain begins to move at the rate the head is moving.

- When the head decelerates or stops altogether, the inertia of the movement keeps the brain moving for a few milliseconds.

- The still-moving brain hits the inside portion of the now rapidly slowed or stationary skull, resulting in another injury to the brain; this injury is called **contrecoup** (pronounced *contra-coo*); thus the coup injury occurs at the point of impact and the contrecoup occurs at the opposite side of the brain.

- Coup and contrecoup injuries cause focal damage to meninges, cortex, and subcortical structures.

- When the brain accelerates and then decelerates, its structures at the base of the cranium rub against sharp bony projections, causing damage to soft tissue. The basal portion of the brain in the frontal and temporal lobes is most likely to sustain the most damage of this kind.

Angular acceleration. A force striking the head off-center will cause the head to move in an angular (nonlinear) direction, known as *angular acceleration.* As it moves, the head rotates away from the blow. Angular acceleration sets off a chain of events as follows:

- The force applied to the head at an angle causes movement and rotation of the head away from the point of impact.

- The same principle of inertia of the brain applies to angular acceleration. For a few milliseconds after the head begins to move, the brain remains still; after the head stops moving, the brain keeps moving for a few milliseconds.

- The brain that remains still when the head began its angular movement sustains twisting and shearing damage. This type of damage is called **diffuse axonal injury,** described later.

- The brain then begins its angular movement in the direction of the skull (away from the point of impact). When the head stops moving, the brain continues its rotational movement, causing additional twisting and shearing damage of the axial structures.

- Because of rotation and twisting forces, angular acceleration produces more severe damage than the linear acceleration.

Deceleration. Although an external force may cause the head to accelerate, structures that hold the head and the neck will cause it to decelerate, or decrease in speed. The rapidly moving head will quickly slow down because of the restraining forces of the vertebrae and neck muscles or because it hits a stationary object (e.g., the windshield in an automobile accident or the ground in the case of a fall). As noted previously, injuries due to initial increasing speed and subsequent slowing down are collectively known as *acceleration/deceleration injuries.*

Impression (impact) trauma. When a moving object strikes the head or the moving head strikes a stationary object, the initial point of contact results in impression or impact trauma, which deforms the skull at the point of impact.

Nonacceleration. Certain other kinds of forces cause neither acceleration nor deceleration of the head and the brain. Nonetheless, such forces cause injuries. Such **nonacceleration injuries** occur when a moving object hits a restrained head. Forces that do not cause acceleration or deceleration of the head deliver a crushing blow. For instance, when a person is standing against a wall, lying on a firm surface, or sitting with a rigid head support, a force may strike the head. Injuries resulting from a workplace accident, such as an automobile crashing on the head of a mechanic lying under it, are examples of nonacceleration injuries. Because there is little or no acceleration of the head in such cases, there usually is no significant deceleration either.

Nonaccelerating injuries occur less frequently than accelerating injuries. Also, such injuries produce less severe consequences for the brain. In many cases, there may be no or only a few neurological symptoms. Skull fractures are the main danger of nonacceleration injuries.

Primary Effects of TBI

The crushing effect or the biomechanical forces that a head receives cause both primary and secondary injuries. The primary effects occur at the time of trauma to the head and include injuries due to linear or angular acceleration, deceleration, and nonaccelerating crushing forces.

The primary effects of trauma to the head include the following:

- *Lacerations or fractures of the skull.* Lacerations are torn or jagged wounds on the skin surface. More serious than lacerations, fractures of the skull are seen in 80 percent of fatal cases. Skull fractures are associated with intracranial hematoma and increased frequency of infections.
- *Diffuse axonal injury.* This is a primary seriously damaging effect that occurs at the moment of closed head injury. **Diffuse axonal injury (DAI)** consists of torn nerve fibers in widespread areas of the brain's white matter. This type of damage is a direct result of the trauma and not a secondary consequence of hypoxia, increased intracranial pressure, or brain swelling. Diffuse axonal injury is typically associated with nonlinear (angular) acceleration/deceleration forces. Focal lesions, especially in the corpus callosum and parts of the brainstem may also accompany DAI. Seen only microscopically, DAI takes three forms, all related to the duration of patient survival (Graham & Gennarelli, 2000):
  - In patients who survive only for a few days, DAI takes the form of axonal bulbs, seen in the white matter of the cerebral hemispheres, cerebellum, and brainstem.
  - In patients who survive for weeks, DAI takes the form of small clusters of microglia (small cell shapes that suggest neural damage) in the white matter of the same structures (cerebral hemispheres, cerebellum, and brainstem).

- In patients who sustain severe disabilities or survive only in a vegetative state, DAI takes the form of degeneration in long neural tracts throughout the hemispheres, the brainstem, and the spinal cord.

- *Primary brainstem injury.* Some patients with TBI may have primary brainstem injury without significant diffuse damage. Other parts of the brain (e.g., the midbrain) may also be involved to some extent. Patients who sustain primary brainstem injury will lapse into a coma at the moment of trauma. Some clinicians consider it a part of the DAI.

- *Diffuse vascular injury.* This involves small and widespread ruptures in the brain's blood vessels. The result is multiple hemorrhages in the brain, some of which may be obvious on autopsy while others need histological examination. Patients with diffuse vascular injury die within hours or even minutes of the trauma (Graham & Gennarelli, 2000).

- *Primary focal lesions (injury).* TBI, depending on the type of force involved, produces focal (restricted, localized) lesions as well. Linear impacts are more likely to produce focal injuries, often described as *contusions,* than are nonlinear impacts. As mentioned previously, the skull may be depressed or fractured at the locus of impact, an example of focal skull damage. Primary focal brain lesions include the following varieties:

  - *Coup injury.* Brain tissue that is damaged just below the skull damage may be focal (coup injury). Focal coup injuries may occur without skull damage, however (Graham & Gennarelli, 2000).

  - *Contrecoup injuries.* Damage that occur on the opposite side of the point of impact (contrecoup) also are focal.

  - *Cranial nerves damage.* Damage to cranial nerves V, VII, X, and XII may cause speech disorders.

  - *Abrading injuries.* The brain tissue in contact with the rough surfaces or projections of the skull may be abraded when the brain accelerates and then decelerates. Such abrading damage is more likely on the orbital and lateral surfaces of the frontal and temporal lobes.

- Other types of primary focal injury include damage to the hypothalamus, corpus callosum, and other specific structures.

In addition to the primary effects of trauma, an injured brain is susceptible to additional effects that further complicate the clinical picture. These somewhat delayed effects are called secondary effects of TBI.

Secondary Effects of TBI

Secondary effects (injuries) are consequences of primary injuries and occur sometime after the trauma has taken place. Prompt and competent management or prevention of secondary effects is crucial for fast recovery and favorable long-term outcome.

The secondary effects or consequences of primary brain injury include the following:

- *Intracranial hematoma.* This is accumulation of blood from hemorrhage within the skull or brain. Intracranial hematoma is more common in patients with fractured skull and is a frequent cause of death. Three types of hematoma produce serious consequences:
  - *Epidural (extradural) hematoma.* Often found in temporal regions of patients with fractured skulls, epidural hematoma is accumulation of blood between the dura mater and the skull. This accumulation is often due to damaged meningeal vessels, resulting in massive bleeding. Automobile accidents frequently cause this type of bleeding. Arterial bleeding causes higher mortality rate (in about 85 percent of the cases) than venous bleeding (in about 15 percent of the cases). Epidural hematoma may be surgically cleared.
  - *Subdural hematoma.* This is accumulation of blood between the dura and the arachnoid. Lacerated cortical blood vessels cause subdural hematoma, which is more common and deadlier than epidural hematoma with a mortality rate that may exceed 60 percent. In most cases, a fall or an assault is the cause of subdural hematoma (Graham & Gennarelli, 2000).

- *Intracerebral hematoma.* This is accumulation of blood within the brain itself. It is a common occurrence in temporal and frontal lobes. Intracerebral hematoma is frequently associated with diffuse axonal injury due to linear acceleration. When combined with axonal injury, it is a frequent cause of coma and death.

- *Increased intracranial pressure.* As a secondary effect, TBI can cause increased intracranial pressure. Accumulation of blood, water, or cerebrospinal fluid causes increased pressure within the cranium. Increased pressure restricts cerebral blood flow; extreme pressures can cause death. Such accumulation causes ventricular enlargement, swelling, and edema. Technically, edema is due to cellular fluid accumulation and swelling is due to blood engorgement of brain tissue (Gillis, 1996). Brain swelling may be limited to a particular area, a single hemisphere, or both hemispheres.

- *Ischemic brain damage.* This is brain damage from lack of oxygen to the tissue (hypoxia) because of reduced or blocked blood supply. Reduced or blocked blood supply to the brain may be caused by:

  - *Breathing difficulties.* These difficulties causes poor oxygenation of blood. Injury to the chest and lungs (as in automobile accidents) and diffuse injury to the medullary respiratory centers in the brain cause breathing difficulty in patients with TBI.

  - *Hypotension (reduced blood pressure).* Heart rate is slow in such cases, causing reduced blood supply to the brain. An injured brain is especially susceptible to reduced blood supply. Hypotension increases the mortality rate in patients with TBI (Tien & Chesnut, 2000).

  - *Constricted cerebral blood vessels.* This condition also results in limited blood supply to the brain.

  - *Cerebral vasospasm.* This is constriction of the muscular layer surrounding blood vessels. Cerebral vasospasm causes restricted blood supply to the brain.

- *Seizures.* Approximately 5 to 7 percent of patients with TBI have seizures as a secondary consequence. The rate is higher in children with TBI (7 to 10 percent of patients) and higher still in soldiers who receive missile injuries in combat (30 to 50 percent). Seizures are more common in cases of severe injuries than in cases of mild injury. Some patients have seizures within the first 24 hours after the injury (more commonly in children), and others have seizures during later recovery from the initial symptoms (more commonly in adults). Repeated seizures cause additional trauma and damage to the brain (Le Roux, 2000).

- *Infection.* Various kinds of infections can threaten the life of a patient with TBI. The head wound (open, depressed, skull fractures) may be infected. Meningitis (inflammation of the membranes of the brain or the spinal cord) may be especially serious. Prompt antibiotic treatment will help control the infectious sequelae.

Variables Related to Recovery

Patients with TBI recover from their symptoms to varying degrees. Because several factors affect recovery, it is difficult to predict its course in individual cases. Some patients recover most of their skills relatively fast whereas others take time. Some patients recover to a greater degree than others do. Advances in emergency medical treatment and trauma management have resulted in lower death rate due to TBI with an attendant better prognosis. Nonetheless, 50 percent of patients who sustain severe head injuries may die. Among those who survive severe head injuries, a significant number may have permanent disabilities that include memory deficits, limited attention span, more or less subtle language deficits, poor emotional control, and drug and alcohol abuse (Andrews, 2000).

We know of several factors that affect the pattern and rate of recovery.

Duration of optimal recovery. Patients who recover most of their functions do so within the first 6 months post-injury.

Severity of injury. As one might expect, patients with more severe injury recover more slowly and to a lesser extent than those with less severe injury.

Type of injury. Patients with diffuse injuries, especially those with diffuse axonal injuries, recover less and slower than those with focal injuries. However, children and adolescents with diffuse injury may have a lower mortality rate than adults with the same kind of injury. TBI resulting in subarachnoid hemorrhage, ventricular compression, and midline shift—more often found in older adults than in younger adults—may be associated with poor prognosis. Surprisingly, persons who sustain head injury in high-speed automobile accidents tend to fare better than pedestrians who get hit by vehicles. Patients with brainstem injuries have a poorer prognosis than those without such injuries. Also experiencing poor outcome are those with intracranial hematoma (formation of a blood pool due to ruptured vessel) and increased intracranial pressure.

Secondary injuries. Patients with secondary injuries recover more slowly and to a lesser extent than those with no such injuries. Those with injuries to the respiratory or circulatory system—resulting in low oxygenation of blood (hypoxia) and lowered blood pressure (hypotension)—fare much worse than those without such systemic injuries. Patients who experience hypothermia (below-normal body temperature) also are likely to have a relatively poor prognosis (Jeremitsky et al., 2003).

Level of consciousness. Levels of consciousness vary depending on the extent and type of injury. Generally, the higher the level of consciousness following TBI, the better the prognosis. Scores on the Glasgow Coma Scale (Teasdale & Jennett, 1976), described in the next chapter, correlate well with recovery and outcome measures.

Duration of coma. Generally, the longer the duration of coma, the lower the level of recovery when it does take place. Some younger patients with prolonged unconsciousness (for more than 30 days) may show functional recovery, however.

Pupillary reactivity at admission. More than 90 percent of patients whose pupils do not react during the first 24 hours of coma either die or become vegetative. Patients with reactive pupils have a 50 percent chance of good recovery or only a moderate disability.

Age of the patient. Older patients have a higher mortality rate and poorer prognosis for recovered functions than younger patients. The mortality rate for patients younger than 21 years of age is 22 percent whereas the same rate for those who are over 65 is 57 percent.

Drug abuse and alcoholism. Patients who were intoxicated or had used illegal drugs before or at the time of accident suffer greater degree of brain trauma, partly due to secondary consequences of edema, cerebral hypoxia, and hemorrhage.

Some factors have no significant effect on prognosis. For example, race and gender of the patient do not seem to be important in recovery.

Variables related to recovery are generally applicable to groups of patients but not necessarily to individual patients whose patterns of symptoms and recovery rates vary significantly.

Neurobehavioral Effects of TBI

Traumatic brain injury produces both immediate and long-term behavioral changes. The behavioral changes depend on the severity of the trauma an individual sustains. Among the more common behavioral effects are the following:

- *Altered consciousness.* Depending on the severity of the injury, various states of consciousness may be observed in patients with TBI. A patient may be simply dazed in the case of mild injury; the patient does not lose consciousness and must be forced to pay attention even for brief periods. **Stupor** is a state in which the patient is generally unresponsive, but pain or other strong stimulus may arouse the patient for a brief period.

Coma is a state in which the patient is unconscious and unresponsive to most or all external stimulation. Coma results from a diffuse trauma to the brain, including the brainstem, and may last a few days or a few weeks. Some patients may die without recovering from coma.

- *Survival with no recovery of consciousness.* Some patients who survive TBI may not recover consciousness at all and exist in a *vegetative state.* In this state, patients are mostly unconscious, although they may experience a sleep-wake cycle. They may even be alert for short periods of time. Reflexive responses may be intact. Anoxia (lack of oxygen to the brain) and diffuse brain injury frequently cause vegetative states. Those who do not recover from a vegetative state within 30 days are said to be in a *persistent vegetative state.* Within the first 6 months, recovery is possible from a persistent vegetative state; adults have a 50 percent chance of recovery while children have a 60 percent chance. Chances of recovery diminish beyond 6 months and are very low after the first year. Those who recover late are permanently disabled.

- *Confusion and disorientation.* Patients in the process of regaining consciousness or who are dazed may experience confusion and disorientation to time and place. Additional symptoms may include headaches, lightheadedness, dizziness, blurred vision, ringing in the ears, fatigue, lethargy, and mood changes. The patient may have difficulty concentrating on events or spoken speech. Thinking may be impaired.

- *Amnesia.* Amnesia is a total loss of memory. Classic amnesic syndromes involve damage to medial temporal lobes and the hippocampus. This type of amnesia is experienced in the absence of confusion and other cognitive deficits. This clinical picture is uncommon in patients with TBI; therefore, the term *amnesia* is less appropriate than *memory problems.*

- *Memory problems.* Patients who emerge from coma are likely to experience loss of memory for events preceding and following the trauma. Patients may fail to register events happening around them. Unlike memory loss found in such patients who have aphasia, patients with TBI experience memory problems mainly associated with either reduced level of consciousness or a state of excessive arousal (delirium). Memory skills are categorized and divided into various components; these are described in the next chapter.

- *Speech disorders.* Patients who are in the process of recovering from TBI may have speech problems, including slurred speech. These problems may be more or less permanent depending on the extent of brain injury. (See the next section for details on speech disorders.)

- *Dysphagia.* At the time of admission to hospitals or emergency rooms, patients with TBI may have difficulty swallowing, known as **dysphagia.** Dysphagia incidence figures vary from around 25 percent to 75 percent of patients with TBI. Greater swallowing problems are related to longer durations of coma, although patients with no coma also may have swallowing problems. Patients with intracranial bleeding, midline shift, and brainstem injury also are likely to experience dysphagia. Such medical treatment or management involving intubation and tracheostomy may worsen the swallowing problem.

- *Other neurological symptoms.* Moderate to severe injury may cause seizures, vomiting or nausea, dilation of pupils, weakness or numbness in the extremities, loss of coordination, restlessness, and agitation. Children may show such additional symptoms as persistent crying and refusal to eat.

- *Behavioral and psychiatric changes.* A variety of behavioral changes have been noted in patients who sustain TBI. Some of these changes may be observed soon after the acute phase and may diminish over time. Other changes may be observed later and persist longer. During subacute recovery, a small percentage of patients may exhibit such psychotic reactions as auditory hallucinations, confabulations, and delusions. Some patients who have had a history of psychiatric problems or substance abuse and have lesions in basal ganglia and subcortical lesions tend to be depressed following TBI. Apathy, a less severe reaction than depression, may be found in some patients.

Brain injured patients, even after functional recovery, may show poor emotional control, social withdrawal, irritability, childishness, and unreasonable behavior.

Communicative Disorders Associated with TBI

Communicative deficits associated with TBI depend on the extent of injury, the brain structures that are injured, and the patient's premorbid communication skills. Most patients with minimal brain injury do not experience significant speech and language problems. They might be dazed and give an occasional irrelevant verbal response, and they may take time to respond verbally (slow verbal reaction time). While generally oriented to place, some may be disoriented to time. Most of these effects may be temporary.

Patients who have moderate to severe injuries may exhibit communication problems. Generally, pure linguistic problems may not be severe in patients with TBI. Grammar may be intact in most patients. Their verbal expressions may be syntactically correct. The patients may experience greater difficulty in achieving effective communication than in producing linguistically accurate sentences. Those who have sustained injury to their cerebellum, brainstem, or peripheral nerves tend to have significant speech problems, described as dysarthria.

Some of the communication problems seen in patients with TBI may be nothing new to them. Due to their educational levels, patients with brain injury may have had limited language skills before the injury. These limitations may be exaggerated after the injury, however.

Patients with severe brain injury experience lasting communication deficits, which include word-retrieval problems that result in paraphasic and circumlocutory speech. These deficits, however, may not be apparent on simple language measures. While phonologically and syntactically correct, language productions of those who have sustained significant brain injury in the past may have subtle problems that are difficult to detect or problems that the traditional tests of speech and language fail to sample (Murdoch & Theodoros, 2000). Timed tests are sometimes useful as the patient tends to do worse under time pressure. Discourse analysis may reveal some of these problems more efficiently than standardized tests. We will address this issue again in the next chapter when we discuss assessment of communicative problems in patients with traumatic brain injury.

Language Problems Associated with TBI

- *Mutism.* Some patients may not talk during the acute stage following injury or recovery from coma. Mutism may last in varying duration across patients. More persistent linguistic deficits are expected if mutism is a result of severe and diffuse TBI.

- *Confused language.* Soon after the injury, patients who are conscious and talking may produce confused language. Though syntactically correct, the patient may speak in an irrelevant, circumlocutory, incoherent, and confabulatory manner.

- *Anomia.* Confrontation naming may be especially difficult for the patient. This difficulty may be due to visual misperceptions (possibly because of inattentiveness) or impulsive responding. Brain injured patients tend to be hasty in naming objects shown, resulting in misnaming. Generally, naming errors are not as prominent or debilitating as in patients with aphasia.

- *Perseveration of verbal responses.* The patient may exhibit multiple repetitions of the same expression.

- *Reduced word fluency.* This problem may be especially evident on a timed test in which the patient is asked to recall as many words as possible in a category (e.g., names of animals). Reduced word fluency may partly be due to naming problems and inattention.

- *Difficulty in initiating conversation.* Spontaneous initiation of social interaction may be limited in some cases.

- *Difficulty in turn taking.* The generally rambling patient may fail to yield to a conversational partner and fail to take turns at appropriate junctures in conversation. The patient also may fail to relate to the previous utterances, thus showing a lack of continuity in conversation.

- *Difficulty in conversational topic selection.* The patient may find it difficult to select appropriate topics for conversation. The patient may talk about inappropriate or irrelevant topics.

- *Problems in maintaining conversational topic.* Although some may have difficulty in shifting from one topic to another, most find it difficult to maintain an extended conversation on a single topic.

- *Lack of narrative cohesion.* Patients with TBI may not provide adequate contextual cues for their utterances, and their narrative may lack cohesion. For example, the referent for the objective pronoun *it* may be unclear in discourse.

- *Problems in being concise and direct.* Patients with TBI tend to speak in vague and inaccurate terms. Frequent circumlocutions may add to this problem.

- *Difficulty in nonverbal communication.* Use of gestures, facial expression, and other nonverbal means of communication may be deficient in patients with TBI. The patient also may have difficulty understanding the meaning of facial expressions and gestures. Some of these difficulties may be due to perceptual or attentional problems.

- *Disturbed social interaction.* Possibly due to severely affected pragmatic use of language and communication, patients with TBI exhibit impaired social interaction.

- *Auditory comprehension problems.* Most patients have trouble comprehending spoken language. Comprehension of complex or abstract material (e.g., comprehension of metaphor or irony) and rapidly spoken material may be especially difficult.

- *Problems in reading and writing.* The patients may have difficulty understanding extended texts they read. Writing problems may be evident especially when the patients are asked to write coherent, precise, and extended paragraphs. Some of these difficulties may reflect the other effects of TBI, such as lack of sustained attention and difficulty following a sequence. Research on reading and writing problems of patients with TBI is extremely limited, however. Obviously, premorbid reading and writing skills are a significant factor to consider in evaluating those skills in patients with TBI.

Speech Problems Associated with TBI

In addition to language problems described, persons with TBI tend to exhibit significant speech problems. In fact, speech problems may be more persistent than language problems in persons with TBI. Speech-language pathologists often spend more time treating speech disorders than treating language disorders of patients with TBI.

- *Dysarthria.* A motor speech disorder, dysarthria refers to a group of oral communication problems due to disturbed muscular control of the speech mechanism. Dysarthria includes a wide range of communication disorders. Respiratory support for speech, articulation, prosody, resonance, voice quality, vocal pitch and loudness, and rate of speech may all be negatively affected in dysarthria. Central neural pathology, peripheral neural pathology, or both may be involved in dysarthria. Roughly 30 to 35 percent of patients with TBI may exhibit dysarthria, although the prevalence may be as high as 65 percent of patients in acute rehabilitation (Beukelman, Burke, & Yorkston, 2003). Murdoch and Theodoros (2001) list the following 10 deviant speech characteristics most frequently noted in patients with TBI:
  1. *Hypernasality.* Up to 98 percent of the patients with dysarthria may exhibit hypernasality that may be rated as mild to moderate in most cases.
  2. *Impaired rate of speech.* Up to 95 percent of patients with dysarthria may speak at a rate that is slower than normal in a majority of patients; this impairment may be mild to moderate in most cases.

3. *Imprecise consonant productions.* Up to 91 percent of patients with dysarthria may speak with imprecise consonant productions; this problem may be rated mild in a majority of patients.

4. *Limited pitch variations.* Up to 88 percent of patients with dysarthria may exhibit limited pitch variations that are rated mild to moderate in severity in a majority of cases.

5. *Reduced breath support for speech.* Up to 88 percent of patients with dysarthria may have limited breath support for speech and may be rated mild to moderate in severity in a majority of cases.

6. *Abnormal stress pattern in speech.* Up to 86 percent of patients with dysarthria may place excess stress on unstressed syllables, rated mild in about half the number of cases.

7. *Reduced phrase length.* Up to 84 percent of patients with dysarthria may speak with short phrases, rated mild to moderate in a majority of cases.

8. *Reduced speech intelligibility.* Up to 79 percent of patients with dysarthria may speak with reduced intelligibility, requiring some effort to understand the speech in a majority of cases.

9. *Prolonged intervals in speech.* Up to 79 percent of patients with dysarthria may have prolonged intervals in speech, rated mild to moderate in a majority of cases.

10. *Limited variations in speech loudness.* Up to 79 percent of patients with dysarthria may speak with limited variation of speech loudness, rated mild to moderate in a majority of cases.

- *Phonatory abnormalities.* Typically a part of dysarthria, may not be a dominant feature of dysarthria in patients with TBI. Thirty to 35 percent of patients with dysarthria due to TBI may exhibit such phonatory abnormalities as harshness, hoarseness, strained-strangled vocal qualities, and glottal fry (Murdoch & Theodoros, 2001).

- *Types of dysarthria.* Among the several types of dysarthria that exist, spastic dysarthria may be more common in patients with TBI.

The spastic type is due to bilateral damage to upper motor neuron and pyramidal and extrapyramidal tracts. Frequent occurrence of frontal lobe damage in patients with TBI account for their spastic dysarthria. The characteristics of this type of dysarthria include abnormal stress patterns, slow rate of speech, imprecise production of consonants and vowels, and a variety of phonatory problems, although phonatory problems are not prominent in dysarthria associated with TBI (Murdoch & Theodoros, 2001). Depending on the nature and locus of brain damage, patients may exhibit any type of dysarthria, including the mixed type.

- *Reduced speech fluency.* Speech dysfluencies may increase in patients with TBI. Rate of speech may be slower with many pauses, or the rate may be normal or faster with many dysfluencies of all kinds. Such deviations may be part of their dysarthria.

- *Impaired prosody.* Prosodic features of speech may be impaired in patients with TBI. Again, such impairments may be part of dysarthria.

- *Impaired thinking, reasoning, and planning skills.* Difficulty in logical thinking, reasoning, and planning is a basic characteristic of brain injury. Generally, the more abstract the reasoning or planning task, the greater the difficulty. The more severe the brain injury, the greater the difficulty with abstraction. In other words, the more severely injured patient is more concrete in thinking than the less severely injured person. Patients with TBI may have difficulty in several thinking and reasoning skills, including the following:

  - Patients may have difficulty in understanding the meaning of proverbs. For example, the meaning of *a stitch in time saves nine* may be fuzzy to a patient.

  - Patients may have difficulty describing similarities and differences between objects or events. For example, the difference between a *table* and a *chair* may be unclear to a patient. Also, the similarity between a *rose* and a *gardenia* may be difficult for the patient to specify.

- When patterns of objects are visually presented in printed form, patients may find it difficult to match geometric patterns, complete incomplete patterns, and sort objects based on shape, color, or other characteristics. See the assessment section in the next chapter for examples of tests that sample such skills.

- Patients may find it difficult to give a reasoned answer when certain situations are described to them. For example, a patient may not answer correctly when asked, "What would you do if you found someone's credit card on the floor of a store?"

- Patients may fail to detect logical inconsistencies in statements. For instance, a patient may be unsure what is wrong with the statement, "She was not hungry so she ate two large sandwiches."

- Patients may be confused in sequentially arranging a storytelling set of pictures presented randomly.

- Patients may find it difficult to point out absurdities in pictures.

- Patients may not be sure what are missing elements in drawings of people or animals.

Communication Problems of Aphasia Versus Those of TBI

It is generally recognized that communication problems associated with TBI are not classic aphasia. In fact, aphasia is not diagnosed in a majority of patients who have TBI. A major difference between communication patterns associated with aphasia and those with TBI is that patients with TBI show more pragmatic problems than patients with aphasia. Language of patients with TBI is more confused or more rambling than that of patients with aphasia. Patients with TBI may be more talkative than most patients with Broca's aphasia. Even though they have better preserved speech and language skills, patients with TBI communicate ineffectively. In contrast, even though their language skills are impaired, patients with aphasia tend to make use of multiple means of expression and thus communicate more effectively.

The pattern of communication found in patients with TBI is similar to that found in patients with right hemisphere syndrome. Predominant frontal lobe damage often found in both the groups may create this similarity. It is often suggested that communication problems found in patients with TBI are due to their cognitive deficits, which include impaired attention, sequencing, memory, and categorization. Patients with TBI tend to be confused, disoriented, disinhibited, and stimulus bound. These neurobehavioral problems affect their communication (Murdoch & Theodoros, 2001).

In summary, patients with TBI exhibit neurological, neurobehavioral, and communicative deficits that depend on the extent and severity of their brain injury. Assessment and rehabilitation of patients, described in the next chapter, should take into consideration all the varied effects of brain injury.

Suggested Readings

Read the following for additional information on TBI:

Cooper, P. R., & Golfinos, J. G. (Eds.). (2000). *Head injury* (4th ed.). New York: McGraw-Hill.

Gillis, R. J. (1996). *Traumatic brain injury: Rehabilitation for speech-language pathologists.* Boston: Butterworth-Heinemann.

Murdoch, B. E., & Theodoros, D. G. (2000). *Traumatic brain injury: Associated speech, language and swallowing disorders.* Albany, NY: Delmar Thomson Learning.

Chapter Outline

- Overview of Assessment
- Assessment of Consciousness and Cognition
- Assessment of Memory and Reasoning Skills
- Assessment of Communicative Deficits Associated with TBI
- Clinical Management of Patients with TBI

Learning Objectives

After reading this chapter, the student will:

- Describe the special parameters of assessment of patients with TBI.
- Describe the assessment techniques used to evaluate consciousness, cognition, memory, and reasoning skills.
- Describe and evaluate techniques for assessing communicative deficits in patients with TBI.

- Give an overview of clinical management strategies to be used with patients with TBI.
- Distinguish between skill management and cognitive rehabilitation.

Overview of Assessment

Assessment of patients with traumatic brain injury (TBI) requires a team effort and continuous monitoring of changes in the patients' neurophysiological, behavioral, and intellectual status. The team of specialists, including the emergency care physician, neurologist, radiologist, speech-language pathologist, physical therapist, nurse, and other professionals, is initially concerned with the patient's general health, levels of consciousness and awareness, and immediate medical or surgical intervention that may be needed. Preliminary assessment of cognitive and behavioral skills and levels is also important at this initial stage. As the patient's physical condition improves, more in-depth assessment of cognitive and behavioral consequences of injury becomes possible. Needed rehabilitation measures become clear through this in-depth assessment.

Because of the varied course of recovery of patients with TBI, assessment is a continuous process. Emphasis of assessment shifts from the urgent need to stabilizing the physical condition of the patient to relatively short-term treatment and then to long-term rehabilitation needs. Methods and instruments of assessment will change as the patient's need changes.

The speech-language pathologist, although mostly concerned with the assessment and treatment of patients' communication skills and dysphagia, needs to have a good understanding of medical assessment and treatment of patients with TBI. The extent and the type of work the speech-language pathologist needs to perform depend on the patient's physical condition, the course of recovery, and the effects of the injury.

All specialists in the team contribute to the initial assessment of patients. The team needs information on the patient and the family. As with any patient, the assessment begins with a quick evaluation of the patient's status and detailed information about the patient, the circumstances of injury, and the family.

> *Case history.* A detailed case history, obtained as soon as it is practical, documents the conditions and events that led to the head trauma. In addition, information is obtained on the patient's premorbid behavior, verbal skills, edu-

cation, literacy skills, employment, family relationship, interests and hobbies, social skills, general health, substance abuse, alcoholism, and long-term prescription medication.

Interviews. At least one member of the patient's family is interviewed to build a premorbid profile of the patient. Person or persons involved with the scene of trauma (e.g., automobile accidents or sport injuries) who could give the details of the incident may be interviewed.

Patient's medical condition. Documentation of the patient's current physical condition, organ injuries, medications, alertness, and responsiveness should be evaluated. This initial evaluation is begun as soon as the paramedical staff finds the patient and continues upon admission to the emergency room.

Medical tests. The physician in charge may order needed laboratory tests to be done as soon as it is practical. Radiological tests, blood tests, brain scanning, and other tests may be ordered to assess the extent of skull and brain injury.

Systematic analysis of the patient's behaviors. During the initial stages of hospitalization the patient's general and communicative behaviors should be systematically analyzed to evaluate the consistency of symptoms over time. If practical, the patient's symptoms may be noted in different situations. This leads to a continuous process of evaluation, as the patient's status is likely to change more or less rapidly, depending on the nature of the trauma.

Assessment of consciousness and cognition. An initial assessment task is to evaluate the patient's level of consciousness and cognition. With the help of standardized scales and systematic analysis of the patient's behavior, the team determines the level of responsiveness to environmental stimuli and the general alertness.

Assessment of memory and reasoning skills. Speech-language pathologists and psychologists evaluate memory, thinking, reasoning, and planning skills of the patient.

Assessment of communication skills. With the help of both standardized and client-specific procedures, the speech-language pathologist evaluates the communication skills of the patient. The emphasis will be on functional communication skills.

Assessment of dysphagia. In most medical settings, assessment of swallowing disorders is primarily the responsibility of speech-language pathologists.

Integration of information. The team integrates information from case history, specific assessment procedures, medical evaluations, communication assessment, and cognitive evaluation.

The initial assessment may be brief or somewhat extended, depending on the medical and behavioral status of the patient. Upon gaining consciousness, the patient may be inconsistent, disorganized, disoriented to time and place (confused), restless, or irritated. In most cases, the initial assessment is done at the bedside to understand these and other aspects of the patient's condition and performance.

Assessment of Consciousness and Cognition

The first task of initial assessment is to evaluate the patient's consciousness, alertness to the surrounding environment, orientation to time and space, and general responsiveness to stimuli and people. Memory skills may be assessed more superficially at the beginning and more in-depth as the patient's consciousness and orientation improve. Some assessment tools concentrate on consciousness, alertness, and orientation, and others include items to assess memory. Several standardized or semistandardized methods are available.

The *Glasgow Coma Scale (GCS)* (Teasdale & Jennett, 1976). This is a commonly used assessment scale to evaluate the patient's condition at this time. It is a subjective rating scale whose results should be interpreted with caution and supplemented with systematic behavioral observations. This scale evaluates three categories of behavior: eye opening, motor responses, and verbal responses. Under each category, a higher score means better response (less severe damage).

Eye opening. The scale evaluates the following: (a) spontaneous eye opening (maximum score of 4); (b) eye opening when verbally commanded (score of 3); (c) eye opening only in response to pain (score of 2); and (d) no response (score of 1).

Motor responses. The scale evaluates the following responses with the specified scores: (a) obeying verbal commands (6); (b) attempting to pull examiner's hand away from painful stimulation (5); (c) pulls the body part in response to pain (4); (d) flexes body part in response to pain (3); (e) extends limbs or increases rigidity in response to pain (2); (f) does not respond (1).

Verbal responses. The scale evaluates the following responses with specified scores: (a) conversing with good orientation (5); (b) conversing though disoriented (4); (c) using intelligible words without engaging in conversation (3); (d) producing unintelligible words (2); giving no response (l).

The total score on the GCS can range from 3 to 15. Based on the scores, brain injury is classified as:

Coma: A score of 8 or less
Severe head injury: 3 to 8
Moderate head injury: 9 to 12
Mild head injury: 13 to 15

The different levels of scores obtained on the GCS, administered 6 hours post-accident, may help predict the outcome or extent of recovery. However, the test is relatively insensitive because it does not allow scoring of untestable behaviors. For instance, a patient may be unable to open eyes because of a bandage or unable to move a limb because of injury. Another patient may be unable to respond verbally because of intubation. Therefore, the test may overestimate the severity of injury.

- The *Glasgow Outcome Scale (CLOCS)* (Jennett & Teasdale, 1981). This test is useful in evaluating outcome for, or course of recovery from, TBI. The scale describes five potential outcomes for patients with TBI.
  - *Death.*
  - *Vegetative state.* As noted previously, patients in a vegetative state give no meaningful

responses although they may open their eyes, track a moving stimulus visually, and have sleep/wake cycles.

- *Severe disability.* With this outcome, patients are conscious but are dependent on caregiver assistance for all daily activities. Cognitive and physical functions may be relatively preserved.

- *Moderate disability.* With this outcome, although they have persistent disabilities, the patients are relatively independent. Patients may continue to work; the level of responsibility they assume may be somewhat lower than those of the premorbid period, however.

- *Good recovery.* With this outcome, patients return to their premorbid functional levels without significant limitations. Mild and persistent neurobehavioral deficits do not affect their work and living activities.

- The *Rancho Los Amigos Scale of Cognitive Levels (RLAS)* (Hagen & Malkamus, 1979; Hagen, 2000) is a widely used assessment procedure to evaluate the cognitive and behavioral levels of patients with TBI. The original scale described behaviors at 8 levels whereas the revised scale (Hagen, 2000) helps rate behaviors at 10 levels.

  1. *No response, total assistance.* The patient does not respond to auditory, visual, kinesthetic, pain, and other stimuli; needs total assistance.

  2. *Generalized response, total assistance.* The patient gives nonspecific and aimless response to stimuli; gives delayed response to pain stimuli; needs total assistance.

  3. *Localized response, total assistance.* The patient blinks, turns toward or away from sound, tracks a visual stimulus that is within the visual field, gives a specific response to sensory stimulation, and may respond to family members but not to others.

  4. *Confused-agitated, maximal assistance.* The patient is highly distractible but pays attention to environmental stimuli; alert and responds to simple commands; easily agitated; exhibits inappropriate or inco-

herent verbal responses; may be uncooperative with treatment efforts.

5. *Confused-inappropriate-nonagitated, maximal assistance.* The patient is alert, relatively calm, though may be agitated when stimulated; confused and still disoriented to time, place, and persons; shows improved attention; has severely impaired recent memory; tries to use everyday objects inappropriately.

6. *Confused-appropriate, moderate assistance.* The patient is inconsistently oriented to place and persons; vaguely recognizes staff; consistently follows simple directions; has impaired recent memory; exhibits some self-care behaviors with assistance and supervision.

7. *Automatic-appropriate, minimal assistance.* The patient is consistently oriented to place and person although may not be to time; attends to familiar task for about 30 minutes; performs daily routines with minimal assistance; lacks insight into one's condition, overestimates personal abilities, fails to plan for the future; may be oppositional and uncooperative.

8. *Purposeful-appropriate with standby assistance.* The patient is oriented to person, place, and time; exhibits generally appropriate and normal behavior; may exhibit low stress threshold and difficulty with abstract reasoning skills; attends to a familiar task for about an hour; can recall past and recent events; can learn new information and generalize it; aware of one's impairments; may be depressed, irritable, easily frustrated.

9. *Purposeful and appropriate, standby assistance on request.* The patient can work for 2 hours at a stretch; capable of shifting back and forth between tasks; completes most familiar tasks but may request help with unfamiliar tasks; aware of impairments; low frustration tolerance, irritability, and depression may still be evident.

10. *Purposeful and appropriate, modified independent.* The patient can handle most tasks with periodic breaks; can initiate and

carry out most daily activities, although may need some extra time. Because the patient knows and anticipates problems, he or she can plan and use compensatory strategies. The patient's social and emotional behaviors are consistently appropriate.

The RLAS scores cannot precisely predict prognosis for patient recovery. Generally, the longer the patient stays in the earlier levels, the poorer the prognosis for recovery.

- The *Galveston Orientation and Amnesia Test (GOAT)* (Levin, O'Donnell, & Grossman, 1979) is used to evaluate patients who are coming out of coma. It consists of 10 questions designed to assess the patient's orientation to time, place, and persons (including self) and memory for events preceding and succeeding the injury. Sample questions include:

  Biographic information. Questions asked of the patient include "What is your name?" "When were you born?" "Where do you live?" and "How did you get here?"

  Orientation. Questions include "Where are you now?" "What time is it now?" "What is the month?" and "What is the year?"

  Memory. Questions asked include "What is the first event you can remember *after* the injury?" "Can you describe in detail (e.g., time, date, companions) the first event you can recall *after* the injury?" "Can you describe the last event you recall *before* the accident?" and "Can you describe in detail (e.g., date, time, and companions) the first event you recall before the injury?"

  The patient is awarded 100 points at the beginning of the test administration and points are deducted for incorrect responses. The scores are interpreted as follows:

  - *Average:* 80 to 100
  - *Borderline cases:* 66 to 79
  - *Impaired:* 0 to 65

Several other tests are available to assess consciousness, cognition, and memory skills. These include the Disability Rating Scale (DAS) (Rappoport et al., 1982) and the Comprehensive Level of Consciousness Scale (CLOCS) (Stanczak et al., 1984). The DAS is more comprehensive and more sensitive to change than the Glasgow Outcome Scale. The DAS rates eye opening, communication ability, motor responses, feeding, toileting, grooming, level of functioning (dependency), and employability. The CLOCS is more comprehensive than the Glasgow Coma Scale and helps assess behaviors in eight categories: posture, resting eye position, spontaneous eye opening, other ocular movements, pupillary reflexes, motor activities, responsiveness, and communicative effort.

Assessment of Memory and Reasoning Skills

In patients with TBI, nonverbal skills (e.g., memory, aspects of perception, drawing, construction, reasoning) tend to be impaired more than verbal skills (e.g., naming, repetition). As noted in Chapter 12, some of the communication deficits of patients with TBI may be due to attentional, perceptual, and memory deficits. Therefore, it is essential to understand these impairments to plan for effective rehabilitation programs.

- *Assessment of memory impairments.* Memory skills have been categorized and broken down into smaller components in numerous ways. The following kinds of memory may be impaired to varying extents in patients with TBI:
  - *Amnesia,* which is a term typically used in medical settings, suggests a failure to remember. Generally, classic amnesic syndromes are associated with damage to medial temporal lobes and hippocampus and involve profound memory loss with relatively intact cognitive functions. Such damage may be uncommon in patients with TBI. Therefore, the term *amnesia* is not frequently used to describe the memory impairments of people with TBI.
  - *Retrospective memory* is memory for past events. This memory component may be subdivided into declarative memory and *procedural memory. Declarative memory* is remembering what has been learned in the past about things, places, and events

in general. The clinician can assess declarative memory by asking questions that test general knowledge. For instance, the clinician may ask a series of questions to test the patient's knowledge of historic, geographic, political, academic, and social events. *Procedural memory* is remembering how to perform actions, such as driving, shaving, and cooking. The clinician may assess procedural memory by asking the patient to describe how he or she would mail a letter, cook a meal, fix a leaking faucet, prepare a lecture outline, send e-mail messages, or plant flowers in the garden.

- *Prospective memory* is remembering to do certain things at particular times. Keeping appointments and checking the mail at a certain time of the day are examples of prospective memory. The clinician can assess this skill by asking questions about such upcoming events as dinner time, doctor's appointment or bedside visits, medication times, and scheduled rehabilitation activities.

- *Posttraumatic memory loss,* also known as *anterograde amnesia,* is difficulty remembering events following the TBI. The clinician can assess this skill by asking client-specific questions about known events that took place after the injury. For instance, the clinician can ask about who brought the patient to the hospital, what was done to him or her soon after arrival in the hospital, activities that followed admission, and events of the day. Interview of family members or police and rescue staff who brought the patient to the hospital will help corroborate the patient's descriptions.

- *Pretraumatic memory loss,* also known as *retrograde amnesia,* is difficulty remembering events that preceded the trauma. The clinician can assess this skill by asking questions about known events that preceded the injury. For instance, the patient may be asked where he or she was or what he or she was doing before the injury. Once again, interview of individuals associated with the patient (e.g., family members) and those associated with the events surrounding the trauma (e.g., other passengers in a car involved in the accident and police or rescue staff who arrived on the accident scene) may provide corroborative evidence.

- *Impaired visual memory* is difficulty in recalling what is seen for a brief duration. To assess this, clinicians show various geometric forms for a brief duration (e.g., a triangle or a circle drawn on a card) and then ask the patient to draw it from memory.

- *Assessment of thinking, reasoning, and planning skills.* Impaired thinking, reasoning, and planning skills, described in Chapter 12, may be assessed informally as well as with standardized instruments. For example:

  - The clinician may assess *verbal abstract reasoning skills* by asking the patient to state the meaning of such proverbs as *a stitch in time saves nine.* The clinician also may ask the patient to state the differences and similarities between objects or words (e.g., "How are *pencils* and *pens* similar? How are they different?" "What is the difference and similarity between a *cabbage* and a *cucumber?*"). Several standardized tests or subtests of other tests also may be used to assess verbal reasoning skills. For instance, some tests of intelligence contain items to assess reasoning skills and ability to detect verbal absurdities. These items may be administered to the patient. Tests that ask the patient to arrange pictures to tell a story are also useful.

  - The clinician may assess *nonverbal abstract reasoning skills* by administering several available tests. A commonly administered test is the *Standard Progressive Matrices* (Raven, 1960). This test consists of black and white incomplete geometric designs and several choices to complete the pattern; the patient makes a choice that completes the pattern. A colored version of the test is also available. Another test that may be administered is the Wisconsin Cord Sorting Test (Grant & Berg, 1948) in which the patient is asked to sort cards on which one or all four symbols (a triangle, a cross, a star, and a circle) are printed. The patient is told "right" or "wrong" at each attempt.

The extent to which reasoning and thinking skills are assessed will depend on the needs of the patient. Extensive assessment of cognitive functions with such standardized instruments as tests of intelligence is performed by a psychologist. Several test batteries, more or less comprehensive in their coverage, are available to assess cognitive and reasoning skills of patients with TBI. These include the Brief Test of Head Injury (Helm-Estabrooks & Hotz, 1991), the Ross Information Processing Assessment–Second Edition (Ross, 1996), the Scale of Cognitive Ability for Traumatic Brain Injury (Adamovich & Henderson, 1992), and the Woodcock-Johnson Psychoeducational Battery–Revised (Woodcock & Johnson, 1989). These and other tests help evaluate memory skills, orientation, reasoning, and thinking.

Assessment of Communicative Deficits Associated with TBI

In assessing communicative deficits of patients with TBI, tests of aphasia have not proven especially useful. However, some clinicians may use certain subtests of aphasia test batteries (e.g., a confrontation naming test, a word fluency test, measures of reading and reading comprehension, and a language comprehension test) to sample responses of interest. Most of the communicative deficits found in patients with TBI require samples of social communication to make a discourse analysis to assess pragmatic communicative deficits that predominate in these patients. Repeated samples of conversational exchanges will be more useful than standardized tests of language skills in assessing the pragmatic deficits as well as deficits in comprehending abstract or complex information and difficulties in understanding humor, proverbs, and implied meanings of statements. Patients' conversation with people other than the clinician is likely to provide more valid information than structured test items (Gillis, 1996).

Assessment of Dysarthria Associated with TBI

Initially, most clinicians may administer a bedside screening test to evaluate speech intelligibility and note the types and frequency of speech production errors. If dysarthria is extensive and persistent after the initial acute stage, clinicians make a detailed assessment. In evaluating dysarthria, clinicians may use both specialized dysarthria test batteries and traditional tests of articulation. Speech samples will be useful as well. Two commonly used tests are:

- *The Frenchay Dysarthria Assessment* (Enderby, 1983). This test helps evaluate respiration, articulation, resonance, phonation, and reflexive aspects of the motor speech mechanism. Altogether, the test evaluates 28 aspects of the motor speech system, including the functioning of the lips, jaw, palate, and larynx. The sampled skills and the neuromuscular system are rated on a 9-point rating scale, with 9 being normal and 1 being severe dysfunction.

- *Assessment of Intelligibility of Dysarthric Speech* (Yorkston & Beukelman, 1981). This test helps evaluate articulation skills and the resulting speech intelligibility, assessed through recorded productions of selected single words and sentences. The recordings are submitted to independent judges who help evaluate speech intelligibility, rate of speech, intelligible and unintelligible words produced per minute, and a communication efficiency ratio calculated by dividing the intelligible words per minute by 190 (which is the normal speech rate).

Articulation skills of patients with TBI also may be assessed with the traditional tests of articulation that typically sample single word productions and limited sentences. The traditional tests, however, may not accurately reflect the articulatory skills of patients with TBI as the tests tend not to give credit for distorted sounds that are still intelligible. Moreover, judges who know the test words may overestimate the patient's articulatory proficiency (Yorkston, Beukelman, & Bell, 1988).

A thorough analysis of dysarthria involves a more detailed assessment of the motor speech system than many standardized tests permit. In addition to evaluating articulation and speech intelligibility, the clinician should make a detailed assessment of:

- *The respiratory system.* The clinician should assess the respiratory support for speech, the smoothness of the inhalation-exhalation cycles, the degree of forced exhalations, and respiratory pressure and flow.
- *The phonatory system.* The clinician should assess the laryngeal muscle function and phonation. Laryngeal muscle weakness may be evident when the patient is asked to cough or produce glottal stops. Such voice quality problems as hoarseness, harshness, and strained and strangled voice should be noted.
- *Resonatory system.* This involves an assessment of the adequacy of the velopharyngeal structures and the resonance aspects of speech production. Hypernasality, hyponasality, and nasal escape of air during speech production should be noted.

A detailed description of the motor speech evaluation is beyond the scope of this chapter. Therefore, the clinicians should consult one of several sources available on diagnosis and evaluation of dysarthria (Duffy, 1995; Freed, 2000; Murdoch & Theodoros, 2001; Yorkston, Beukelman, Strand, & Bell, 1999).

Assessment of Language Skills

As summarized in Chapter 12, various neurobehavioral effects of TBI complicate language deficits. Inattention, confusion, perceptual problems, impulsiveness, emotionality, lack of judgment, reasoning problems, and difficulty with abstract concepts affect communication skills. Also, as noted, many standardized tests of language skills, especially those used to assess patients with aphasia, do not capture the unique pragmatic communication deficits of patients with TBI. Because of the changing nature of the patient's physical and behavioral condition, assessment should be continuous and adaptive.

Assessment should include systematic and continuous analysis of the patient's physical and behavioral condition, communication and cognitive functions, and general improvement or lack of it. Initial language assessment will be brief and informal, and subsequent assessment will be in-depth and both informal and formal.

Systematic and continuous analysis. The initial condition of the patient may be coma, confusion, or various levels of consciousness. Systematic and continuous analysis of the patient's actions will help document the changing condition of the patient's general behavior, attention and alertness, and communicative attempts. Depending on the results of observation, various aspects of language assessment may be implemented.

Analysis of language and communication in the initial stages. In the initial stages, and especially when the patient recovers from coma or altered levels of consciousness, the patient may be mute or may exhibit confused language. However, as the patient's physical condition improves, the mute patient may begin to talk and confused language may clear up. Frequent observation; attempts at simple conversation; and questions about orientation to time, place, and persons will help document the initial communicative status of the patient and subsequent changes.

Assessment of language comprehension (receptive language). During the acute stage of injury when the patient may be confused, simple conversational exchanges may give an idea of the patient's comprehension of spoken language. As the patient's confusion subsides and alertness improves, formal assessment of language comprehension will be productive. The clinician may administer the Peabody Picture Vocabulary Test (Dunn & Dunn, 1981) to assess comprehension of single words. Conversational exchanges may be continuously used to assess improvement in language comprehension. The original Token Test (DeRenzi & Vignolo, 1962) and the Revised Token Test (McNeil & Prescott, 1978) may be used to assess language comprehension. Token tests give a series of commands to assess language comprehension. Although not standardized on children, the

Test for Auditory Comprehension of Language, Third Edition (Carrow-Woolfolk, 1999) may be useful in assessing significant impairments in language comprehension. A reading test, passages from newspapers or magazines, or printed stories—all specifically selected for the given patient—may be used to assess comprehension of silently or orally read material.

Assessment of verbal expression. Various aspects of verbal expression, including naming, word fluency, picture description, and story narration, may be assessed either with client-specific procedures or standardized tests. (See Chapter 8 on assessment of aphasia for some of the tests.) Conversational speech samples may be recorded to make an analysis of such pragmatic skills as turn taking, topic initiation, appropriate topic selection, topic maintenance, conversational repair, social appropriateness of speech, rambling, logical sequencing of events, and appropriate use of gestures. A writing sample will help analyze difficulties in letter formation and word and sentence writing.

Assessment of Dysphagia

Although assessment of dysphagia in patients with TBI is a primary responsibility of speech-language pathologists, space here will not permit a detailed description of the procedures; the reader should consult other sources (Murdoch & Theodoros, 2001). It may be noted that the assessment may require both a clinical bedside evaluation of swallowing and radiological procedures. An initial bedside evaluation will take note of any problem the patient has in swallowing by conducting a few feeding trials and observing the patient during typical feeding times.

Among several formal procedures, the **videofluoroscopy** (*videofluoroscopic swallowing study*)—a radiological method for examining the physiological processes involved in swallowing—is the most useful and commonly used procedure. In this procedure, the patient is asked to drink or swallow various boluses of foods impregnated with barium (to enhance contrast on X-ray pictures). The swallowing movements and any problems (especially aspiration) are noted and the reasons for the problems are analyzed (Logemann, 1998; Murdoch & Theodoros, 2001).

Ethnocultural Considerations in Assessment

There is little or no research on ethnocultural issues in the assessment of patients with TBI. However, the issues are not likely to be different from those raised in the assessment of aphasia or any other disorder of communication. General guidelines available in the literature on the assessment of clients with varied ethnocultural backgrounds apply (Battle, 2002; Payne, 1997; Screen & Anderson, 1994).

Suggestions offered in the assessment of aphasia in ethnoculturally diverse clients are applicable for patients with TBI. A client-specific approach; minimal dependence on standardized tests that may not be relevant to the patient's ethnocultural background; detailed information on family's ethnic, cultural, and linguistic background; an understanding of the patient's and the family's view of the disability; and expectations of the patient and family regarding rehabilitation will help make an appropriate assessment of ethnoculturally diverse patients with TBI. See Chapter 8 for details.

Clinical Management of Patients with TBI

Clinical management of patients with TBI is a team effort. The rehabilitation concerns of patients change as the time passes. The initial concern is to stabilize the patient's physical condition and improve the chances of survival. Emergency medical treatment may be the immediate priority. Depending on the severity of the injury, medical and surgical treatment may be necessary to stabilize the patient and prevent additional secondary injuries to the brain.

Soon, the concern is shifted to stabilizing or improving the patient's level of consciousness, alertness, orientation, and attention. As the patient improves, communication, memory, and continued physical recovery are the main concerns. As the patient's condition improves and permits, formal communication treatment along with physical therapy and other rehabilitative measures are implemented. Eventually, promoting community reentry, planning resumption of education or occupation, and teaching compensatory strategies to handle any residual deficits will be the main tasks.

Establishment of trauma facilities, safety education programs offered to the public, and prompt medical and surgical treatment of patients with TBI have resulted in reduced mortality rates. The head injury mortality rate was 22 per 100,000 in the 1970s. The recently reported rate is around 15 per 100,000 injuries (Wilberger, 2000).

Medical and Surgical Management of Patients with TBI

Patients with TBI may be initially treated in emergency departments and acute care facilities. Soon, they may be transferred to rehabilitation units. Depending on the severity of the brain injury and its consequences, the patient may undergo a variety of medical and surgical treatments. The speech-language pathologist working with patients with TBI in the initial stages of acute care and rehabilitation should be familiar with these treatments and their effects on overall rehabilitation plans.

The kinds of treatment offered depends on the timing and the stage of TBI. During the **acute stage,** the initial period following TBI, the goal of surgical and medical treatment is to stabilize the patient. Some of the common surgical and medical treatments offered in the acute stage include the following (Cooper & Golfinos, 2000; Tien & Chesnut, 2000):

- The very first medical treatment may involve efforts to save the patient by unblocking the patient's airway, keep the blood circulating, and assist breathing. Cardiopulmonary resuscitation may be necessary.
- Within hours or days of TBI, surgical procedures may be performed. For instance, a

blood clot in the brain may be removed with surgery. Intracranial pressure due to subdural hematoma and intracerebral hemorrhage also may be controlled through surgical means.

- To monitor brain tissue swelling (edema), neurosurgeons may insert to the brain (through the skull) an intracranial pressure (ICP) monitor. If the monitor shows too high intracranial pressure due to edema, drugs may be administered to draw fluid out of the brain and into the bloodstream to relieve ICP. In an extreme case of edema, a portion of the skull may be temporarily removed to prevent damage to the brain tissue.

- To ensure adequate supply of oxygen to the brain, which promotes healing, the patient may be placed on a **ventilator** (respirator).

- To remove the excess fluid that may accumulate and block and expand the ventricles, neurosurgeons may insert a tube called a **shunt** to drain the fluid (hydrocephalus) and allow the ventricles to shrink to normal size.

- To facilitate feeding in a patient who has swallowing difficulties, a nasogastric tube may be inserted through the nose to the stomach.

- To continuously measure and monitor a patient's blood pressure, **arterial lines** (tubes) may be inserted into the arteries.

- To measure the blood oxygen levels, a **pulse oximeter** may be clamped on to a patient's toe, finger, or earlobe.

- To control seizures that are a serious consequence in TBI, most patients may be given anticonvulsant drugs for at least the first few weeks.

- To stabilize the levels of sodium, calcium, sugar, and other blood substances, patients may receive a variety of other medications.

- To control such likely infections as pneumonia and urinary tract infection, additional medications may be administered.

- Depending on the additional symptoms a patient may exhibit, such other medications as analgesics (to reduce pain), antianxiety agents (to reduce fear, anxiety, and nervousness), anticoagulants (to prevent blood clotting), antidepressants (to control depression), antipsychotics (to control combativeness, hostility, and hallucinations), sedatives (to induce sleep or calm the patient), and stimulants (to improve attention and alertness) may be administered.

During the **subacute stage,** the goal of treatment is to detect and treat complications, facilitate neurological and functional recovery, and prevent additional injury. During this stage, the patient may receive the following kinds of treatment (Cooper & Golfinos, 2000; Tien & Chesnut, 2000):

- To detect complications, the medical staff watch for and treat bedsores, muscle contractions, infections, and fluid accumulations in the brain.
- To facilitate neurological and functional recovery, the rehabilitation team, including physicians, nurses, speech-language pathologists, occupational therapists, physical therapists, psychologists, and other professionals, implements its specialized programs. The medical staff continue to monitor the patient's progress and administer additional medications as necessary.

Speech-language pathologists and other rehabilitation specialists need to take into consideration the various surgical and medical treatment the patient has received or is currently receiving. The clinician should be aware of the side effects of medications the patient is on. For instance, a patient who is highly sedated may not be alert in communication treatment. A patient who has nasogastric tubes or is placed on a respirator may not be in a position to perform various assessment and treatment tasks.

Communication Treatment for Patients with TBI

Direct behavioral treatment of communication problems of patients with TBI is known to be effective (Deaton, 1990; Marquardt, Stoll, & Sussman, 1990). For example, by giving immediate, response-contingent corrective feedback, it is possible to reduce perseverative responses, inappropriate laughter, interruptions, and failure to maintain a topic during conversation. It is possible to teach self-monitoring skills to patients to make them more effective communicative partners.

Communication and behavioral self-management are the two pressing skills for which patients need help. From the standpoint of speech-language pathologists, direct work on communication and related behavioral self-management should be the primary concern. Unfortunately, research on direct communication training is extremely limited, partly because of the strong belief among professionals that it is important to remediate underlying cognitive deficits that will then automatically help improve communication and behavioral self-management. A later section contains critical discussion of cognitive rehabilitation.

Treatment of patients with TBI is similar to the treatment of patients with right hemisphere injury (see Chapter 11). Patients in both categories show similar communication deficits and related behavioral deficits.

With medical and rehabilitative efforts, many patients with mild TBI recover from their most disabling symptoms and resume normal or near-normal lives. However, most patients with moderate to severe TBI may be left with residual symptoms that last a lifetime. In such cases, initially the clinician teaches specific communicative behaviors and eventually teaches compensatory skills and strategies to minimize the effects of residual problems.

Ethnocultural Considerations in Treatment

There is little or no empirical data on treating ethnoculturally varied clients who have TBI. In the absence of specific data, the clinician can follow general guidelines considered appropriate for treating communicative disorders in ethnoculturally varied clients (Battle, 2002; Payne, 1997; Screen & Anderson, 1994). While watching for treatment efficacy studies involving patients of varied ethnocultural backgrounds, the clinician may follow general guidelines on treating ethnoculturally varied patients with aphasia and other communication disorders. Please see Chapter 9 for details.

Basic Treatment Principles

The following treatment principles help direct efforts at increasing more appropriate communication and teaching compensatory skills.

- Select client-specific and functional treatment goals that help improve immediate communication, orientation to the environment (including time, place, and person), memory for events and persons, and those that help reduce confusion. Use the functional communication skills of the kind Hartley (1995) summarizes under specific life domains (e.g., under the domain *home,* she summarizes such skill areas as personal health care and safety, family life and social interactions, and housekeeping and maintenance; the other two domains are *community* and *work*).

- Include the client and his or her family members, peers, and, when practical, colleagues or teachers from the beginning of treatment. Let the client and others help select treatment targets that are meaningful and functional to the patient and to themselves. Let the patient build a hierarchy of skills he or she would like to master.

- Structure the initial treatment environment to facilitate learning. Avoid distractions, noise, and potential for social embarrassment.

- Initially, emphasize effectiveness of communication instead of syntactic or semantic accuracy of expressions. Initially, the client is likely to use gestures, phrases, or grammatically inaccurate structures to indicate needs. Accept such communicative attempts and reinforce them.

- Simplify the treatment tasks. This initial simplicity will help establish basic communication skills upon which to build more complex skills. Increase the complexity of treatment tasks only as the patient learns to reliably produce simpler functional skills.

- Target a variety of treatment tasks to avoid boredom. In the initial stages, do not overwhelm the client with a bewildering array of activities, however. When the patient appears bored or fatigued, switch to a different task or simplify the task.

- Increase the duration of treatment sessions gradually. Note that initially, more frequent but brief sessions may be helpful.

- Integrate such skills as orientation, attention, and memory skills into direct communication training. Avoid meaningless drills or nonspecific sensory stimulation that do not directly contribute to communication or living activities.

- Select treatment stimuli and activities that are personally relevant to the client. Select music, pictures, and stories (to be read to the client) based on the client's premorbid preferences or experiences. For instance, music the client preferred or pictures of family members may be more relevant than some arbitrarily selected music or pictures.

- Select effective reinforcers. Use tangible reinforcers when necessary. Some patients with TBI may not respond to verbal reinforcers in the early stages of recovery; in such cases, use food, drink, and small gifts to reinforce target behaviors. Always measure the target behaviors to ensure that the selected consequences are working.

- Train caregivers (institutional and family) in promptly reinforcing desirable behaviors and communicative attempts.

- Move treatment from a more structured situation to progressively less structured and more naturalistic situations. Offer treatment in varied settings, including areas of daily living activities.

- Design an environmental control program to give the client a stable and predictable living arrangement. Minimize environmental control and rigid routines as the client's functioning improves.

- Assess the need for compensatory strategies to be taught. Train compensatory behaviors to reduce the effects of residual deficits.

- Use strategies that promote maintenance in natural settings of clinically reestablished skills. Teach self-monitoring and self-evaluation skills. See a later section on various maintenance strategies.

- Design and implement a community reentry program. Facilitate reentry to academic, occupational, and social situations. See a later section for suggestions.
- Work closely with other health care professionals to coordinate the efforts and to use an integrated plan of rehabilitation for the patient.

Basic Treatment Targets and Strategies

- *Flexible therapeutic environment.* For the initial stages of treatment, design a controlled therapeutic environment with reduced variability in activities and schedules. Create a simple, structured routine for the patient with few activities. Hold treatment and other activities at the same time, with the same clinicians and caregivers. Increase the number of activities and their complexities as the patient can tolerate them. Introduce variety and variability as the patient's medical condition stabilizes and behavior improves.
- *Orientation to place, person, and time.* Increase a client's orientation to place, persons, and time as an initial step of treatment. Use certain questions, modeled responses, and positive reinforcement as the main treatment techniques.
  - Ask such questions as "Where are you now?" "Who am I?" "Who is this person?" "Is this morning or evening?" "What time is it?"
  - Model the answers if the patient does not respond or responds incorrectly. For instance, soon after asking "Where are you now?" model the response, "Say,'I am in the hospital.' "
  - After a few correctly imitated responses, withdraw modeling and prompt the correct response. For instance, after asking relevant questions, give such prompts as "This is not afternoon, but this is . . ."; "I am your speech . . ."; "You are in a medical setting, and it is called a . . . "; "This is not your son, but this is your . . ."
  - Promptly reinforce all correct or approximately correct responses that were successful in communicating a message.

- Post such written signs as the day of the week, date, and month, and the name of the hospital to further promote orientation. Post them within the client's visual field and frequently point them out to the client.
- *Attention to the surroundings and communication partners.* Increase the patient's attention to the surroundings, especially to communication partners.
  - Frequently draw the patient's attention to surrounding events and persons.
  - Frequently name the persons, including the health care staff persons, while talking to the patient.
  - Ask the patient questions about the surrounding events and persons to encourage the patient to talk or comment about them.
  - Verbally reinforce any attempts at paying attention or saying something relevant.
- *Alternative or augmentative devices.* During the initial stages of rehabilitation, provide for needed alternative or augmentative assistive devices to establish a basic mode of communication.
  - Select a simple and effective device that helps communicate the patient's basic needs. For instance, teach the client to use a communication board to express needs.
  - Fade the use of the device as the patient's oral communication improves.
  - Continuously assess the need for alternative or augmentative devices and provide for them in later stages of therapy as the need becomes evident because of residual deficits.
- *Memory for daily routines.* As the patient's orientation and alertness improve, begin work on improving the patient's memory for daily routines.
  - Make a list of daily routines and scheduled activities for the patient.
  - Post written signs or the list of activities to remind the patient of daily routines. Reinforce the patient for frequently consulting the signs or the list.

- Go over the list with the patient and ask the person to describe the events or routines he or she is expected to follow.

- Ask the patient to write a list of daily activities from memory. Prompt the name and the correct sequence of the activities.

- Ask the patient to silently read the list and then describe the activities without looking at the written material. Prompt and reinforce the correct responses.

- *Memory for the names of significant persons.* Improve memory for names of health care staff and family members.

  - Have the family members bring their pictures to treatment sessions; frequently show them and ask the patient to name them; initially model or prompt the correct names.

  - Holding informal treatment sessions during daily care activities, repeat the names of the health care staff and ask the patient to name them. Prompt the names and reinforce the correct responses.

  - Have the patient write the names of family members and caregivers; expand the repertoire by including the names of friends, colleagues, and significant others.

- *Comprehension of spoken language.* Increase the patient's attention to communication partners and topics to promote better comprehension of spoken language.

  - At the beginning of a conversational exchange, draw the patient's attention with cues such as "Listen carefully, now," "I want to say something to you," and "Are you listening?"

  - Repeat such statements throughout conversational exchanges as necessary.

  - Fade such statements as the patient's attention to conversational topic improves; reinforce the client for paying attention to conversation.

  - Give introductions to new topics to help retain communicative attention. Do not abruptly introduce topics; tell the patient you are going to change the topic or will be talking about something different. Name the new topic or subject; repeat instructions to pay attention, if necessary.

- Assess comprehension of spoken speech as a part of treatment. Ask the patient to re-state what you just said, to give the main points of a discussion, or to summarize the conversation. Prompt the patient to mini-mize errors and reinforce the client.

- Reinforce behaviors that suggest compre-hension or engagement in conversation. For example, reinforce eye contact, smil-ing, and nodding; however, frequently as-sess comprehension to ensure appropriate reinforcement.

- Teach the client to ask questions when something said is not understood. Give complex instructions and then model such questions as "What do you mean?" "I do not understand that," and "Tell me more about that," for the patient to imitate. Again, say something you know the pa-tient cannot understand and immediately prompt a question. Reinforce the ques-tion-asking behavior.

- *Irrelevant, inappropriate, or tangential re-sponses.* Withhold attention from such re-sponses to decrease their frequency.

  - Without responding to such responses, change the topic. Ask a simple question for which a more relevant response is likely.

  - Reinforce all desirable responses.

  - Use time-out to decrease irrelevant, inap-propriate, and tangential behaviors by looking away from the patient whenever he or she produces such behaviors.

- *Speech production problems (dysarthria).* Treat dysarthria and related speech production problems depending on the assessment re-sults and the type of dysarthria present. Treatment of dysarthria is complex because all aspects of speech production (respiratory, phonatory, articulatory, resonatory, and prosodic features) may have to be modified. Therefore, consult other sources for details (Hegde, 2001b; Murdoch & Theodoros, 2001; Yorkston, Beukelman, & Bell, 1988).

  - Consider not treating mild dysarthria with a minimal effect on speech intelligibility if the patient's occupation is unlikely to be affected by it.

- Treat moderate and severe forms of dysarthria as it is likely to affect speech intelligibility.
- Improve respiratory support for speech. For instance, require and support good body posture during speech; teach fast inhalation but slow and controlled exhalation; provide abdominal support for exhalation by pushing against the abdomen during exhalation; and shape progressively longer utterances per breath.
- Improve the laryngeal functions. Reduce laryngeal hyperabduction by such methods as gentle voice onset.
- Increase vocal fold abduction by such techniques as pulling, pushing, and lifting exercises during phonation.
- Modify voice quality deviations with the help of such instruments as VisiPitch®, VisiSpeech®, and SpeechViewer®.
- Modify speech resonance problems by improving velopharyngeal function; consider fitting the patient with prosthetic devices as a palatal lift to improve velopharyngeal closure; teach increased vocal effort to achieve better approximation of the velopharyngeal port; use such instruments as the Nasometer® to give feedback on nasal-oral resonance.
- Improve articulation by (a) prescribing exercises that increase or reduce the muscle tone (depending on whether the patient has hypotonia or hypertonia); (b) providing biofeedback through electromyography to increase muscle tone and strength; (c) giving visual feedback on tongue placement through electropalatography; (d) shaping progressively more intelligible speech through repeated discrete trials and positive reinforcement; and (e) reducing the rate of speech.
- *Narrative and other pragmatic language skills.* Teach narrative skills in graded steps. Integrate such pragmatic skills as topic maintenance and topic initiation into narrative skills teaching.
  - Tell a brief and simple story and ask the patient to retell it. Prompt the responses as well as correct temporal sequence of events.

- Increase the length and complexity of the stories told in gradual steps. Frequently assess comprehension of stories or episodes told to the patient.

- Ask the patient to describe such events of common knowledge as fixing a breakfast, planning a vacation, buying a gift for someone, or going on a camping trip. Prompt the words and names the patient has difficulty with; reinforce correct narratives.

- Ask the patient to describe personal experiences. Gradually reduce the frequency of prompting. Continue to reinforce acceptable responses. Withhold attention from inappropriate responses.

- Prompt the patient to "Say more," or "Give details" to extend the narration on a topic. Give such hints as "What about this . . .?" or "What about that . . .?" to suggest missing details.

- Prompt new topics for conversation to teach topic initiation. Fade such prompts as the patient begins to initiate new topics for conversation.

- Teach turn taking in conversation by ignoring interruptions and reinforcing the patient for speaking at appropriate times in conversation. Use such verbal devices as "It is your turn" and "It is my turn."

- Integrate work- or school-related words, phrases, and narratives into communication training at all levels. Determine client-specific work or school-related vocabulary and expressions and make them a part of such skill training as discourse and narration.

- *Stimulus control.* To bring the target behaviors under the control of natural stimuli, fade special stimuli that control behaviors.

  - Pair the written signs, prompts, and modeling with natural stimuli for behaviors: typical reminders, questions, and natural conversational exchanges.

  - Fade the written signs, prompts, and modeling while maintaining the behaviors with typical stimuli.

- *Self-monitoring skills.* To promote better maintenance of target skills, teach self-monitoring skills at all levels of training.

- Teach the patient to catch himself or herself when attention wanders.
- Teach the patient to self-reinforce when he or she gives correct, relevant, or extended responses.
- Teach the client to stop talking when confused about something.

Teaching Compensatory Strategies

The clinician should assess the need for compensatory strategies when communication training effects have reached a plateau and the residual deficits need compensation. Some severely impaired persons may benefit from augmentative and alternative communication forms (AAC). See Chapter 9 for an overview of AAC strategies that might be used with patients with aphasia as well as those with TBI.

Analyze the patient's residual deficits to select compensatory strategies. The deficits may be found in verbal expression, speech intelligibility, and memory skills.

Teach the patient to write down steps involved in performing an action. For example, teach the client to use written directions to fix a breakfast.

Teach the patient to request information. For instance, teach the client to request information about time, date, and unclear statements.

Teach the patient to request others to modify their speech. For example, teach the client to request others to speak slowly and repeat statements.

Teach the patient to rehearse important information. For instance, teach the patient to first *self-talk* about how to perform such activities as fixing a breakfast or to think of steps involved in performing them.

Teach the patient to write down important information. For instance, teach the client to write down instructions, appointments, daily schedules, medications, directions to shopping centers, maps of important places, and phone numbers.

Teach the patient to ask others to give written instructions. For example, teach the patient to ask for phone numbers or appointments in writing.

Teach the patient to use electronic devices. For instance, teach the patient to use (a) digital watches that display time and date and signal appointment times and important actions with alarms; (b) databank watches that store messages and appointments; (c) electronic pill boxes that have alarm reminders for taking medications; (d) microcassette recorders to record lectures, directions, and even discourse; (e) handheld electronic spell checkers; (f) notebook computers for more complex information management; and (g) any other assistive device that may be useful in compensating for a specific residual deficit.

Teach the patient to establish consistent, manageable routines. For example, teach the patient to initially simplify daily routines; let the patient gradually increase the variety and complexity of routines.

Teach the patient to limit distractions or modify the environment. For example, ask the patient to find a quiet space to study; alternatively, change the work environment to suit the need for a quiet place.

Teach the patient to keep possessions at specific places. For instance, teach the patient to have an invariable place for such personal belongings as car and house keys, pens, shoes, and jackets.

Teach the patient strategies of self-cuing. For example, teach the client to use alarms as reminders of appointments and notes placed at prominent places in the house as reminders of activities.

Management of Dysphagia

Although it is not our purpose to address dysphagia management in this chapter, it is important to note that when such problems exist in a patient with TBI, the speech-language pathologist will design and implement a swallowing treatment plan. The reader is referred to other sources on dysphagia management and treatment (Logemann, 1998; Murdoch & Theodoros, 2001).

Skill Maintenance Program

A carefully designed and implemented program is essential to promote skill maintenance in natural settings. Functional skills that are useful in everyday living and those required in educational and occupational settings are more likely to be maintained than those that are selected arbitrarily. Skills consistently reinforced in everyday situations also are more likely to be maintained than those that are not reinforced. Skills that are self-monitored are more likely to be maintained than those that are not self-monitored. Finally, clients who receive follow-up and booster treatment maintain their skills better than those who do not receive booster support when needed.

Teach family members and peers to prompt, model, and reinforce desirable behaviors to sustain them in natural environments. Teach this to all who regularly interact with the client, including friends, teachers, and colleagues. Monitor the skill with which family members and others recognize and reinforce target skills. Give feedback to improve their performance.

Shift training to more natural settings. Move treatment out of the therapy room and into more informal settings. If practical, hold informal training sessions in the client's home, classroom, or workplace.

Use such natural reinforcers as verbal praise, a smile, and informative feedback (e.g., a chart showing progress made in treatment). Work with family to obtain natural and valuable consequences (e.g., a desired gift that the family can provide for certain skills maintained at home).

Teach self-monitoring skills to promote greater independence. For instance, have the client count his or her appropriate and inappropriate communicative or noncommunicative behaviors in treatment sessions. Have the client keep a notebook in which he or she makes entries of successful or failed attempts at communication in natural settings.

Arrange for regular follow-up and booster treatment. Measure response maintenance during follow-up sessions. If the measures suggest deterioration in skills, offer booster treatment.

Group Therapy

Group treatment is a typical part of rehabilitation for patients with TBI. Group sessions may help ease the transition into community reentry by emphasizing social skills. Group therapy is advocated on the assumption that it provides social support, helps dispel feelings of social isolation, creates a structure for teaching such pragmatic skills as conversational turn taking and topic initiation, and offers an opportunity for self-evaluation of strengths and limitations.

Although group therapy may be beneficial to some or most patients, there is little controlled empirical research to show that it does (Brookshire, 2003; Deaton, 1990). Therefore, clinicians who use group therapy should carefully measure the frequency of behaviors they target for treatment in the group format. Group therapy format may prove to be useful if the sessions are used to manage behavioral contingencies. That is, systematic reinforcement of appropriate behaviors in the group setting may help establish the skills in social settings. Group therapy with no contingency on social skills is of questionable value.

Promoting Community Reentry

Rehabilitation of individuals with TBI should end with a program of community reentry. To facilitate a relatively smooth transition from rehabilitation settings to home, school, and office, the clinician needs to prepare both the patient and the people in the natural environment for reentry. The reentry program will be individualized and may include the following steps:

- Analyze the skills that are needed or are still deficient that will make community reentry difficult. An analysis of educational, social, and occupational demands made on the patient will help determine the nature of the reentry program.

- Prepare the patient for reentry. In the final stages of treatment, emphasize self-help skills and independent living skills. Stimulate the patient's interest in academic, professional, social, and domestic activities. Incorporate discussions of such activities in discourse training.

- Educate family members, teachers, and supervisors about the patient's current status. Help the significant others understand what the patient can and cannot do, the kinds of compensatory strategies the patient uses, and the kinds of support he or she needs.

- Teach family members, teachers, colleagues, and supervisors to change their style of communication if necessary. For instance, they may have to speak slowly, speak in simple sentences, repeat instructions, give instructions in writing, post signs, and remind the person about appointments and tasks.

- Modify teacher or supervisor demands if necessary. For instance, the teacher may have to give reduced amounts of homework or extra time to take a test; the supervisor may have to refrain from assigning new tasks until the client can handle new challenges.

- Teach family members and others to recognize reasons for oppositional behaviors so they can take appropriate actions. For instance, many oppositional behaviors may be due to difficult task demands; if the task is simplified, more appropriate behaviors may follow.

Cognitive Rehabilitation for Patients with TBI

In the clinical management of patients with TBI, the approach of *cognitive rehabilitation* raises some important clinical issues. While such other professionals as psychologists may implement cognitive rehabilitation as an entity unto itself, whether speech-language pathologists should do the same is debatable. Whether to combine cognitive rehabilitation with communication training also is debatable.

Although cognitive rehabilitation is a widely used approach, there are questions about its validity. All cognitive rehabilitation programs teach some directly observable behavioral skill. For instance, treatment aimed at improving memory often is described as cognitive rehabilitation. However, to improve a patient's memory (e.g., remembering appointments), various environmental cues such as calendars, logbooks, and clocks are typically used. Except by manipulating external variables (stimuli that prompt an action), affecting some observable behavior (e.g., keeping an appointment), and systematically reinforcing that action, there is no way to directly affect cognition. If cognition ever is affected, it is known only by observable actions. The question then is whether it is valid or necessary to presume that some underlying cognitive process has been modified (Fordyce, 1991). What has been clearly modified is an observable action, a useful clinical outcome. What has been used to achieve that outcome also is observable clinical manipulation of target response antecedents (stimuli) and consequences (reinforcers). The presumably intervening cognitive processes do not add much to theoretical rigor or clinical efficiency. The construct of *cognitive processes* does not describe treatment targets that cannot be identified with behavioral observations and assessments. Such processes do not provide any treatment techniques that cannot be deduced from behavioral approaches.

Cognitive rehabilitation is a superfluous concept until it is demonstrated that:

- Cognitive processes are not simply presumed from behavioral observations.
- When a specific skill is taught, a presumed underlying cognitive process has been changed.
- Cognitive rehabilitation results in improved, functional communication.
- Cognitive rehabilitation is a prerequisite for communication treatment.

There is no controlled data to show that cognitive rehabilitation that *does not* include teaching specific, observable, communicative behaviors either results in improved communication or is a prerequisite for communication training.

Among the specific aspects of cognitive rehabilitation, *component training* has been popular. Specific components typically trained include attention, visual processing, and memory. Theoretically, these components are thought to underlie cognitive and communicative skills and hence are necessary to train those skills.

Training attention is based more on theoretical models than on controlled evidence supporting its usefulness. There is no convincing and experimentally controlled evidence that such activities as asking the patient to push a button every time a number is heard or backward counting of numbers result in meaningful gains in personal, social, or communicative skills.

Training visual processing involves such activities as copying geometric shapes from memory or scanning an array of symbols to match a target. It is not evident that such drills result in improved functional skills.

Memory training programs include drills to remember letters, numbers, pictures, geometric shapes, or even isolated words. However, such drills have proven ineffective in producing meaningful changes that translate into functional skills in everyday life. Therefore, the most productive approach might be to use behavioral management techniques that are known to be effective in teaching functional communication skills that seem also to improve memory (Marquardt, Stoll, & Sussman, 1990). For instance, when a patient keeps an appointment because he or she has been taught and reinforced to use an alarm watch, the patient is said to have improved memory for such tasks.

Attempts to improve attention may be better handled in the context of communication training. For example, in treating such functional communication skills as maintaining eye contact during conversation, reading printed material, and talking on a topic for an extended duration, reinforcement may be made contingent on paying attention to the task at hand for increasingly longer durations (Giles & Clark-Wilson, 1993; Hartley, 1995). In all sessions involving communication treatment, paying attention to instructions, suggestions, modeling, and various treatment tasks should be highlighted and frequently reinforced.

In essence, speech-language pathologists may be effective in their rehabilitation work if they incorporate skills that reflect memory and visual and auditory attention into their communication training. Drills that reflect presumed cognitive processes may not contribute much to functional and social skill acquisition.

Suggested Readings

Read the following for additional information on assessment and clinical management of patients with TBI:

Bigler, E. D. (Ed.). (1990). *Traumatic brain injury.* Austin, TX: Pro-Ed.

Cooper, P. R., & Golfinos, J. G. (2000). *Head injury* (4th ed.). New York: McGraw-Hill.

Deaton, A. V. (1990). Behavioral change strategies for children and adolescents with traumatic brain injury. In E. D. Bigler (Ed.), *Traumatic brain injury* (pp. 231–249). Austin, TX: Pro-Ed.

Gillis, R. J. (1996). *Traumatic brain injury: Rehabilitation for speech-language pathologists.* Boston: Butterworth-Heinemann.

Logemann, J. A. (1998). *Evaluation and treatment of swallowing disorders* (2nd ed.). Austin, TX: Pro-Ed.

Marquardt, T. P., Stoll, J., & Sussman, H. (1990). Disorders of communication in traumatic brain injury. In E. D. Bigler (Ed.), *Traumatic brain injury* (pp. 181–205). Austin, TX: Pro-Ed.

Murdoch, B. E., & Theodoros, D. G. (2000). *Traumatic brain injury: Associated speech, language and swallowing disorders.* Albany, NY: Singular Thomson Learning.

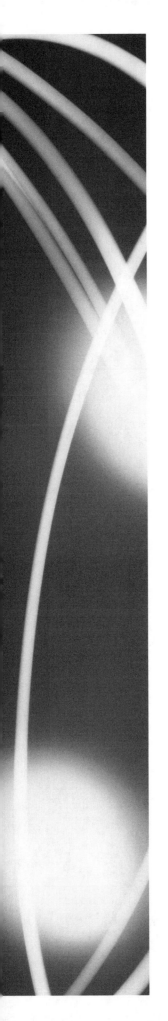

PART IV

DEMENTIA

14 DEMENTIA OF THE ALZHEIMER'S TYPE

Chapter Outline

- Incidence of Dementia

- Ethnocultural Factors and Dementia

- What Is Dementia?

- Reversible Dementia

- Progressive Dementia

- Dementia of the Alzheimer's Type

Learning Objectives

After reading this chapter, the student will:

- Define dementia and describe reversible and progressive forms of dementia.

- Discuss the ethnocultural variables that affect dementia and its management.

- Describe the neuropathology of dementia of the Alzheimer's type.

- Specify the general and speech-language characteristics of patients with the Alzheimer's type of dementia.

Incidence of Dementia

Dementia, characterized by a general decline in intellectual functions caused by acquired neurological diseases, is a major health problem affecting older persons (Bayles & Kaszniak, 1987; Cummings & Benson, 1992; Lubinski, 1995; Payne, 1997; Ripich, 1991; Shadden & Toner, 1997). It is estimated that 6 to 20 percent of people in nursing homes may have dementia. In the over-65 population in all settings, the prevalence of dementia may be as high as 25 percent (Cummings & Benson, 1992). The higher the age group, the greater the prevalence of dementia. After age 65, the prevalence of dementia doubles every 5 years. While the prevalence rate for people in their 60s is less than 1 percent, the same for those 85 and older is 30 percent (Ritchie & Lovestone, 2002). Among those who have dementia at a relatively younger age, patients with acquired immune deficiency syndrome (AIDS) are a significant number.

As the U.S. population is getting older, the incidence of dementia is expected to increase significantly. By 2030, the number of older individuals who may have geriatric psychiatric disorders, including dementia, may exceed 15 million. In fact, as people live longer because of improved health care, the incidence of dementia is expected to be the main public health problem in most societies (Kapp, 2002).

Dementia is an expensive health problem because patients need constant care over a protracted period of 6 to 8 years. The need for such expensive care often ends only with the death of the patient. The health care cost associated with dementia was in excess of $30 billion a year in the previous decades.

Ethnocultural Factors and Dementia

Data on ethnocultural factors that affect prevalence of dementia are limited as well as difficult to interpret. Recent data on the possible genetic basis of some forms of dementia (e.g., dementia associated with Alzheimer's disease) suggest that ethnicity may be a contributing factor. Some data suggest that there is no difference in the prevalence of dementia in different societies and ethnocultural groups; in one study, whites and African Americans and men and women had roughly the same prevalence rate (Schoenberg, Anderson, & Haerer, 1985). Other studies have suggested that dementia, especially of the Alzheimer's type (DAT), may be more common in whites than in African Americans, Asian Americans, or Hispanic Americans (Ritchie & Lovestone, 2002; Yeo & Gallagher-Thompson, 1996). However, limited data suggest that DAT may be uncommon in African people living in Africa; the disease is said to be nonexistent in Nigerians (Ritchie & Lovestone, 2002). See Payne, 1997, for a review of studies and their critical evaluation.

Some data suggest that late onset dementia may be more common in African Americans than in whites. Studies also have suggested that vascular dementia, described in a later section, is more common in African Americans and Asian Americans than in the Hispanic or white elderly (Yeo & Gallagher-Thompson, 1996).

In Japan, vascular dementia is more common than other forms. In Caucasians living in Europe and the United States, vascular dementia is less common than dementia of the Alzheimer's type.

Cultural and social factors and factors that affect health care access may influence the accuracy of counting people who have dementia. In certain cultural groups, early signs of dementia may be thought of as the inevitable result of the aging process. More nonwhite elderly than the white elderly may receive care at home and may not use mental health services. These factors may lead to an underestimation of dementia in nonwhite populations (Payne, 1997).

What Is Dementia?

Dementia is an acquired neurological syndrome associated often with progressive deterioration in intellectual skills and general behavior.

In most cases, and especially in its well-known forms, dementia is persistent and progressive. In other cases, dementia may be reversible.

Cummings and Benson (1992) define dementia as an "acquired persistent impairment of intellectual function with compromise in at least three of the following spheres of mental activity: language, memory, visuospatial skills, emotion or personality, and cognition (abstraction, calculation, judgment, executive function, and so forth)" (pp. 1–2). This definition differs from the widely used definition given in the fourth edition of the *Diagnostic and Statistical Manual of Mental Disorders* (DSM-IV) (American Psychiatric Association, 1994) and its 2000 text revision (American Psychiatric Association, 2000), which *requires memory impairment* in addition to at least *one* of the following: aphasia (language disturbances), apraxia, agnosia, or impaired executive functions. Executive functions include abstract thinking and planning, initiating, monitoring, and stopping complex actions and action sequences.

The psychiatric definition requires that the impairments should be serious enough to affect occupational and social life. The definition does not allow a diagnosis of dementia based on cognitive impairments due to **delirium** (impaired consciousness associated with cognitive deficits), although a patient may have both dementia and delirium. Delirium has a relatively quick onset and may be somewhat temporary (as in head trauma or substance intoxication) or relatively permanent (as in chronic schizophrenia, a severe form of psychiatric disorder in which the person is not oriented to reality).

Cummings and Benson (1992) think memory impairment is not a basic feature of dementia because such an impairment is not common in early and middle stages of dementia associated with Pick's disease. Also, according to the psychiatric definition, dementia in people with limited social and occupational demands would be hard to diagnose.

Dementia is distinguished from congenital mental retardation or developmental disabilities by its acquired pathology. Also, the onset of dementia is preceded by normal intellectual function unless its onset is documented in persons with developmental disabilities.

Dementia's persistent quality distinguishes it from such transient states as confusion due to acute cerebral trauma, metabolic disorders, and toxicity.

Dementia is distinguished from aphasia by its more diffuse cerebral pathology. Also, the typical onset of persistent dementia is gradual whereas that of confusion and aphasia is more acute. In addition, dementia includes deterioration in most aspects of intellectual functioning; aphasia does not.

Dementia is a generic term that includes multiple causes and possibly different combinations of symptoms. There is no consensus on the classification of dementia. Cummings and Benson (1992) suggest the following three major types of dementia: cortical, subcortical, and mixed. The mixed variety is associated with cortical and subcortical pathology.

Some experts have described DAT and dementia due to Pick's disease as *cortical* dementias, whereas dementias associated with such diseases as Parkinson's disease and human immunodeficiency virus have been classified as *subcortical*. Generally, intellectual deterioration, including language disturbances, appears before motor deficits in cortical dementias. To the contrary, motor symptoms (e.g., tremor, rigidity, myoclonus) appear first in subcortical dementias and intellectual deterioration only in later stages.

The *DSM-IV* of the American Psychiatric Association describes dementias based on their etiology, without a specific categorization. Currently, the cortical–subcortical classification is controversial because most dementias seem to share certain neuropathology and neurochemical deficiencies. For instance, the neurochemical cholinergic may be deficient in the subcortical structures of patients with DAT. Neurofibrillary tangles and neuritic plaques, considered diagnostic of DAT (cortical) are also found in the cortical regions of Parkinson's patients (subcortical). Nonetheless, the distinction may help make differential diagnosis because of certain behaviors and symptoms are different in cortical versus subcortical dementias. We will take note of the distinction as we describe the different forms of dementia.

Reversible Dementia

Most cases of dementia are persistent or progressive; however, there are notable exceptions. Because of these exceptions the *DSM-IV* definition of dementia does not suggest a course of the disorder; accordingly, dementia may be reversible, relatively static, or progressive (irreversible).

In about 10 to 20 percent of cases, dementia may be reversible to varying degrees (Molloy & Lubinski, 1995; Bourgeois, 2005). Reversible dementias are due to treatable diseases or disorders. For instance, nutritional deficiencies, especially vitamins B_1 and B_{12} deficiency, may lead to dementia. Several metabolic disorders may be associated with dementia. Both low sodium or calcium and high calcium may lead to dementia. Chronic renal failure may cause a form of dementia called *uremic encephalopathy.* Longstanding lung disease, cardiac disease, and anemia may cause chronic *anoxia* (oxygen deficiency) that may lead to **postanoxic dementia.** In some patients, prolonged dialysis is associated with *dialysis dementia.*

Such endocrine disorders as hypothyroidism, hyperthyroidism, and hyperparathyroidism also may cause dementia in some cases.

Dementia due to toxicity include several varieties. *Drug-induced dementias* are varied and may be the result of several prescription drugs. Many drugs used to treat mental disorders (e.g., lithium carbonate, used to treat manic-depressive disorder, and tricyclic antidepressants), known as *psychotropic agents,* can cause dementia in some individuals. Anticonvulsants (used to treat seizure disorders) and some antibiotics (e.g., penicillin) may cause dementia. *Toxic metal exposures,* including lead and mercury, also can cause dementia. *Alcoholism* is another toxic factor that may induce dementia.

Various infections also can cause dementia. Some kinds of untreated or not promptly and effectively treated infections (e.g., syphilis) may lead to dementia. Two major kinds of infectious dementias—AIDS dementia complex and Creutzfeldt-Jakob disease—are described in a separate section.

If the underlying disease that causes dementia is diagnosed early and treated effectively, the course of dementia may be reversed or significantly improved. At the least, the patients' cognitive and behavioral condition may be stabilized. When stabilized, the patients may have varied levels of relatively static dementia (Bhatnagar, 2002; Cummings & Benson, 1992).

Progressive Dementia

Several forms of dementia are progressive. Among these forms, dementia due to Alzheimer's disease is the most common. Other progressive dementias include those associated with Parkinson's disease, Pick's disease, and Huntington's disease.

Dementia of the Alzheimer's Type (DAT)

Alzheimer's disease is the most common cause of dementia. Roughly 50 percent of all reported dementias are attributed to Alzheimer's disease, although this number may be an overestimate. Dementia of the Alzheimer's type is classified as a cortical form of dementia (Cummings & Benson, 1992).

DAT has been known since late 1906 when the German neuropsychiatrist Alois Alzheimer (1864–1915) described the clinical condition of a 51-year-old woman who was in a Frankfurt asylum for the insane. Alzheimer's description of the woman's symptoms included jealousy toward her husband, rapidly deteriorating memory skills, disorientation even within her own apartment, and various symptoms of paranoia. The woman had no motor dysfunction; her gait, coordination, and reflexes were normal. She died after 4½ years of sickness. An autopsy revealed extensive cortical cell loss and what later came to be called *neurofibrillary tangles* and *neuritic plaques.*

To the surprise of Alzheimer, his mentor, the eminent German psychiatrist Emil Kraepelin coined the term *Alzheimer's disease* in 1910. A professor of psychiatry in Breslau, Poland, Alzheimer was only 51 when he died in 1915.

Incidence and Prevalence of DAT

- Though the prevalence rates differ widely across studies, it is estimated that 2 to 3 percent of persons under 75 years of age, 6 percent of those between 75 and 84 years, and nearly 15 percent of those 85 or older may have DAT; uncommonly, onset during the 40s has been reported.

- More women than men are diagnosed with DAT, not because of higher prevalence in women but because of their longevity, which puts them in older age groups with greater risk.

- DAT is more commonly associated with a family history of Down syndrome; older Down syndrome patients show brain morphologic changes associated with DAT.

- A higher familial incidence than that in the general population has been reported.

- Unless effective treatments are developed, the incidence of Alzheimer's disease will quadruple by year 2047. In the United States, 2.3 million people were affected in the late 1990s; in 2047, the incidence is expected to be 8.64 million people (Larkin, 1998).

Etiology of DAT

The causes of DAT are not known precisely, but recent research has strongly suggested several potential causes, especially genetic factors:

- Genetic factors are the most strongly suggested etiologic factors (Jacques & Jackson, 2000; Simon, Aminoff, & Greenberg, 1999; Weiner, 1996). Familial Alzheimer's disease is thought to have an autosomal dominant inheritance. The prevalence rate among the first-degree relatives of patients with DAT is about 50 percent. However, different kinds of genetic abnormalities may be involved in familial Alzheimer's disease.

- In some early onset familial cases, mutations affecting the gene for amyloid precursor protein may be evident in chromosome 21.

- Mutations on chromosome 14 may be involved in other familial cases, resulting in an early onset dementia. The protein involved in this gene is called presenilin 1.

- In still other cases, abnormalities on chromosome 19, affecting apolipoprotein E (ApoE) may be involved, especially in the late onset dementia. ApoE is a protein that metabolizes and transports fats in the body. ApoE has three gene variants, ApoE2,

ApoE3, and ApoE4. Among these, the presence of ApoE4 poses increased risk for dementia of the Alzheimer's type whereas the presence of ApoE2 may be protective.

- More recently, chromosome 12 has been found to be involved in certain cases of late onset familial dementia of the Alzheimer's type.

- Studies also have suggested that a gene on chromosome 3 (called the *K variant*) may increase the risk of developing Alzheimer's disease.

- In a small number of people of Volga German descent, highly prevalent familial Alzheimer's disease has been linked to a protein called presenilin 2 on chromosome 1. Yet another protein, called microtubule-associated protein tau, found on chromosome 17 may be associated with familial dementia of the Alzheimer's type. Research has shown that an area on chromosome 10 (D10S1423) may increase the susceptibility to the late onset dementia of the Alzheimer's type (Butcher, 2000; Frankish, 2001).

- Other genetic abnormalities that may explain DAT in many cases include mutations in mitochondria (structures in the cytoplasm of cells responsible for cell metabolism), although it is not clear whether such mutations are inherited or occur anew in each case or generation.

- **Trisomy 21,** which causes Down syndrome, also is associated with an increased risk of Alzheimer's disease. Trisomy 21 is a genetic condition in which three free copies of chromosome 21 are involved. Alzheimer's disease in people with trisomy 21 is likely to manifest in the fourth decade of life.

- Disturbed immune functions, documented in several cases, may be one of the causes, although research to date has not clarified their precise role (they may be causes, associated pathologies, or consequences of DAT).

- Viral infections have been hypothesized, but the evidence has not been convincing.

Beyond known genetic factors, an increased risk of developing DAT is associated with:

- Old age
- Family history of DAT

- Down syndrome
- Family history of Down syndrome
- History of head trauma (20 or more years before the onset of DAT)
- Limited education and limited intellectual activity
- Reduced cerebral blood flow
- Vascular diseases
- Inflammation

Observational evidence suggests the following factors may reduce the risk of Alzheimer's disease:

- Estrogen intake
- Apolipoprotein E2
- Nerve growth factors
- Antioxidants
- Sustained intellectual activity
- Cholesterol-lowering drugs and activities
- Physical activity
- Control of factors that lead to vascular diseases (e.g., hypertension)
- Anti-inflammatory drugs (e.g., aspirin)

Neuropathology of Alzheimer's Disease (DAT)

Neuropathology of DAT is better understood than its etiology. Definitive evidence of neuropathology underlying DAT can be obtained only through autopsy because there are no conclusive laboratory findings that help make a diagnosis of DAT.

Routine blood, urine, and cerebrospinal fluid examinations, though showing certain abnormalities, do not help make a definitive diagnosis of DAT. Even the various brain imaging techniques (see Chapter 3) do not produce strong evidence for an unequivocal diagnosis of DAT, although such techniques often are used to obtain supportive evidence.

A variety of neural and neurochemical pathologies, including cerebral atrophy, ventricular dilation, neuronal degeneration, neurofibrillary tangles, senile plaques, white matter changes, and depletion of neurotransmitters, are associated with DAT. These changes are most evident in the temporoparietal-occipital junctions and the inferior temporal lobe. Relatively spared are the frontal lobe, motor and sensory cortices, the occipital lobes, the cerebellum, and the brainstem.

There is some evidence to suggest that damage may extend to deeper structures in the brain. Some of the cell bodies that produce such neurotransmitters as acetylcholine (ACh) are in the nucleus basalis of Meynert, a structure deep in the middle portion of the hemispheres (Bhatnagar, 2002).

Since the 1990s, researchers also have found that cerebral inflammatory processes may be at work in Alzheimer's disease (Jones, 2001). In most cases, inflammation is limited to cerebral, not peripheral, structures.

Currently, most experts think that neurofibrillary tangles, neuritic plaques, and neuronal loss are the three dominant structural neuropathologies associated with DAT. Neurochemical changes, probably a consequence of structural changes, significantly contribute to the clinical picture.

Neurofibrillary Tangles

Neurofibrils are filamentous structures in the nerve cell's body, dendrites, and axons. In patients with DAT, these neurofibrils are thickened, twisted, and tangled. They form unusual loops and triangles. The pyramidal neurons of the cortex, the hippocampus, and the amygdala are the most frequent sites of tangled neurofibrils.

These tangles may be found in other neurological diseases (e.g., postencephalitic Parkinson's disease and progressive supranuclear palsy), older persons with Down syndrome without dementia, and apparently healthy older persons.

Neuritic Plaques

Neuritic (senile) plaques are minute areas of cortical and subcortical tissue degeneration. These plaques destroy synaptic connections and thus disturb neuronal transmission of messages. The primary sites of these plaques are the cerebral cortex and hippocampus (a structure deep within the brain presumably concerned with memory), although they also may be seen in the corpus striatum, amygdala, and thalamus.

Alzheimer had noted that a "peculiar substance" had accumulated in the cortical regions of his patient. This substance is now recognized as the main chemical constituent of neuritic plaques and is called the β-*amyloid protein.* This protein may be found in the cerebral and meningeal blood vessels as well. β-amyloid protein concentrations suggest a potential metabolic impairment that may contribute to the cerebral pathology in patients with Alzheimer's disease.

Neuritic plaques also are found in persons with Down syndrome, patients with Creutzfeldt-Jakob disease, lead encephalopathy, and apparently healthy older persons.

Neuronal Loss

The cerebral cortex of patients with Alzheimer's disease shrinks in size because of neuronal loss. The ventricles of the brain enlarge as the brain tissue is atrophied or shrunk. The shrinkage is most common in the cerebral hemispheres, especially in temporal and parietal lobes.

Recent studies of brain structures with serial magnetic resonance imaging have documented the details of neuronal loss in patients with Alzheimer's disease (e.g., Fox et al., 2001). Studies of high-risk individuals with no symptoms have shown that neuronal loss may begin several years before the onset of cognitive decline becomes evident. The loss tends to begin in the hippocampus and surrounding areas and spread to other structures.

Neurochemical Changes

Such brain chemicals that facilitate neural transmission as acetylcholine, somatostatin, vasopressin, β-endorphin, and corticotropin are severely depleted in patients with Alzheimer's disease. This depletion may be due to selective neuronal death, but many cognitive deficits are probably due to this reduced amount of neurotransmitters.

As noted before, β-amyloid, a form of protein, tends to accumulate in the neuritic plaques as well as in cerebral and meningeal blood vessels. Some experts think that this accumulation may be responsible for certain cell death (Simon, Aminoff, & Greenberg, 1999).

Parkinsonian Symptoms in Alzheimer's Disease

Some patients with Alzheimer's disease may develop symptoms consistent with Parkinson's disease. Patients with neurofibrillary tangles in substantia nigra are likely to exhibit Parkinson's symptoms. Such patients also are known to face higher mortality rate (Bennett et al., 1998).

Symptoms of DAT

DAT begins with mild symptoms that intensify over the years. Additional symptoms appear as the disease progresses (Bayles & Kaszniak 1987; Bourgeois, 2005; Cummings & Benson, 1992; Hamdy, Turnbull, Edwards, & Lancaster, 1998; Jacques & Jackson, 2000; Kempler, 1995; Lubinski, 1995; Rabins, Lyketsos, & Steele, 1999; Simon, Aminoff, & Greenberg, 1999).

THE EARLY STAGE OF DAT

In the early stage, the symptoms are mild. The person's behavior does not show radical changes. Motor functions are typically normal.

In the early stages, the patient may exhibit:

- *Subtle memory deficits.* The patient may experience memory problems, including mild impairment in remote recall of events and more pronounced difficulty in new learning or recalling more recent events. Generally, only the family members may notice these problems. The patient may be aware of these memory problems and may try to cope with them by taking certain steps (e.g., writing down things to remember).

- *Impaired visuospatial skills.* The patient may have difficulty in copying three-dimensional drawings, constructing block designs, or lacing his or her shoes. Simultaneous execution of multiple tasks (e.g., adjusting the controls on the tape recorder and the tuner at the same time) may be impaired.

- *Poor reasoning and judgment.* The patient may show poor judgment in social and personal situations. The patient may forget to pay bills or pay the same bill repeatedly. More than any other symptom, poor judgment may alert family members to a serious problem.

- *Behavioral changes.* Personality or behavioral changes noted in the early stages may be subtle or somewhat compensated. The patient may avoid certain difficult tasks (e.g., cooking, knitting, or reading books). The patient may ask someone else to perform certain tasks (e.g., a tennis player may ask the partner to keep score). Self-neglect may be another significant behavioral change. Patients stop taking care of themselves and do not care how they appear to or make an impression on others.

- *Disorientation.* In the early stages, disorientation and confusion may be limited to new surroundings.

- *Depression.* Awareness of some initial difficulties may depress the patient. Frequent mood changes and some indifference also may be evident.

- *Subtle language difficulties.* Although they may not be apparent to others, patients may have subtle language problems even in the early stages. (Please see the next section for details.)

A sudden decline in cognitive functions may occur even in the earliest stage of Alzheimer's disease if it is combined with cerebrovascular disease. In more advanced stages of Alzheimer's disease, the presence of cerebrovascular disease does not seem to make a significant difference.

Latter Stages of DAT

As the disease progresses, the early stage symptoms intensify and additional symptoms emerge:

- *Profound memory loss.* Both recent and remote recall may be severely affected.

- *Severe visuospatial problems.* The problems of the early stage tend to intensify. In the more advanced stages of the disease, most automatic skills are impaired. Such routine skills as dressing and undressing, eating, walking, and bathing may be severely impaired.

- *Generalized intellectual deterioration.* Debilitating problems in managing daily activities, including cooking, shopping, and taking care of personal or family finances, become evident. Difficulty integrating new information and problems in making rational decisions will be obvious.

- *Restlessness, agitation, and hyperactivity.* These reactions may include purposeless pacing, ritualistic or meaningless handling of objects, and picking things.

- *Acalculia.* Difficulty with arithmetic and mathematical calculations becomes more acute in the later stages.

- *Profound disorientation.* Patients may get lost in their own home or other familiar surroundings. Patients may wander off. Eventually, they may lose all sense of orientation to time, place, and person.

- *Agnosia.* Eventually, patients are not just unable to name objects or persons but fail to identify them. They may mistake a fork for a spoon or, in more advanced stages, mistake a pencil for a fork and try to eat with it. Family members may find themselves in a most distressing situation when the patient stops recognizing them and even begins to accuse them of being strangers or intruders.

- *Delusions of persecution.* Patients may believe that family members and other caregivers are conspiring to harm them.

- *Aberrant behaviors.* Patients may act on their delusions, make baseless accusations, steal or hide things, and rummage through rooms of other people. Patients may show a variety of uninhibited behaviors, including inappropriate humor and incongruous laughter, urinating at inappropriate places, and masturbating in public places. Emotional outbursts, called *catastrophic reactions,* may be observed during apparently trivial incidents.

- *Loss of initiative.* Patients may be unmotivated, show a lack of affect, or even be clinically depressed. Patients may talk about distressing experience with no emotion.

- *Periodic incontinence.* Lack of control of urinary function becomes evident in more advanced stages.

- *Problems of language and communication.* (Please see the next section for details.)

- *Physical deterioration.* Motor and physical problems appear only in the most advanced stage. Patients may experience generalized muscle rigidity or spasticity. Unstable gait and frequent falls may force them to spend more time sitting or lying down. A bewildered facial expression may be evident. When mostly bedridden, patients may assume the fetal position, have seizures, exhibit grasping and sucking reflexes, lose weight, and become urine- and feces-incontinent.

In most cases with Alzheimer's disease, death is due to aspiration pneumonia, heart failure, or infection.

Communication Problems of Patients with DAT

In the early stages, language is not as affected as cognition. As with other aspects of dementia, language skills show a progressive deterioration. Articulation is preserved until the very late stage (Bayles & Kaszniak, 1987; Bourgeois, 2005; Cummings & Benson, 1992; Kempler, 1995; Lubinski, 1995; Mentis, Briggs-Whittaker, & Gramigna, 1995; Orange, Lubinski, & Higginbotham, 1996).

LANGUAGE PROBLEMS OF THE EARLY AND MIDDLE STAGES INCLUDE THE FOLLOWING:

- *Anomia.* Mild naming problems are among the very early signs of dementia. Initially anomia is more pronounced with low frequency words. Patients may perform poorly on such tasks as generating a list of words that start with a specific letter. Being aware of the problem, patients may try to compensate by paraphasic speech.

- *Verbal paraphasia.* Alzheimer himself noted circumlocution (describing an object without naming it) and verbal paraphasia in his first patient who said *milk pourer* when shown a jug. Presumably, anomia leads to such paraphasic expressions.

- *Language comprehension deficits.* Unless professionally evaluated, subtle problems in comprehending abstract, implied, or proverbial meanings and humor may go undetected. Comprehension of concrete language may be intact in the early stages.

- *Impaired picture description.* Anomia may affect picture description, resulting in paraphasic and circumlocutory descriptions.
- *Difficulty in topic maintenance.* The patients may shift topics abruptly and lose track of what they were saying.

In the early stages, most other aspects of language, including articulation of speech sounds, voice, syntactic aspects, rhythm and intonation, and gestures that accompany speech are unaffected, as is automatic speech.

Reading aloud and writing also may be intact in early stages of dementia.

Speech of patients with DAT is more fluent, resembling the speech of those with transcortical sensory aphasia. Patients with DAT do not show agrammatic and effortful speech of Broca's aphasia.

LANGUAGE PROBLEMS OF THE LATER STAGES INCLUDE THE FOLLOWING:

- *Literal (phonetic) paraphasia.* The patient may substitute one sound for the other (e.g., *Lamerican* for *American*) or add a sound to the word (e.g., *Amelrican* for *American*).
- *More frequent circumlocution.* The patient may beat around the bush instead of using direct expressions. Many patients fail to use the correct pronouns.
- *Jargon and empty speech.* Repetitious, paraphasic, and jargon-filled speech may be devoid of meaning to the listeners.
- *Hyperfluency.* In some cases, speech, though lacking meaning, may be extremely fluent and flowing.
- *Incoherent speech.* In the latter stages, speech may be completely incoherent with disorganized thought processes.
- *Impaired conversational skills.* Most pragmatic language skills may be impaired, resulting in severe problems in maintaining a conversation.
- *Impaired comprehension.* This deficit will be more pronounced as the disease advances. The impaired comprehension is more evident for complex spoken material (e.g., sequential instructions given for task performance).

- *Impaired reading comprehension.* The problems in reading may parallel progressive deterioration in comprehending spoken speech.
- *Impaired oral reading.* This skill may be better preserved until the late stage.
- *Poor letter formation and other writing problems,* as seen in aphasic patients.
- *Echolalia, palilalia, and logoclonia.* The patient may repeat what is heard (echolalia), repeat one's own utterances (palilalia), or repeat the final syllable of words (logoclonia).
- *Difficulty initiating conversation.* Patients may be somewhat reluctant to initiate social interaction.
- *Inattention to social conventions.* The patient may neglect to greet people and bid farewell.
- *Lack of meaningful speech.* In the final stages of the disease, speech is uninterpretable largely because of many paraphasias and confused language.
- *Complete disorientation.* In the final stage, the patient may be completely unaware of time, place, self, and other persons.
- *Articulatory problems.* Generally, articulation is preserved in patients with dementia. However, other complicating neuropathological conditions that superimpose a dysarthria on dementia may lead to articulatory problems. In many patients, speech may be slurred in the final stage.
- *Mutism.* Repetition of nonlanguage sounds or complete mutism may be found in the terminal stage.

Some studies have suggested that a few patients with DAT may have visual problems that may account for confrontational naming problems. Ideomotor apraxia (difficulty performing an act on command that is performed spontaneously) and ideational apraxia (difficulty demonstrating a sequence of movements, such as filling a glass with water) may be seen in a majority of patients in the later stage.

Suggested Readings

Read the following for additional information on DAT:

Bourgeois, M. (2005). Dementia. In L. L. LaPointe (Ed.), *Aphasia and related neurogenic language disorders* (3rd ed., pp. 199–213). New York: Thieme.

Clark, C. M., & Trojunowski, J. Q. (2000). *Neurodegenerative dementias.* New York: McGraw-Hill.

Cummings, J. L., & Benson, F. D. (1992). *Dementia: A clinical approach.* Newton, MA: Butterworth-Heinemann.

Jacques, A., & Jackson, G. A. (2000). *Understanding dementia* (3rd ed.). New York: Churchill Livingstone.

Lubinski, R. (Ed.). (1995). *Dementia and communication.* San Diego, CA: Singular Publishing Group.

Simon, R. P., Aminoff, M. J., & Greenberg, D. A. (1999). *Clinical neurology* (4th ed.). Stamford, CT: Appleton & Lange.

Weiner, M. F. (1996). *The dementias: Diagnosis, management, and research* (2nd ed.). Washington, DC: American Psychiatric Press.

Chapter Outline

Learning Objectives

After reading this chapter, the student will:

- Describe how frontotemporal dementias and Pick's disease are related.

- Distinguish both the neuropathology and behavioral symptoms (include communication deficits) found in patients with Pick's disease, Parkinson's disease, and Huntington's disease.

- Describe how one might distinguish dementias associated with progressive supranuclear palsy, infectious dementias, and vascular dementia from each other.

- Describe dementia associated with TBI and specify its unique characteristics.

Overview of Other Forms of Dementia

Although dementia of the Alzheimer's type is the most common and the most researched, information on other forms of dementia is increasing at a rapid rate. Several neurological diseases are associated with these varied forms of dementia.

In this chapter, we will learn about the following kinds of dementias and their associated neuropathologies:

- Frontotemporal dementia (including Pick's disease)
- Parkinson's disease
- Huntington's disease (HD)
- Progressive supranuclear palsy
- Infectious dementias
- Vascular dementia
- Dementia associated with traumatic brain injury
- Other dementia syndromes

Frontotemporal Dementia (Including Pick's Disease)

In 1892, Arnold Pick (1851–1924), a psychiatrist in Prague, described a man with marked language problems and dementia. Pick described two kinds of neuronal abnormalities in his patients. One kind involved dense intracellular formation in the neuronal cytoplasm, later named *Pick bodies,* and the other kind involved inflated neurons, later named *Pick cells.* The syndrome he described came to be known as **Pick's disease** (PiD), which results in a form of cortical dementia (Rossor, 2001). In about 20 percent of cases, PiD is familial, suggesting autosomal dominant inheritance (Dickson, 2001).

The typical age of onset of PiD is between 40 and 60 years. Patients survive for 6 to 12 years. Some data suggest that men may be more prone to develop PiD than women.

Currently, PiD is considered a member of a group of diseases called **frontotemporal syndrome** or **fron-**

totemporal dementia (FTD), associated with degeneration in frontal and temporal lobes. As early as 1848, even before Pick's 1892 description, profound behavior and "personality" changes following frontal lobe damage were known (Morris, 2001). Until recently, PiD was thought to be a rare degenerative disease of the brain. However, the expanded diagnostic category of FTD is more common than the classic form of PiD. Some evidence suggests that FTD may be found in 12 percent of cases of dementia diagnosed in people younger than 65 (Rossor, 2001). It is now considered a major form of non-Alzheimer type dementia (Morris, 2001).

FTD is a heterogeneous group of diseases sharing certain common features (Hodges, 2001). The diagnostic categories within FTD are still evolving, and different diagnostic classifications are advocated in the medical literature (Dickson, 2001). Furthermore, FTD, especially PiD, is often undiagnosed or confused with the Alzheimer's type (Perry & Miller, 2001).

FTD is associated with behavioral (personality) changes and social conduct; affected people become entirely different persons with previously nonexistent profanity, irresponsibility, irreverence, and disregard for social conventions (Morris, 2001). Some evidence suggests abnormalities in chromosome 17 as the cause of the disease. One potential diagnostic feature of patients with frontotemporal dementia is their tendency to imitate gestures of others even when told not to imitate. This imitative behavior has been called *obstinate imitation* (Shimomura & Mori, 1998).

Neuropathology of Frontotemporal Dementia

The general neuropathology is degeneration of cells in the left and right frontal and temporal lobes (Morris, 2001). The atrophy is evident in the temporal lobe in about a quarter of patients and in the frontal lobe in another quarter. The rest have atrophy in both the lobes. When both the right and left sides of the brain are affected, some patients have a predominantly left degeneration while others have a predominantly right degeneration. Somewhat different clinical pictures emerge from the differential involvement of the right and left sides and temporal and frontal lobes.

In the *classic form of PiD* (in some sources, Type A Pick's disease), specific neuropathology includes the following (Dickson, 2001; Hodges, 2001; Morris, 2001; Rossor, 2001):

- Presence of relatively focal atrophy in the anterior temporal and frontal lobes, the orbital frontal lobe, and the medial temporal lobes. The posterior superior temporal gyrus and precentral and postcentral gyri are typically normal.
- Presence of **Pick bodies** (dense intracellular formations in the neuronal cytoplasm), especially in nonpyramidal cells in the cerebral layers 2, 3, and 6.
- Presence of **Pick cells** (ballooned, inflated, or enlarged neurons), especially in the lower and middle cortical layers. Pick cells, however, are not crucially diagnostic as they are found in other neurodegenerative diseases (e.g., Creutzfeldt-Jakob disease and progressive supranuclear palsy).
- Such other abnormalities as dilated lateral ventricles and atrophy of the caudate nucleus may be present.
- Atrophy may be worse on the left (dominant) hemisphere.

Neuropathology in the other forms of FTD is characterized by the following:

- Absence of the Pick bodies and the Pick cells in some variant of FTD
- Atrophied, gliosed, and swollen brain cells (**Gliosis** is an excess accumulation of astrocytes (neuroglia cells) in the atrophied regions of the brain in other variant of FTD.)
- Atrophy in the frontotemporal regions with no distinctive histology in yet another variant of FTD

Some experts describe a frontal variant (FvFTD) and a temporal variant (TvFTD) of frontotemporal dementia; the temporal variant also may be described as *semantic aphasia* (Hodges, 2001), although this term might be somewhat confusing with classic syndromes of aphasia. As the terms suggest, a predominant degeneration of the frontal cortex characterizes patients with FvFTD and a predominant degeneration of the temporal lobe characterizes patients with TvFTD.

Some investigators emphasize that the varied symptom complex found in FTD, including the classic form of PiD, may be better understood in terms of the differential atrophy of the left or the right hemispheres. Whether atrophy is concentrated in the left or right frontal lobe or the left or right temporal lobes makes a difference in the symptom complex. Evidence also suggests that FTD is primarily a neurobehavioral disorder in the sense that behavioral changes are diagnostic of the disease. Because of the predominant behavioral symptoms, patients in initial stages of FTD may be diagnosed with such psychiatric disorders as schizophrenia and depression (Mychack, Kramer, Boone, & Miller, 2001; Perry & Miller, 2001).

General Symptoms of Frontotemporal Dementia, Including PiD

Frontotemporal dementia is characterized by dramatic behavior changes, including certain speech-language behaviors (Dickson, 2001; Hodges, 2001; Morris, 2001; Rossor, 2001):

- Insidious onset of the disease; difficult to establish the time of onset.
- Behavioral changes that are often the initial and presenting symptoms; behavior changes are marked in patients with predominantly right-sided atrophy. Patients with left-sided atrophy initially present fewer or less serious behavior symptoms but more marked language disturbances.
- Uninhibited behavior, including inappropriate social behavior, uncharacteristic sexual jokes, and socially inappropriate comments.
- Depression characterized by withdrawal, irritability, atypical mood fluctuations, and reduced speech output; however, depression of patients with AFT is not associated with guilt or suicidal ideation.

- Euphoric symptoms, including elevated mood, excessive jocularity, and exaggerated self-esteem; these symptoms provide a paradoxical contrast to their depression at other times.
- Apathy in many patients with FTD; the patients may be cold and unconcerned about the feelings of people around them.
- Delusions without persecutory thoughts in some patients; auditory hallucinations are absent.
- Intellectual deterioration, including impaired judgment and insight and impaired constructional ability, planning, and abstraction; this is opposite of what happens in DAT. In FTD, including PiD, the behavioral changes precede intellectual deterioration.
- Difficulty recognizing names, faces, and voices of known people; especially noted in patients with predominantly right-sided atrophy.
- Repetitive and meaningless behaviors in many patients; the patients may compulsively and repeatedly fold napkins, brush teeth many times, perform bathroom routines all the time, count and hoard food items constantly, check clocks and doors endlessly, and insist on eating the same food at precisely the same time every day.
- Excessive eating and weight gain; patients may develop a craving for carbohydrates; in later stages, the patients may eat bizarre combinations of foods or even try to consume nonedible substances.
- Lack of insight into one's own condition, an early symptom of FTD.

Language Disorders Associated with Frontotemporal Dementia (Including Pick's Disease)

- Language disturbances are among the early symptoms in patients who have a predominantly left temporal lobe atrophy; in such patients, behavioral disturbances are less marked than they are in patients with right-sided atrophy. Until the final stages, patients with left-sided atrophy remain socially appropriate.

- Unlike in DAT, memory and orientation are better preserved, but language disturbances are predominant.

- Anomia (word-finding problems and impaired confrontation naming) is more pronounced in patients with left temporal lobe atrophy; this difficulty may be serious and limited to naming; the patient's speech may be relatively fluent. The naming problem is thought to reflect a loss of meaning and knowledge that underlie words and concepts. Therefore, some use the term *semantic dementia* to describe the language problems of patients with left temporal lobe atrophy (Hodges, 2001).

- Progressive shrinkage in expressive vocabulary may lead to verbal paraphasia, circumlocution, and use of general words (e.g., *this thing, that thing*) instead of specific words. Because the grammatical and phonological aspects of language may be better preserved in the early and middle stages, progressively shrinking vocabulary may not be apparent until much later.

- Severe impairment may be noted in word definition tasks and category-specific word list generation tasks (e.g., giving the names of animals); these problems are especially dominant in patients with temporal lobe pathology.

- Spontaneous conversation is reduced, but no severe naming difficulty occurs in patients with predominantly frontal atrophy; such patients may do well on visual object and space perception tasks and on Mini-Mental State Examination.

- Patients exhibit echolalia and verbal stereotypes, meaningless repetition of phrases, and monotonous recall of the same anecdotes or stories (*gramophone syndrome*). These characteristics are more noticeable in advanced stages of the disease.

- Comprehension of spoken and printed material is impaired; these problems become progressively worse.

- Speech is nonfluent with notable phonological problems; these difficulties are noted in a group of patients who have Pick-like pathology, but without Pick bodies or Pick cells.

These patients may not show significant behavioral changes or language comprehension problems in the early stages of the disease (Hodges, 2001).

- Muteness may be complete in the final stage of the disease; profoundly impaired memory and orientation, combined with confusion, lead to severe dementia.

Some patients with PiD may retain reading, writing, and visuospatial skills until the final stages.

Death of patients with PiD often is due to aspiration pneumonia or infection (as in DAT).

Medical Management of Patients with Frontotemporal Dementia

Very few studies have been published on medical management of patients with FTD. Some evidence suggests that treatment with seratonergic drugs may be beneficial, especially in patients with frontal lobe pathology who typically show reduced amount of seratonin. Seratonergic drugs reduce depression, apathy, and violent behaviors (Litvan, 2001).

Dopamine treatment for patients with FTD is controversial. It is not clear whether all or most patients with FTD have reduced amounts of dopamine (Litvan, 2001).

Behavioral Management of Patients with FTD

Behavioral management of patients with FTD is similar to the course to be described in the next chapter. Generally, clinical experience suggests that both the patient and the caregivers need behavioral treatment. Caregivers of patients with dementia are severely stressed, and the degree of stress they feel is correlated with nursing home placement of patients. The stress caregivers experience is physically harmful: Their immune response is impaired, resulting in vulnerability to infections. Studies have shown that treatment (especially emotional and social support) offered to caregivers improves the functioning of their immune system (Litvan, 2001).

Caregivers should be (a) educated on the disease and its inevitable progression, (b) closely monitored to detect depression or other psychiatric problems they may experience, (c) promptly offered counseling and psychiatric treatment, (d) provided social and emotional support, and (e) offered respite care of patients.

Parkinson's Disease

James Parkinson (1755–1824), an English physician, first described in 1817 the degenerative brain disease that now bears his name (Olanow, Watts, & Koller, 2001; Rajput, 2001). Ironically, neither Parkinson nor other experts thought that dementia was a part of this neurological disease. Since the 1980s, there has been general agreement that Parkinson's disease can cause dementia. Some experts classify dementia associated with Parkinson's disease as *subcortical* (Cummings & Benson, 1992).

Parkinson's disease (PD) is more common in males than in females (Cummings & Benson, 1992). Its prevalence rate is relatively uniform around the world (Simon, Aminoff, & Greenberg, 1999). Prevalence of the disease escalates with age: Its general prevalence is 106 per 100,000 individuals, but it afflicts 1 in 100 after age 50. About 1 million people in the United States have PD, and about 60,000 new cases are reported each year (Olanow, Watts, & Koller, 2001). The average age of onset is 60 years, although a juvenile form exists. Most patients survive for about 8 years postonset, longer if the disease is diagnosed in younger people.

The term **Parkinson's disease,** also known as *paralysis agitans,* refers to a single disease entity. Traditionally, it has been described as *idiopathic* because its causes are unknown, although research continues to shed more light on its pathology and potential causes. The term *parkinsonism* refers to a group of neurologic disorders with hypokinesia, tremor, and muscular rigidity, but these disorders may have different causes (e.g., *postencephalitic parkinsonism, drug-induced parkinsonism*). A *parkinsonian* disease may refer to any one of these diseases. Unfortunately, sources are not consistent with each other or with themselves in the use of these terms.

The reported incidence of dementia in patients with PD is highly variable across studies. A review of studies suggests that 35 to 55 percent of patients with PD may develop dementia (Cummings & Benson, 1992). Parkinson's patients for whom the diagnosis of dementia is not applied may still show mild cognitive deficits.

Etiology of Parkinson's Disease

Although the etiological factors are not well understood (hence the term *idiopathic* in most cases), recent research suggests the importance of genetic factors in some cases. An autosomal dominant pattern of inheritance has been identified in a familial form of the disease.

An autosomal recessive form of inheritance has been identified in cases with a relatively early onset of the disease. Mutations in the gene on the long arm of chromosome 6 have been noted. The gene encodes a protein called *parkin* (Olanow et al., 2001).

Parkinson's disease that begins after age 50 may be associated with such environmental factors as exposure to pesticides and herbicides, rural living, and drinking well water. In the majority of cases, a genetic susceptibility and exposure to environmental toxins may be involved (Olanow et al., 2001).

Neuropatholgy of Parkinson's Disease

Parkinson's disease (paralysis agitans or shaking palsy) is a slowly progressing disease characterized by the following (Giasson et al., 2001; Olanow et al., 2001; Rajput, 2001; Subramanian, 2001):

- *Degeneration of nuclei.* This is evident especially in the brainstem.
- *Widened sulci.* This is evident especially in the frontal region.
- *Loss of cells from the substantia nigra.* Most severe changes occur in this structure. Less severe loss may be found in other parts of the brainstem and diencephalic nuclei.
- *Neurofibrillary tangles and neuritic plaques.* These cortical abnormalities, typically found in patients with Alzheimer's disease, may be

found in the cortical regions of many patients with PD (Olanow et al., 2001).

- *Presence of Lewy bodies.* Known as intraneural inclusion granules, these Lewy bodies are found in the basal ganglia, brainstem, spinal cord, and sympathetic ganglia (see "Dementia of Lewy Body Type" in a later section for more on Lewy bodies).

- *Reduced dopamine levels.* Depleted levels of this inhibitory neurotransmitter are especially evident in the basal ganglia. Other brain chemicals, including norepinephrine, glutamate decarboxylase, and seratonin, also may be depleted. The loss of neurochemicals is attributed to neuronal cell loss. Depleted levels of dopamine cause a lack of inhibitory potential, leading to excessive cholinergic excitation and consequent motor symptoms of Parkinson's patients.

Movement Disorders in Parkinson's Disease

Movement disorders are the main motor symptoms of patients with PD.

Bradykinesia. Also known as *hypokinesia* or *akinesia,* bradykinesia refers to immobility or slow voluntary movements. Diminished facial expression and decreased spontaneous eye blinking give the appearance of a mask-like face.

Tremor. Most frequent in resting muscles, these are the 4-, 6-, or 8-Hz tremors. Starting with the hand or foot, they may spread to all four limbs. The tremors are exacerbated with stress and diminished during voluntary activity.

Rigidity. Increased tone and resistance to movement are evident in the muscles of limbs and trunk; if severe, tremors may be absent.

Disturbed gait and posture. A standing flexed position is typical. Difficulty standing up from a sitting position, small and shuffling steps, forward leaning, absence of hand swinging while walking, and festinating gait (taking short, accelerating, involuntary steps while walking) characterize these disturbances.

Falls. Because of their motor dysfunction, patients with PD are prone to fall frequently.

Freezing. Patients with PD tend to freeze during movement—their feet "stick" to the ground. Freezing is more common when initiating walking or while passing through a doorway.

Swallowing disorders. Dysphagia, which occurs in 40 percent of patients, may be more severe during periods when the levodopa is not effective (see the section on medical treatment). The patient may drool because of swallowing problems.

Dementia and Related Problems Associated with Parkinson's Disease

Dementia found in patients with PD is typically mild to moderate in severity. Roughly 30 to 40 percent of patients with PD may develop dementia, although across studies, the prevalence rates vary from 20 to 50 percent (Simuni & Hurtig, 2001). Dementia is more likely if Parkinson's disease had its onset after age 60. Communication and related deficits in patients with Parkinson's disease and dementia have been documented in recent years (see Murray, 2000, and Murray & Stout, 1999, for reviews). The various characteristics of patients with dementia associated with Parkinson's disease include the following (Giasson et al., 2001; Murray & Stout, 1999; Olanow et al., 2001; Rajput, 2001; Simuni & Hurtig, 2001):

- *Memory problems.* Deterioration in memory skills is evident as in other forms of dementia. Some evidence suggests that unlike those with Alzheimer's disease, patients with PD may find it especially difficult to recall dates more so than events.

- *Naming problems.* The more advanced the dementia, the greater the extent of naming problems. To the contrary, patients with Alzheimer's disease may have mild dementia and yet have severe naming problems.

- *Impaired wordlist generation.* However, Parkinson's patients are less impaired in this skill than are Alzheimer's.

- *Impaired discourse comprehension.* Although patients with mild or no dementia may comprehend the main points of discourse, they still may miss detailed or implied aspects of what is said during conversation.

- *Impaired visuospatial perception.* Atypical of patients with subcortical dementia, those with Parkinson's disease may have difficulty with angle matching, figure-ground discrimination, perception of spatial position, constancy of shape and size, and touching their own body parts shown on a diagram.

- *Voice problems.* Monopitch and monoloudness are the two major and common voice problems. Hoarseness, breathiness, and roughness also may be observed. Some patients may be hypernasal.

- *Increased duration and frequency of pauses.* Hesitations and pauses may be more evident at the beginning of sentences.

- *Dysarthric speech.* Nearly half of all patients with PD show motor speech disorders. Parkinson's disease is the most common cause of *hypokinetic dysarthria* (Yorkston, Miller, & Strand, 2003). The speech rate may be slowed, increased, or festinating. Reduced speech, short phrases, short rushes of speech, and imprecise production of consonants are other dominant features of hypokinetic dysarthria. Repetitions of phonemes also may be a feature of this speech disorder.

- *Apathy and depression.* Patients with PD tend to show apathy (flat affect), social withdrawal, anxiety, and depression.

- *Confusion, hallucination, and delirium may be observed in some patients.* Visual hallucinations are more common than auditory hallucinations. The patients are unlikely to report their hallucinations to their caregivers (Korczyn, 2001). These symptoms may be aggravated by antiparkinsonian medications.

- *Sleep disturbances.* More than 75 percent of patients with PD may have difficulty falling asleep, daytime sleepiness, and fragmented sleep. Nightmares and disturbingly vivid dreams may aggravate sleep disturbances. Possibly related to levodopa, some patients may suddenly fall asleep (*sleep attacks*).

- *Micrographia.* Writing in extremely small letters is a feature of patients with PD, which is not a dominant feature of patients with Alzheimer's disease.

Symptoms of aphasia, agnosia, and severe amnesia are rare in patients who have dementia associated with Parkinson's disease.

Medical Treatment of Parkinson's Disease

Levodopa, a neurotransmitter, is the most commonly prescribed drug treatment for patients with PD. This neurotransmitter reduces some neurological symptoms, especially the movement disorders. To control nausea and vomiting that levodopa tends to induce, the drug is usually combined with another, called *decarboxylase inhibitor* (Olanow et al., 2001; Rascol, Goetz, Koller, Poewe, & Sampaio, 2002; Colcher & Stern, 2001). Some improvement in intellectual functions has been associated with levodopa treatment.

Long-term administration of levodopa is associated with serious motor and neuropsychiatric complications. Motor complications include motor fluctuations and dyskinesia. Motor fluctuations consist of cyclic periods during which the patient either responds to treatment with reduced movement problems or fails to respond with increased problems. In addition to motor fluctuations, the patient also may experience fluctuations in mood and cognition. Long-term use of levodopa may aggravate cognitive impairment and confusion, if already present.

Dyskinesia associated with long-term use of levodopa includes involuntary, choreiform, or dance-like movements, involving the head, neck, torso, limbs, and respiratory muscles.

Another class of drugs used to treat patients with PD is known as *dopamine agonists,* which directly stimulate dopamine receptors and minimize the motor complications associated with dopamine treatment. For this reason, they often are combined with levodopa. However, dopamine agonists tend to induce such psychiatric symptoms as hallucinations.

Because of persistent and worsening motor complications and dyskinesia associated with drug treatment, neurosurgical alternatives have been researched. There are three techniques, all grouped under *functional neurosurgery,* designed to destroy overactive brain tissues. In **thalamotomy,** the ventral intermediate nucleus of the thalamus is surgically ablated, resulting in reduced frequency and magnitude of tremors. In **pallidotomy,** the internal segments of the globus pallidus is ablated. Finally, in **subthalamic nucleotomy,** the subthalamic nucleus is ablated. In addition to reducing tremors, the latter two procedures help minimize akinesia, rigidity, gait problems, and postural disturbances (Olanow et al., 2001; Rascol et al., 2002). All surgical ablative procedures run the risk of destroying neighboring tissue, causing such additional problems as dysarthria, dysphagia, and cognitive deficits. Therefore, an alternative to surgical ablation of target structures is to use a procedure called **high-frequency deep brain stimulation (DBS),** which does not ablate brain tissue but simulates the effects of ablation. The DBS procedure requires the implantation of electrodes in target brain cells. The electrodes are connected to an externally controllable pulse generator placed over the chest wall, just below the skin.

Fetal transplantation of aborted embryonic dopaminergic tissue into the brain of patients with PD is currently an experimental procedure (Colcher & Stern, 2001; Subramanian, 2001). Animal studies and postmortem examinations of implanted patients' brains have shown that implanted embryonic nigral cells innervate, grow, and begin to function in brain regions affected by the disease. The procedure needs additional research to determine the best implantation sites (Lindvall, 2001).

Another experimental procedure is to implant **stem cells,** which are precursor cells that can differentiate into virtually any kind of cell, into the patient's affected brain sites (Lindvall, 2001). Human embryonic stem cell implantation has shown some promise.

Transplantation of fetal brain tissue or embryonic stem cells needs additional research for its efficacy and long-term benefits. The procedures have lead to ethical controversies.

In some cases, levodopa and other antiparkinsonian drugs may have to be reduced or withdrawn to control hallucinations. **Antipsychotic** (also called *neuroleptic*) **drugs** may be necessary to reduce confusion and hallucinations. Antidepressant medications also may be necessary for some patients.

No current treatment procedure can reverse the course of the disease. All medical treatments are designed to control or minimize the effects of the disease until it progresses to a stage where the treatment's effects begin to diminish (Cummings & Benson, 1992).

Huntington's Disease (HD)

In 1872, George Huntington (1850–1916), an American physician, described the case of a Long Island family with an idiopathic degenerative disease of the brain characterized by chorea, psychiatric problems, and cognitive decline. The disease now bears his name (Hake & Farlow, 2001). Previously, the disease also was known as *Huntington's chorea.* Because chorea may not be present in some patients, the term *Huntington's disease* is currently preferred.

Huntington's disease is a genetic (inherited) neurodegenerative disease. With autosomal dominant inheritance, half the offspring of an affected person may have the disease. The genetic mutation causing Huntington's disease occurs on the short arm of chromosome 4 and results in dozens of copies of the DNA sequence CAG (cytosine-adenine-guanine). CAG codes for the amino acid type of neurotransmitter called *glutamate* (Glu). Such repeated CAG sequences cause the symptoms, with a greater number of repeats causing more severe symptoms and earlier onset of the disease (Haines, 2004; Simon, Aminoff, & Greenberg, 1999). This mutation is thought to have originated in Britain and spread to other parts of the world because of British colonization (Harper, 1996). A destructive product of the gene mutation is called *huntingtin,* a malformed protein that kills the brain cells that control movement and memory. The huntingtin protein negatively affects mitochondrial membranes of cells. A genetic test is available and provides for accurate diagnosis of the disease.

The incidence of Huntington's disease is about 40 to 70 per million persons with equal male-female distribution. The typical age of onset is between 35 and 40 years. In about 5 percent of the cases, the disease begins before age 20 (Harper, 1996).

Some experts classify dementia associated with HD as *subcortical* (Cummings & Benson, 1992).

Neuropathology of HD

The general neuropathology found in patients with HD is loss of neurons primarily in the basal ganglia. Neuronal loss is striking in the caudate nucleus and the putamen in the basal ganglia. Neuronal loss may be found in the globus pallidus to a lesser extent. Atrophy may be evident in the prefrontal and parietal lobes as well. The extent of cortical cell loss in Huntington's disease is controversial (Klein, Ferrante, & Ball, 2001).

The neuronal loss in the basal ganglia results in reduced levels of such inhibitory neurotransmitters as GABA (gamma-amino butyric acid) and acetylcholine. In contrast to Parkinson's disease, HD is not associated with dopamine depletion. Inhibitory neurotransmitters help regulate movement.

Dementia and Related Problems Associated with HD

Communication patterns of patients with HD are similar to those of patients with Parkinson's disease (Murray, 2000; Murray & Stout, 1999; Yorkston, Miller, & Strand, 2003). Generally, patients with HD tend to exhibit the following kinds of deficits:

- Behavioral changes, including excessive complaining, nagging, eccentricity, irritability, emotional outbursts, and a false sense of superiority, are among the earliest signs of the disease and precede chorea in a majority of cases.
- Serious psychiatric disturbances such as mood swings (depression and euphoria) and schizophrenic-like behaviors (paranoia, persecutory delusions, and hallucinations) characterize patients in more advanced stages. Suicide accounts for approximately 8 percent of deaths of patients with HD, and attempted suicide is common. Psychiatric disturbances precede chorea in about one-third of patients.
- **Chorea** is the major neurological symptom of HD; it is the irregular, spasmodic, involuntary movement of the limbs, neck, head,

and facial muscles. The initial form of chorea may be mere restlessness and fidgeting, eventually developing into grossly abnormal chorea.

- Various ticlike movement disorders, including transient facial grimaces and head nodding, are among the early neurological symptoms. These movements become increasingly uncontrollable.

- Gait disturbances typical of patients with HD include alternating hand extension-pronation and flexion-supination while walking. These movements, when combined with lurching, halting, and faltering movements give patients the appearance of dancing while walking.

- Slow movements characterize the advanced stage of the disease. In the final stages, the patient may exhibit little voluntary movement.

- Rigidity, an atypical form of movement disorder that typically characterizes patients with Parkinson's disease, may be seen in 12 to 14 percent of patients. This condition is known as the *Westphal variant,* which is more commonly seen in HD of juvenile onset (onset before age 20) and frequently associated with epilepsy.

- Impaired memory for both recent and remote events, attentional deficits, and slowness at all intellectual activities follow the onset of chorea.

- Communication deficits that become evident only in later stages of the disease include impaired word-list generation, mild naming difficulties (especially in recalling low-frequency words), shorter or simpler utterances, fewer grammatically correct utterances, and difficulties in comprehending subtle and implied aspects of discourse.

- Dysarthria is a prominent characteristic of patients with HD (Yorkston, Miller, & Strand, 2003). Choreiform movements of the lips and the tongue affect speech articulation, resulting in dysarthria of the hyperkinetic type. Such movements of the respiratory muscles and larynx cause other symptoms of hyperkinetic dysarthria, including excess variations in speech loudness, monoloudness, short phrases, monopitch, and harsh voice quality.

- The patient may be mute in the final stage of the disease. Extreme intellectual deterioration typically accompanies muteness.
- In the final stages, the patient may experience incontinence, sleep disturbances, dysphagia, and sleep reversal. Some patients may be violent and extremely confused. Patients are prone to diabetes, heart disease, lung disease, and infections of various sorts. Typically, death comes within 10 to 20 years postonset.

Medical Treatment of Huntington's Disease

Although no cure exists, symptomatic treatments are available to manage the neurological and psychiatric problems of patients with HD. Such tranquilizers as phenothiazine and haloperidol are frequently prescribed to control the abnormal movements. Some GABA-ergic drugs have also been shown to be beneficial for some patients. Unlike patients with Parkinson's disease, levodopa treatment is contraindicated; it worsens the choreiform movements.

Psychiatric problems may be controlled by psychotropic drugs. Antidepressants, for example, will help minimize depression, and neuroleptic agents may help control irritability and angry outbursts (Cummings & Benson, 1992).

Several newer treatments for HD are currently being investigated. Because the patients are known to have mitochondrial energy deficits, one line of treatment research is examining the usefulness of a nutritional supplement known as *co-enzyme Q*. Some cell death is a product of overstimulation. Therefore, drugs are being tested to reduce such harmful stimulation of target cells.

Surgical treatment under investigation includes transplantation of fetal stem cells or fetal basal ganglionic cells into the affected areas of patients' brains (e.g., the putamen and the head of the caudate nucleus). Preliminary results have shown improvement or stabilization in motor and cognitive functions in some patients (Lindvall, 2001; Lindvall & Bjorklund, 2000; McMurray, 2001). It is not clear whether any of these treatments will eventually stop or reverse the course of the disease.

Progressive Supranuclear Palsy

Progressive supranuclear palsy (PSP) is a degenerative neurological disorder whose symptoms are similar to those found in Parkinson's disease. PSP is an extrapyramidal disorder with typical onset in the sixth or seventh decade of life. A relatively rare disorder, PSP affects more males than females.

Neuropathology of PSP is largely limited to the basal ganglia and the brainstem, sparing mostly the cortical structures. General neuronal loss, neurofibrillary tangles, granulovacuolar degeneration, demyelination, and gliosis are frequently noted (Greenberg, Aminoff, & Simon, 2002). Neurochemical deficiencies include depleted levels of dopamine and impaired cholinergic system.

The neurological symptoms of PSP include rigidity, slowness of movement (bradykinesia), and impaired balance, which also characterize patients with Parkinson's disease. A differential diagnostic sign is that patients with PSP do not exhibit tremors that characterize patients with Parkinson's disease. Additional symptoms of PSP include impaired eye movements, a thrust-back head position, masklike face, jerky movements of the face and jaw, dysphagia, and drooling. Ophthalmic deviations are an early symptom of PSP. Impaired downgaze appears early. Unable to look down while walking, the patient tends to fall down. Later, upward and lateral eye movements are also affected.

Dementia due to supranuclear palsy is classified as a form of subcortical dementia (Cummings & Benson, 1992). The symptoms of dementia include apathy, depression, slowness of thought processes, and forgetfulness. Frightening visual hallucinations and delusions based on those hallucinations may also be present. Generally, intellectual deterioration is not severe until the later stages of the disease.

Communication problems associated with PSP include dysarthria, which may be one of the earliest speech disorders to be noted. Patients with PSP may exhibit a variety of dysarthria types, including hypokinetic, mixed hypokinetic-spastic, and mixed hypokinetic-spastic-ataxic dysarthrias. Typically, dysarthria associated with PSP includes monopitch, hoarseness, nasal emission, excess and equal stress, hypernasality, and imprecise articulation (Duffy, 1995).

Language skills are not affected until the final stages of PSP. With worsening dysarthria, the patient becomes unintelligible. Eventually, the patient becomes mute.

Medical management of PSP is limited to controlling depression and apathy with psychotropic drugs. Levodopa treatment has been found to be beneficial in controlling the motor symptoms in some patients (Cummings & Benson, 1992). All medical treatments lose their effects as the disease progresses.

Infectious Dementias

Several infections can lead eventually to dementia. These include dementia due to HIV infection (Larsen, 1998) and that due to Creutzfeldt-Jakob disease (Cummings & Benson, 1992).

AIDS Dementia Complex (Human Immunodeficiency Virus Encephalopathy)

Human immunodeficiency virus (HIV) infection and the resulting acquired immune deficiency syndrome (AIDS) terminates in a form of subcortical dementia and death. This has been a more recently found, and currently the most frequently reported, variety of infectious dementia (Larsen, 1998).

HIV infection is under control in the United States and other western industrialized countries. Since 1995, there has been a decline in the incidence of the infection in the United States. The incidence of the disease is still high in many Asian and African countries. It is estimated that worldwide, some 30 million people may have been affected (Rabins, Lyketsos, & Steele, 1999).

HIV-1 infection causes a variety of symptoms, including many associated with various neurologic diseases. Because of the reduced efficiency of the body's immune system, various *opportunistic infections,* which are infections that invade the weakened body and produce their own variety of symptoms, also occur. For example, HIV-infected people are especially prone to such opportunistic brain infections as cryptococcal meningitis—causing language disturbances, affective disorders, and problems in executive functions—and toxoplasmosis—causing a subcortical form of dementia.

Even without opportunistic infections, HIV infection itself affects the brain and causes dementia. Known as *HIV encephalopathy, AIDS dementia complex,* or *HIV-1-associated dementia,* the disease has a slow progression although the terminal stage is characterized by rapid deterioration resulting in death. Most patients with HIV infection will develop dementia to varying degrees and at varying intervals; in some individuals, diagnosis of dementia may *precede* the diagnosis of full-blown AIDS.

Encephalopathy is a general term that refers to any disease of the brain; most are degenerative. HIV encephalopathy causes degeneration of subcortical white matter, basal ganglia, and eventually, cortical layers (Cummings & Benson, 1992).

Symptoms of AIDS dementia complex include the following:

- Neurologic symptoms may, with some variability across patients, consist of gait disturbances, tremor, headache, seizures, ataxia, rigidity, motor weakness, myoclonus, facial nerve paralysis, and incontinence.
- Dementia symptoms may consist of forgetfulness, impaired concentration, slow thinking, apathy, loss of interest in work, diminished sex drive, social withdrawal, depression and mania, confusion, hallucinations, and delusions. Memory loss may intensify as the disease progresses; language problems may become less prominent although mutism is evident in the final stage.

Medical management of HIV infection has progressed significantly during the past decade. Treatment with a combination of drugs known as highly active antiretroviral therapy (HAART) has been effective in (a) reducing the HIV viral load in the body, (b) minimizing the number of symptoms or their severity, (c) prolonging the life of patients, (d) decreasing the incidence of opportunistic infections, (e) reducing the mortality rate, and (f) lessening the incidence of AIDS dementia complex by about 50 percent. Unfortunately, HAART induces some toxic effects that are on the increase as a progressively higher number of patients have received the treatment over longer periods of time (Sacktor, 2002).

Creutzfeldt-Jakob Disease

Named after two German psychiatrists, Hans Creutzfeldt (1885–1964) and Alfons Jakob (1884–1931), the **Creutzfeldt-Jakob disease** is thought to be caused by a viral infection. It is a rare disease, with an incidence of 1 in a million, that is associated with dementia.

Although no virus has been microscopically identified, an unconventional infectious agent called *prion,* which stands for proteinaceous infectious particle (a form of protein), has been proposed because traces of prion have been demonstrated in the brains of patients who have had the Creutzfeldt-Jakob disease. Therefore, dementia due to Creutzfeldt-Jakob disease is sometimes referred to as a form of *prion dementia.* The disease does not produce inflammation or an immune response, but it leads to widespread development of a spongiform state in the brain.

Typical onset occurs when the individuals are in their 60s or 70s, although the age range of onset is 60 to 82 years. A positive family history is found in about 10 percent of cases. The gender distribution of the diseases is roughly equal. Although considered infectious, human-to-human transmission is rare. Human-to-animal transmission of the disease has been experimentally demonstrated, however.

Unlike most other dementias, this form shows a more rapid course with certain fatality. Most patients die within 12 to 18 months postonset; the mean duration of illness is 7 months. No treatment is available for this disease.

A new form of Creutzfeldt-Jakob disease is known as *bovine spongiform encephalopathy* because the infection is thought to be transmitted from cows (bovine) to humans. The mean age of onset is about 30 years, and the course of disorder is more prolonged than in the classic Creutzfeldt-Jakob disease. Early symptoms include depression and behavioral changes.

Neuropathology associated with the Creutzfeldt-Jakob disease include the following:

- There is diffuse and varied loss of neurons in many cortical areas, the basal ganglia, the thalamus, the brainstem, and the spinal cord.
- There is spongiform states (soft and spongy tissue) in the brain, especially in the cerebral cortex, thalamus, caudate, and putamen. Spongiform states are due to empty spaces, called *vacuoles,* that form within brain cells.

Symptoms of Creutzfeldt-Jakob disease include the following:

- Initial symptoms include physical discomfort, fatigue, apprehension, sleep disorders, forgetfulness, and impaired concentration.
- Soon, such signs of dementia as memory problems, difficulty in reasoning, and impairment in problem solving tend to appear.
- Psychiatric symptoms that appear include anxiety, euphoria, depression, hallucinations, and delusions.
- Additional neurologic symptoms that appear include cerebellar ataxia, tremor, rigidity, chorea, athetosis, and visual problems.
- Inevitably, the disease leads to generalized and profound intellectual deterioration (dementia).
- The vegetative final stage of the disease is characterized by stupor, mutism, myoclonus, and seizures. Most patients die from such diseases as urinary tract infection and aspiration pneumonia.

Vascular Dementia

Vascular dementia is associated with a variety of diseases that affect the cerebral vascular system. Dementia due to vascular diseases that cause widespread, bilateral damage may be subcortical,

cortical, or both (mixed). Vascular disease also contributes to Alzheimer's disease. Vascular dementia is the second most common form of dementia, the first being the Alzheimer's type.

Some recent research has questioned the traditional thinking that dementia of the Alzheimer's type is distinct from vascular dementia. A few studies have suggested that an undiagnosed dementia of the Alzheimer's type probably existed when a vascular dementia was diagnosed following a stroke. The symptoms of an underlying dementia may become exacerbated following a stroke, thus leading to a diagnosis of vascular dementia (Jagust, 2001).

Vascular dementia is more common in men than in women and is associated with a history of hypertension. Compared to patients with DAT, those with vascular dementia are typically younger and die sooner. However, aggressive treatment for hypertension may reduce the incidence of dementia as well as the mortality rate.

Compared to whites, African Americans have a greater tendency to have the highest prevalence of high blood pressure, cerebrovascular diseases, and stroke. Therefore, vascular dementia is more common in African Americans than in whites.

Unlike most other forms of dementia, the onset of vascular dementia is relatively sudden, although dementia due to degeneration of subcortical white matter has a more gradual onset. The course of dementia fluctuates, and the patient experiences increased confusion during the night.

Vascular dementia is a heterogeneous syndrome, and there exists some disagreement in describing or classifying its varieties. The three commonly described varieties of vascular dementia are *multiple bilateral cortical infarcts, lacunar state,* and *Binswanger's disease.*

Multiple Bilateral Cortical Infarcts

Multiple bilateral cortical infarcts produce a variety of mixed dementia with both cortical and subcortical pathology. Dementia is the result of bilateral, multiple (repeated) cerebrovascular accidents due to thrombosis or embolism (see Chapter 3).

Most etiologic factors that cause cerebrovascular accidents resulting in aphasia (see Chapter 3) also can cause cerebrovascular dementia. While a single infarction produces focal damage and the classic syndromes of aphasia, multiple infarctions tend to result in diffuse damage and eventual dementia, often called **multi-infarct dementia (MID).**

Symptoms of MID depend on the frequency of infarcts and the areas they damage and include the following:

- Multiple neurological symptoms associated with MID include bilateral pyramidal and extrapyramidal symptoms consisting of limb rigidity, spasticity, hyperflexia, gait abnormality, hemiparesis or hemiplegia, and incontinence.

- Communication deficits depend on the type, frequency, and location of lesions and may include symptoms of aphasia and apraxia. Unlike patients with dementia of the Alzheimer's type, those with MID may retain some insight into their condition and an ability to respond emotionally. Consequently, their communicative failures and other problems may frustrate and distress them.

- Symptoms of dementia include a gradual deterioration in intellectual functions, inconsistent memory loss, poor judgment, deterioration in thinking, abstraction, and behavioral deterioration.

- The general course of slow decline may be interrupted by a sudden decline due to a major stroke. Immediately following such a major episode, the patient may experience delirium or acute confusion. Subsequently, intellectual functions may improve, although not to the previous levels.

Lacunar State

Lacunar states refer to a special type of neural atrophy associated with a variety of subcortical dementia. A **lacuna** is a hollow space, cavity, or gap in an anatomic structure. Cerebral lacunar states are created by *lacunae,* which are due to ischemic infarctions. Such infarctions occur within the deep structures of the brain because of the occlusion in small-end arterial branches of the middle cerebral, posterior cerebral, and basilar arteries. Multiple, small infarcts in the basal ganglia, thalamus, midbrain, and brainstem are common. Prolonged hypertension is significantly associated with lacunar states.

Symptoms of lacunar states include the following:

- Initially, the patient may have a stroke, hemiplegia, and related symptoms from which recovery is common. A long-standing history of hypertension characterizes these patients.
- Repeated infarcts result in persistent neurologic symptoms, including rigidity, plasticity, pseudobulbar palsy, and limb weakness.
- Dysarthria and swallowing problems may characterize most patients.
- Symptoms of dementia, found in 70 to 80 percent of cases, are not specific; the symptoms do not appear until the late stage of the disease.
- Language problems also do not appear until the late stage.
- Psychiatric symptoms include apathy, disinhibition (socially inappropriate behavior), and frequent mood swings.

Binswanger's Disease

Binswanger's disease, sometimes referred to as subcortical arteriosclerotic encephalopathy, is associated with *leukoareosis,* which is atrophy of the subcortical white matter. This kind of atrophy produces another variety of subcortical vascular dementia. This condition is due to multiple infarcts. Lacunar infarctions also are common in the basal ganglia and thalamus of patients with Binswanger's disease. Cortical structures are mostly spared. A history of long-standing and acute hypertension is associated with the disease.

Symptoms of Binswanger's disease, which resemble those of lacunar states, include the following:

- Acute strokes that eventually lead to a slow accumulation of focal neurologic symptoms
- Significant motor problems, including pseudobulbar palsy
- Intellectual deterioration and eventual dementia

Dementia Associated with Traumatic Brain Injury

Repeated brain injury is a cause of dementia in some cases. Severe forms of open or closed head injuries (see Chapter 12 for details) can cause dementia. Head injuries that cause prolonged periods of unconsciousness are especially likely to cause dementia. Other dementia risk factors associated with traumatic brain injury include older age at the time of injury, slower recovery from injury (longer hospital stays), limited premorbid intellectual status, presence of brain lesions prior to injury, and high velocity closed head injuries.

Depending on the site and extent of damage, traumatic brain injury may cause cortical, subcortical, or mixed types of dementia. Aphasic symptoms may be present in 30 percent of patients who sustain traumatic brain injury. Significant memory problems are a common problem. The patient may be unable to remember events preceding the trauma (retrograde amnesia) and may have difficulty learning or remembering new information (anterograde amnesia).

Dementia following traumatic brain injury also may be associated with such psychiatric symptoms as confusion, anxiety, withdrawal, depression, and poor attention.

A variation of posttraumatic dementia—seen in professional boxers who sustain repeated head injuries—is called **dementia pugilistica** ("punch drunk"). Dementia noted in boxers who have stopped boxing for years is characterized by intellectual slowness, memory deficits, irritability, gait disturbances, dysarthria, and parkinsonian symptoms. Paranoia, euphoria, and depression may be found in some cases.

Additional Dementia Syndromes

There are many other syndromes of dementia, and space will not allow a complete description of them. However, a few additional dementias are defined here to suggest the wide range of conditions that can cause dementia (American Psychiatric Association, 2000; Cummings & Benson, 1992).

Pseudodementias

Pseudodementias are dementias associated with psychiatric disorders. Cognitive and behavioral problems associated with such psychiatric disorders as depression, mania, and schizophrenia may be described as forms of dementia. Most patients who are diagnosed with pseudodementia are clinically depressed. Therefore, pseudodementia also may be described as *dementia associated with mood disorders.*

Differential diagnosis is important because some poststroke patients and patients with several other forms of dementia (e.g., those with Parkinson's disease) also may be depressed. Generally, pseudodementia due to psychiatric reasons has a more rapid onset than those that are due to degenerative diseases. Various test performances also may help distinguish true dementia from pseudodementia. Patients with true dementia are more stable in their test performance whereas those with pseudodementia are highly variable.

Dementia due to mood disorders is more effectively treated than those with degenerative diseases. Antidepressant drugs combined with behavioral or psychological methods may be beneficial in most cases.

Dementia Associated with General Medical Conditions

Various general medical conditions may be associated with dementia in certain cases. For instance, primary or secondary brain tumors may block the flow of cerebrospinal fluid and cause hydrocephalus dementia. Subdural hematoma, electric shock to the head, intracranial radiation, and multiple sclerosis (MS, a demyelinating disease of the white matter of the brain) may also lead to dementia.

Dementia of Lewy Body Type

Lewy body dementia is a relatively new diagnostic category. **Lewy bodies,** also known as intraneuronal cytoplasmic inclusions, are small pathologic spots within the damaged nerve cells, typically found in the substantia nigra, a structure at the top of the brainstem. This neuronal pathology is named after the German-born American neurologist Frederick Lewy (1885–1950).

Lewy bodies are usually found in the substantia nigra of patients with Parkinson's disease. In recent years, patients with a specific set of dementia symptoms who have Lewy bodies in cortical regions have been described. (Lewy bodies are not common in the cortical regions of patients with PD.) The disease is characterized by visual and auditory hallucinations, paranoid thoughts, mild features of Parkinson's disease (e.g., muscular rigidity and slowness of movement), and transient changes in consciousness leading to repeated falls. Unlike other dementias, visual and spatial skills, especially in the early stages, may be more severely involved than memory skills. A critical feature of these patients is a hypersensitivity to antipsychotic drugs, which may be prescribed because of the patients' hallucinations. Negative reaction to such drugs may be so severe as to cause death in some cases (Jacques & Jackson, 2000; Weiner, 1996).

Some experts think that Lewy body dementia is a variant of Alzheimer's disease because roughly a third of autopsied patients with Alzheimer's disease may have Lewy bodies in their cortical regions. Others believe that it is a separate disease with a unique course. Patients with Lewy body dementia are reported to deteriorate more rapidly than those with the Alzheimer's type (Jacques & Jackson, 2000; Weiner, 1996).

Dementia Due to Multiple Causes

In some cases, dementia may be due to multiple causes. For instance, dementia in some cases may be due to head trauma as well as Alzheimer's disease. In other cases, drug abuse and Parkinson's disease may both underlie dementia.

Suggested Readings

Read the following for additional information on other forms of dementia:

Clark, C. M., & Trojanowski, J. Q. (2000). *Neurodegenerative dementias.* New York: McGraw-Hill.

Dickson, D. W. (2001). Neuropathology of Pick's disease. *Neurology, 56* (Suppl 4), S16–S18.

Hodges, J. R. (2001). Frontotemporal dementia (Pick's disease): Clinical features and assessment. *Neurology, 56*(Suppl 4), S6–S9.

Jagust, W. (2001). Understanding vascular dementia. *Lancet, 358,* 2097–2098.

Larsen, C. (1998). *HIV and communication disorders.* Albany, NY: Thomson Delmar.

Litvan, I. (2001). Therapy and management of frontal lobe dementia patients. *Neurology, 56*(Suppl 4), S41–S44.

McMurray, C. T. (2001). Huntington's disease: Expanding horizons for treatment. *Lancet, 358*(Suppl), S37.

Rascol, O., Goetz, C., Koller, W., Poewe, W., & Sampaio, C. (2002). Treatment interventions for Parkinson's disease: An evidence based assessment. *Lancet, 359*(9317), 1589–1598.

Sacktor, N. (2002). The epidemiology of human immunodeficiency virus-associated neurological disease in the era of highly active antiretroviral therapy. *Journal of Neurovirology, 8*(Suppl 2), 115–121.

Yorkston, K. M., Miller, R. M., & Strand, E. A. (2003). *Management of speech and swallowing in degenerative diseases* (2nd ed.). Austin, TX: Pro-Ed.

CHAPTER 16

ASSESSMENT AND MANAGEMENT OF PATIENTS WITH DEMENTIA

Chapter Outline

- Assessment of Dementia
- Clinical Management of Dementia

Learning Objectives

After reading this chapter, the student will:

- Summarize accurately the various medical, neurological, laboratory, and family assessment parameters in evaluating patients with dementia.

- Give a brief description of procedures to assess mental status, cognitive functions, and intellectual levels of patients with dementia.

- Describe the procedures and tools of communication assessment.

- Specify the various management strategies implemented by different members of the dementia management team.

- Describe procedures designed to manage the communication and behavioral deficits of patients with dementia.

Assessment of Dementia

As noted in the previous chapter, extensive research on dementia done during the past few years has greatly advanced our understanding of this disease, leading to more accurate diagnosis. Although experimental research on clinical management techniques is still limited, many behavioral and medical strategies are now described in the literature.

Assessment of patients with dementia is a team effort. Both medical and nonmedical specialists contribute to the assessment process. As the disease has many facets, a comprehensive assessment can be both time consuming and expensive. In many cases, differential diagnosis among the varieties of dementia can be difficult. The final confirmation of a specific diagnosis of dementia may require neuropathological evidence from an autopsy.

The diagnosis of dementia is made on the basis of information collected from a variety of sources. A comprehensive assessment of impaired and spared skills is needed to design a management plan for each patient (Tomoeda, 2001). Assessment results reported by medical specialists, speech-language pathologists, psychologists, and other specialists need to be integrated to arrive at a diagnosis of dementia and develop a treatment plan.

The symptoms of moderate to severe dementia are easily recognized. Therefore, assessment of moderate to severe dementia poses no serious challenge, although a detailed documentation of behavioral deterioration is necessary for differential diagnosis. Diagnosis of mild dementia often requires a careful analysis of higher intellectual and language functions. Verbal description of common objects, immediate and delayed recall of events, and word fluency (asking the patient to say all the words that he or she can think of that start with the letter *t*) are three tasks that are especially helpful in diagnosing mild forms of dementia. Pointing to stimuli and automatic speech tasks are least sensitive in diagnosing early and mild forms of dementia. A speech-language pathologist may play a significant role in this diagnosis.

Most patients do not receive an early diagnosis because the patient and the family members tend to attribute such early symptoms as memory problems to normal aging. Family members may request an assessment only when a patient begins to exhibit dangerous behaviors or causes a crisis (Rabins, Lyketsos, & Steele, 1999). Early diagnosis is important because it might identify a reversible form of dementia that may be effectively treated. Even in cases of nonreversible dementia, an early diagnosis can help minimize the effects or stabilize the patient to the extent possible.

The goals of assessment are to make a diagnosis of dementia; measure intact and impaired skills; establish a baseline of skills against which improvement associated with intervention can be assessed; and design an intervention plan for the patient and a counseling and training plan for the caregivers. Because dementia is an age-related deterioration in skills and general behaviors, it is essential to distinguish negative changes associated with aging from a progressive disease process (Clark, 2000; Tomoeda, 2001).

Assessment of dementia requires the diagnostic team to collect information from the following sources:

- Case history
- Parameters of assessment
- Physical and neurological examination
- Laboratory tests
- Assessment of mental status, cognitive functions, and intellectual skills
- Communication assessment

Case History

A carefully obtained case history, especially when multiple family members are interviewed, will help assess the patient's premorbid skills and behavior patterns and initial signs of dementia the family members may have noticed. The clinician should seek information on a variety of issues, including the following:

- The reasons for seeking help (the current problems the patient, family members, or both see)
- Mode of onset of the symptoms that prompted consultation (sudden, gradual, constant, or variable)

- General health of the patient and any chronic diseases; medical and surgical treatment received
- Family constellation and current living conditions (information on caregivers, financial situation of the patient or family, any legal issues)
- Family history of dementia
- Educational and occupational history of the patient, including information on hobbies, leisure activities, religious faiths, and typical daily activities
- The time when family members noticed a change in the patient's behavior or intellectual functioning
- Medical conditions that could explain the changes, including:
  - Strokes (single or multiple), brain tumors, head injury, or other neurological problems
  - Infections (especially AIDS), high fever, convulsions, or other medical conditions that might suggest a reversible form of dementia
  - Alcoholism and other drug abuse along with prolonged use of anticonvulsants and certain antibiotics (e.g., penicillin)
  - Prolonged dialysis for kidney problems
  - Vitamin deficiencies (especially the B1 and B12 deficiency) and endocrine disorders
  - Long-standing lung and cardiac diseases, anemia, and anoxia
  - Neurological symptoms (e.g., tics, tremors, rigidity, facial gestures, gait disturbances) and the timing of their onset
  - History of Down syndrome in the family
- Long-standing signs of psychiatric problems (e.g., schizophrenia and associated delusions, hallucinations, paranoia, anxiety, depression, mania) that may have existed prior to the onset of dementia
- Changes in behavior (e.g., eating and sleeping problems, emergence of irritability, eccentricity, emotional outbursts, all forms of atypical behaviors, deterioration in memory and other intellectual tasks, and deterioration in self-care and in such daily activities as driving, cooking, and shopping)

- Changes in speech, language, communication, reading, and writing

A detailed case history will make a preliminary diagnosis of dementia and possibly suggest a differential diagnosis. A more firm diagnosis requires the completion of other aspects of assessment, however.

Parameters of Assessment

After taking a detailed case history, the clinician should select parameters (specific behaviors or skills) for assessment. In making a complete assessment, the following aspects of patients' skills, levels of functioning, or characteristics should be evaluated (Clark, 2000; Cummings and Benson, 1992; Tomoeda, 2001):

- *State of awareness.* Whether the patient is fully awake, aware of surroundings and questions asked, aware but depressed, not awake at all (mostly sleeping), or awake but confused should be evaluated.
- *Mood and affect.* Whether the patient feels depressed, feels optimistic about the future, or exhibits flatness of emotions should be evaluated.
- *Speech and language skills.* These are the skills that speech-language pathologists evaluate fully and provide extremely sensitive information for a differential diagnosis; the clinician should assess the presence of aphasia, apraxia, agraphia, alexia, and dysarthria in a total evaluation plan. In evaluating language, the clinician should sample spontaneous verbal output, comprehension of spoken language, repetition of spoken words, naming, reading, and writing. Speech and language assessment is further discussed in a subsequent section (see Communication Assessment).
- *Memory skills.* Whether the patient can learn new material, recall past events, and recall the most recent events should be assessed; whether the patient confabulates also should be assessed.
- *Other cognitive functions.* Such other functions as calculating arithmetic, understanding proverbs, and stating similarities and

differences between concepts or objects (e.g., "how are apples and bananas alike?") should be assessed.

- *Thought, belief, and judgment.* Presence of abnormal thinking, hallucinations or delusional beliefs, evidence of poor judgment, or lack of insight should be assessed.
- *Visuospatial skills.* Whether the patient can copy simple and three-dimensional drawings and construct block designs should be assessed.

Physical and Neurological Examination

Comprehensive physical and neurological examinations are necessary. The physical examination helps assess the patient's general health. A complete neurological examination helps assess sensory systems (e.g., visual and auditory sensations), cranial nerve functioning, muscle strength and tone, and movement disorders, including gait problems and tremors.

Comprehensive medical and neurological tests encompass a variety of laboratory tests, including routine X-rays and brain imaging, described in the next section on laboratory tests.

Laboratory Tests

Some laboratory tests (e.g., blood and urine) may be normal in DAT and other idiopathic progressive neurological diseases. However, blood, urine, and spinal fluid analysis may be helpful in diagnosing infectious diseases (such as AIDS) that are associated with dementia. Elevated levels of a protein called tau (hyperphosphorylated tau) in the cerebrospinal fluid (CSF) is thought to be a biochemical marker of neurofibrillary tangles. Therefore, a laboratory analysis of CSF tau levels is often done (Clark, 2000).

Other laboratory tests include electroencephalogram (EEG), skull X-ray, and various brain imaging techniques that were described in Chapter 3. Computed tomography (CT) or magnetic resonance imaging is considered usually sufficient to visualize brain atrophy and related problems by examining the skull, brain, ventricles, and various gyri and sulci. Magnetic resonance imaging (MRI) is helpful in visualizing cortical and subcortical structures, including the basal ganglia and hippocampus. In addition to atrophy, various imaging techniques may also reveal malignant growth, cerebral bleeding, and other abnormalities (Clark, 2000).

Functional imaging of the brain offers additional information on the integrity of visualized structures. Degenerative diseases affect cerebral metabolism, which can be studied by such techniques as positron emission tomography (PET), which helps assess glucose metabolism, and single-photon-emission computed tomography (SPECT), which helps assess regional cerebral blood flow. Unfortunately, these techniques may not detect mild cerebral hypometabolism associated with the early stage of dementia.

Assessment of Mental Status, Cognitive Functions, and Intellectual Skills

Supplemented with a carefully taken case history, an assessment of mental status and cognitive functions is the most crucial element of dementia diagnosis. Several assessment tests and batteries are available. The following are among the commonly used instruments:

- *The Mini-Mental State Examination (MMSE)* (Folstein, Folstein, & McHugh, 1975). This brief screening test of general mental state is useful to identify possible dementia. The test does not measure specific behaviors in detail, however. With a normal score of 30, a score below 25 is considered clinically significant. The test asks simple questions to assess orientation (e.g., asking "what is the date?"), "registration" (e.g., asking "name three objects"), attention and calculation (asking the patient to count backward by 7 or to spell a word backward), recall of names tested earlier, basic language skills (e.g., asking the patient to point to selected objects, repeating phrases, following commands, and writing a sentence), and figure copying. A modified Mini-Mental State Examination (Teng & Chui, 1987) is available with expanded items and a wider range of scores (0–100 as against 0–30 in the original).

- *The Blessed Dementia Scale* (Blessed, Tomlinson, & Roth, 1968). This is a widely used rating scale. Based on information provided by family members, professional caregivers, and medical records, the clinician rates changes in performance in everyday activities (e.g., inability to perform household tasks or to find way about indoors) and a variety of changes in habits (e.g., eating, dressing, sphincter control, emotional control). Scores are specified for *no impairment* (below 4), *mild impairment* (4 to 9), and *moderate to severe impairment* (10 and higher with a maximum possible score of 28).

- *The Global Deterioration Scale (GDS)* (Reisberg, Ferris, DeLeon, & Crook, 1982). This is another frequently used 7-point rating scale to measure deterioration in behavior and intellect. The GDS requires information gathered from a variety of sources, including the patient's complaints and reactions (e.g., subjective feelings of memory loss) on levels of functioning ranging from *no cognitive decline* to *very severe decline*. Clinically significant scores on the GDS range from 3 (mild cognitive impairment) through 4 (mild dementia), 5 (moderate dementia), 6 (moderately severe dementia), and 7 (severe dementia). This scale has been widely used in treatment efficacy research studies (Ferris & Mohs, 2000) although it is known to be relatively insensitive to pharmacological effects unless the effects are large.

- *The Progressive Deterioration Scale (PDS)* (Dejong, Osterlund, & Roy, 1989). This scale helps assess changes in activities of daily living (ADL) that help document deterioration over time. ADL scales generally evaluate a patient's personal care tasks (e.g., eating, dressing) and skills required to live independently (e.g., managing money, using the telephone or other household appliances, being able to live alone). The PDS consists of 27 questions answered by caregivers and measures functional decline in patients. This scale also has been found to be useful in assessing treatment efficacy in patients with dementia.

- *The Clinical Dementia Rating Scale (CDR)* (Morris, 1993). The CDR is similar to the GDS in that both result in a global rating of skills and behaviors from information gathered through structured interviews of the patient and caregivers. It helps assess six categories of cognitive functions: memory, orientation, problem solving and judgment, community affairs, home and hobbies, and personal care. A patient's degree of impairment may be rated as follows: 0 for *none,* 0.5 for *questionable,* 1 for *mild,* 2 for *moderate,* and 3 for *severe.* Although used in treatment research, the CDR, like the GDS, is somewhat insensitive to small pharmacological effects.

- *Alzheimer's Disease Assessment Scale (ADAS)* (Rosen, Mohs, & Davis, 1984). Another assessment scale more widely used in medical settings, the ADAS helps assess both noncognitive and cognitive behaviors and their deterioration over time as a consequence of Alzheimer's disease. This scale was especially designed to assess patients enrolled in drug trials (experiments) and provides alternative forms for repeatedly assessing the patients. The 40-item scale includes 11 items to assess cognitive skills. The scale helps assess memory, orientation, attention, reasoning, language skills, and motor performance. It yields a range of scores from 0 (no impairment) to 70 (profoundly impaired). This scale has emerged as the preferred instrument to assess improvement or effectiveness associated with pharmacological treatment effects in randomized clinical trials (Thomas, 2000).

- *Dementia Deficits Scale (DDS)* (Snow et al., 2004). This newer scale seeks to assess self-awareness of deficits in patients with dementia because lack of self-awareness of deficits may lead to dangerous behaviors. A multidimensional assessment instrument, the DDS evaluates self-awareness of cognitive, emotional, and functional deficits. The patient, clinician, and an informant may fill out separate, but parallel, forms. The instrument helps assess discrepancy between the deficit scores of the patient and the clinician and the patient and the informant. The greater the discrepancy, the lower the patient's self-awareness of deficits.

- *Activities of Daily Living Questionnaire (ADLQ)* (Johnson, Barion, Rademaker, Rehkemper, & Weintraub, 2004). This newer scale that targets daily living skills of patients with dementia is administered with the help of an informant who has observed the patient. The questionnaire targets six functions: self-care, household care, employment and recreation, shopping and money, travel, and communication. The ADLQ helps assess decline in daily living skills over time.

- *Specific memory tests.* Although scales of dementia assess memory skills to some extent, specific tests may be used to assess memory skills in detail. In assessing dementia, assessment of anterograde memory or recent memory for recently learned information is especially important. Several tests of memory are available. For instance, the Wechsler Memory Scale—Revised (Wechsler, 1987) helps assess immediate recall of digits or narratives, immediate recognition of figures, and so forth. Other tests include the Memory Assessment Scales (Williams, 1991) and the Benton Visual Retention Test (Benton, 1992). In the latter test, such visual memory as immediate reproduction of various stimulus cards is assessed.

- *General tests of intelligence.* Psychologists may administer tests of intelligence to evaluate the patient's general intellectual level. Such intelligence tests as the Wechsler Adult Intelligence Scale–III (WAIS–III) have been used in assessing patients with dementia (Wechsler, 1997). Some normative information is now available for persons who are 74 years old and older. Some subtests of the WAIS–III are especially relevant for evaluating intellectual deterioration due to dementia. Performance on the block design, digit symbol, and similarities tests shows greater degree of deterioration than that on the vocabulary and picture completion tests.

In administering tests and using the rating scales, the clinician needs to make many subjective judgments. Also, as noted in a later section, many tests and test batteries are not standardized on representative samples that include women, minority groups, and people of varied educational and socioeconomic backgrounds. Therefore, the results of such instruments should be interpreted with caution. Test and rating scale results should supplement detailed behavioral observations and in-depth assessment of specific skills (e.g., memory loss or language deterioration).

Communication Assessment

Changes in language skills are an important and often early indication of dementia. Changes in memory skills—another important early sign—may be evident during communication assessment. Therefore, a careful assessment of communication skills will help make a diagnosis of dementia, especially in its early stages. Communication assessment, when combined with the results of memory, intellectual (cognitive) functioning, and medical evaluation (including laboratory tests) will provide a comprehensive picture of the patient. Both informal and formal (standardized) procedures, as the following descriptions show, may be useful:

- *General picture description.* Pictures that depict a story or an event may be used to evaluate various aspects of language skills, including memory for words, temporal sequence, logical connections, antecedents and consequences, grammaticality of sentence structures, and topic maintenance. Many clinicians use the "cookie theft" picture of the Boston Diagnostic Aphasia Examination (Goodglass, Kaplan, & Barresi, 2001), but other similar pictures may be just as appropriate.

- *The Arizona Battery of Communication Disorders of Dementia* (Bayles & Tomoeda, 1991). This test is especially relevant for assessing dementia associated with Alzheimer's disease because the test was standardized on 50 patients with Alzheimer's disease and 50 normal adults matched for age. The battery consists of 4 screening subtests of speech discrimination, visual perception and literacy, visual fields, and visual agnosia and 14 subtests to assess mental status, linguistic expression, linguistic comprehension, and visual-spatial construction.

- *Various tests of aphasia.* In addition to instruments standardized on patients with dementia, speech-language pathologists can use various tests of aphasia, described in Chapter 8, to assess specific language impairments of patients with dementia. Some aphasia tests are not standardized on patients with dementia, although two of them—the Western Aphasia Battery (Appell, Kertesz, & Fishman, 1982) and Communicative Abilities in Daily Living (Fromm & Holland, 1989)—have been used with dementia patients with some normative information being made available. To test memory for names, appropriate subtests of an aphasia test or the Boston Naming Test (Kaplan, Goodglass, & Weintraub, 2001) may be used. Clients may be asked to give as many names as possible either within a category (e.g., food items or clothing items) or those that start with a given letter. Generally, patients with early stages of dementia recall more names starting with a given letter than those within a category. When their results are cautiously interpreted, tests of aphasia help identify communication and memory deficits.

- *Various tests of language comprehension.* Tests that include complex syntactic structures may be administered to detect changes in patients with early-stage dementia. Such instruments as the Test for Auditory Comprehension of Language (Carrow-Woodfolk, 1999) and Discourse Comprehension Test (Brookshire & Nicholas, 1993) may be administered. The latter test may be especially useful as it evaluates comprehension of main ideas, implied details, and stated details. Patients with mild dementia may have a marked deficiency recalling implied details offered during discourse. Both delayed storytelling tasks in which the patients recall details of brief stories told to them and the Peabody Picture Vocabulary Test (Dunn & Dunn, 1981) are known to detect memory changes in patients who are in their early stages of Alzheimer's disease.

Ethnocultural Considerations in Assessment

Research on ethnocultural issues in the assessment of patients with dementia is limited. The issues are similar to those raised in the assessment of aphasia. To interpret the results of assessment tests and batteries administered to patients with dementia requires normative data. Normative data on normal intellectual decline in older individuals are emerging. Nonetheless, normative data are established on a relatively small number of individuals who are not representative of diverse populations. Lack of ethnocultural balance in normative samples is still a troubling issue. In addition, test standardization samples do not adequately represent people of different socioeconomic levels, gender, educational backgrounds, and rural populations (Ogrocki & Welsh-Bohmer, 2000).

The clinician should follow general guidelines available in the literature on the assessment of clients with varied ethnocultural background apply (Battle, 2002; Payne, 1997; Screen & Anderson, 1994). Suggestions offered in the assessment of aphasia in ethnoculturally diverse clients are applicable to patients with dementia. See Chapter 8 for details.

Clinical Management of Dementia

Although there is no cure for dementia, interest in developing pharmacological, behavioral, and communication treatment strategies are on the increase. Until recently, controlled experimental research on communication and behavioral treatment of patients with dementia has been limited, possibly because of the poor prognosis for neurodegenerative diseases. Fortunately, the idea that it is of no value to treat patients with progressive brain disorders is rapidly changing (Bayles & Kim, 2003; Bourgeois et al., 2003; Hopper, 2003). Based on some of the treatment studies done to date, clinicians and clinical researchers now believe that well developed treatment procedures may prove useful to both the patients and their caregivers. Patients with dementia have been shown to be capable of new learning that generalizes to other situations and is maintained over time (Bourgeois et al., 2003; Camp, Bird, & Cherry, 2000).

Systematic behavioral interventions that include family or caregiver training combined with pharmacological treatment for the patient may hold the greatest promise for improving skills or slowing functional deterioration in patients with dementia (Abrahams & Camp, 1993; Arkin, 1998, 2001; Bayles & Kim, 2003; Bourgeois & Mason, 1996; Bourgeois et al., 2003; Camp et al., 1996, 2001; Chapman et al., 2004; Mahendra, 2001; Mahendra & Arkin, 2003; Mahendra & Arkin, 2004; Quayhagen & Quayhagen, 1989, 2001). In both medical and behavioral treatment research, dementia of the Alzheimer's type has received much attention, partly because of its high prevalence.

There is intense interest in developing and testing newer and more effective pharmacological treatments for patients with dementia. With increased funding made available for treatment research, many investigators are at work to develop new medical and nonmedical strategies of treatment or clinical management.

Measuring the Effects of Dementia Intervention Strategies

Although treatment research studies are on the increase, measurement of treatment effects in patients with dementia poses special challenges. Because age is a natural and uncontrollable variable inducing deficits that are exaggerated in dementia, treatment research has to separate the effects of aging from those of the special disease process—a task that is riddled with methodological complications (Ferris & Mohs, 2000; Thomas, 2000).

Even in new drug treatment evaluation studies, the effects are measured only on behaviors because there is no way of measuring the biological effects of medications (Ferris & Mohs, 2000). Thus, the question of what is a treatment effect in dementia may be answered in many ways. Short of a complete cure, which is many years away, one gets what one can get out of treatment. In the order of most desirable to minimally acceptable effects, one might expect: (1) a reversal of the deteriorating process and recovery of normal skills (cure); (2) partial recovery of most skills; (3) partial recovery of some skills; (4) reduction in the severity of symptoms while the progression of the disease is slowed; and (5) reduction in the severity of symptoms while the rate of deterioration is unabated. At least one of these outcomes must be realized to document treatment effects.

To reduce variability in what is measured and how it was measured in pharmacological treatment efficacy studies, the U.S. Food and Drug Administration (FDA) helped develop guidelines on what should be measured and how to document the effects of new drug treatments for dementia (Ad Hoc Dementia Assessment Task Force, 1991). The guidelines require that treatment efficacy studies show improvement in two independent outcome measures: (1) a measure of cognitive function and (2) a clinical measure based on the patient's overall (global) improvement in behavior that is obvious to trained clinicians.

Although comparable FDA guidelines are lacking for behavioral (including communication) treatment studies, one might suggest that personally and socially significant improvement in behaviors should be documented by increased frequency of desirable skills and decreased frequency of problem behaviors. Such improvements should be sustained in natural settings for at least some time following the termination of treatment.

Components of a Management Plan

A team of specialists designs a program to manage the client, help the family cope with the disease and its effects, and stabilize the client to the extent possible. Clinical management of patients with dementia is multifaceted. Therefore, clinical management involves a multidisciplinary approach. Different specialists help manage different sets of problems patients with dementia exhibit.

While medical treatment seeks to improve brain function that affects behavior and cognition, behavioral treatments concentrate on manipulating the environmental variables to control behavioral deficits.

An overriding concern of management is that family members and other caregivers need help with coping and management strategies. Professionals should minimize the devastating effects of dementia on both the patient and the caregivers while giving adequate support to all. Therefore, continuous counseling and increasing support for the caregivers as the patient's disease progresses are an essential component of a management strategy.

Research on dementia suggests that it is important to pay attention to risk factors that predispose people to dementia (Doody, 2000). As reviewed in previous chapters, many lifestyle factors affect the chances of developing dementia. Therefore, reducing the risk factors is also a part of a comprehensive management plan.

A comprehensive and multifaceted treatment approach includes (a) management of risk factors to reduce the prevalence of dementia; (b) medical treatment to control dementia patients' neurological symptoms, psychiatric problems, and cognitive decline; (c) caregiver education, training, and support in managing patients with dementia; (d) general behavioral management programs to control behavioral problems; (e) management of cognitive deficits; (f) management of communication problems; and (g) environmental modifications to improve patient safety and health.

Management of Dementia Risk Factors

Evidence is accumulating that certain steps that people can take might help reduce the risk of dementia or postpone its onset (Coulson, Strang, Marino, & Minichiello, 2004; Doody, 2000). Reducing the risk factors requires public education, preventive medical treatment, and behavior modification.

Educating people to change the pattern of their unhealthy behaviors is the essence of public education and prevention. People who avoid factors that predispose them to heart diseases and stroke may reduce the chances of dementia later in life. There is evidence that the risk of heart disease, stroke, and eventual dementia may be reduced by:

- *A healthy diet.* Several studies have suggested that the so-called Mediterranean diet, which reduces saturated fats and includes fruits and vegetables, monounsaturated fats, and moderate drinking of alcohol may slow age-related cognitive decline. A combination of such a healthy diet and regular exercise helps decrease blood cholesterol with a concomitant decrease in risk for vascular disorders and eventual stroke and other conditions that are associated with dementia (Solfrizzi, Panza, & Capurso, 2003; Solfrizzi et al., 2005).

- *Regular exercise.* The benefits of regular physical exercise in keeping fit, controlling weight gain, reducing stress, and promoting physical and emotional well-being are common knowledge. Research has demonstrated that people who walked 2 miles a day experienced a reduced risk of developing dementia (Abbot et al., 2004). Several studies have shown that even in patients who already have dementia, regular physical exercise has been shown to improve cognitive skills (see Heyn, Abreu, & Ottenbacher, 2004, for a review and meta-analysis of research).

- *Prompt and effective treatment of high blood pressure.* There is evidence that reducing hypertension in the elderly can reduce the risk of Alzheimer's diseases and vascular dementia (Sys-Eur Investigators, 1998).

- *Controlling high cholesterol levels.* Research has shown that a group of drugs known as statins, effective in reducing high levels of cholesterol, may reduce the risk of Alzheimer's and vascular types of dementia (Hick, Zornberg, Jick, Seshadri, & Drachman, 2000).

- *Use of anti-inflammatory drugs.* Regular use of aspirin (and ibuprofen) may help reduce the risk of strokes and thus the risk of dementia (Jacques & Jackson, 2000).

- *Reducing the chances of head injury.* Head injury earlier in life is a factor known to predispose people to dementia later in life. Steps taken to prevent head injury (e.g., wearing seat belts in automobiles) may help reduce the risk of later dementia (Doody, 2000).

- *Sustained intellectual activities.* Compared to people who are illiterate or have low levels of education, those who obtain higher education or engage in regular reading and writing experience a lower risk of developing dementia (Doody, 2000; Friedland, 1993). By implication, a preventive strategy is to maintain a high level of intellectual and literacy activities throughout life to reduce the risk of dementia.

Medical Treatment of Dementia

Much research has been devoted to finding the genetic basis of dementia. As specific genes are found for different forms of dementia, new treatments are expected to emerge.

Medical treatment is most effective in the case of reversible dementia. As noted in Chapter 12, if the underlying disease can be effectively treated, the risk of eventual dementia may be avoided. For instance, vitamin B12 deficiency, renal diseases, and other such endocrine disorders may be treated effectively if diagnosed early to prevent subsequent dementia.

Although research on pharmacological treatment of dementia continues, no treatment has been successful in completely reversing or stopping the course of dementia (Ferris & Mohs, 2001). Nonetheless, drug treatment has been important in achieving certain short-term goals of improving or stabilizing the neurological symptoms and the behavioral or cognitive levels of patients with dementia.

Chapters 14 and 15 offer information on various medical treatments available for symptomatic treatment of cognitive deficits seen in specific types of dementia. The cholinergic group of drugs that help improve neural transmission (hence called *neurotransmitters*) have effected modest levels of improvement in cognitive and behavioral symptoms of patients with dementia (Erkinjuntti et al., 2002). As noted in Chapter 15, levodopa, a precursor of dopamine, has a favorable effect not only on movement disorders in patients with Parkinson's disease but also on cognitive deficits.

Improved cognitive function and reduced psychiatric and behavioral symptoms are associated with enhanced levels of the neurotransmitter acetylcholine (Ach). It is well known that reduced amounts of Ach lead to memory loss. Unfortunately, Ach cannot be directly administered to patients because it is very short-lived. Among several approaches taken to increase or maintain the Ach level in the brains of patients, the one designed to reduce its naturally occurring breakdown has been more successful. An enzyme called acetylcholinesterase (AchE) breaks down acetylcholine in the brain. Drugs that inhibit AchE can increase or maintain the levels of Ach in the brain. Cognitive as well as behavioral improvements have been noted in patients with mild to moderate Alzheimer's disease who have been administered AchE inhibitors (Doody et al., 2001).

Several other kinds of drugs are being researched. Some animal research has shown promise for human application in the future. A pharmacological agent known as *beta-sheet breaker peptide* has been successful in preventing plaques in rat brains. Researchers are pursuing several leads, including ways to prevent cortical cell death, modulation of neuroprotective glial-cell function, and inhibition of monoamine oxidase type-B to develop more effective treatments for dementia.

Medical treatment of psychiatric symptoms has been widely available. Specific medications include antipsychotic drugs that have been used to treat various forms of psychosis, including schizophrenia. Some antipsychotic agents are effective in reducing hallucinations and delusions found in patients with dementia, especially dementia of the Alzheimer type. Some antipsychotic medications increase such parkinsonian symptoms as tremor and slowness. Long-term use of antipsychotic drugs may lead to tardive dyskinesia, which is characterized by involuntary movements, especially of the face, cheeks, tongue, and limbs. Therefore, they may not be appropriate for patients with Parkinson's disease.

Several other types of drugs are used to treat the behavioral and psychiatric symptoms of patients with dementia. These drugs help control depression, violent behavior, emotional explosiveness, irritability, euphoria, and agitation. Still other kinds of medications are useful in reducing sleep disturbances and anxiety.

The movement disorders found in patients with dementia, especially in Alzheimer's disease, Parkinson's disease, and Lewy body dementia, are treated with levodopa and such dopamine agonists (agents that stimulate dopamine) as amantadine.

Surgical treatment for certain kinds of dementia have been researched as well. As noted in Chapter 15, such surgical procedures as fetal transplantation of stem cells or aborted embryonic dopaminergic tissue into the brains of patients with Parkinson's disease are in the experimental stage.

Caregiver Education, Training, and Support

Most patients with mild to moderate dementia are cared for in their homes. Family members take care of their loved ones with dementia from 2 to 15 years. Patients are likely to be institutionalized only when the family cannot cope with the ever-escalating demands of taking care of the patient. After spending some time in a nursing home, most patients enter an extended care facility during the final stage of the disease.

Clinicians know that both the patient and the caregivers need behavioral treatment. Patients' family caregivers are severely stressed and the degree of stress they feel is correlated with nursing home placement of patients. It is known that the stress the caregivers experience physically harms them: their immune response is impaired, resulting in vulnerability to infections. Studies have shown that treatment, especially emotional and social support, offered to caregivers improves the functioning of their immune system (Litvan, 2001). Furthermore, effective support offered to family caregivers delays nursing home placement of patients by 12 to 24 months (Doody et al., 2001).

Family caregivers should be (a) educated on the disease and its inevitable progression, (b) closely monitored to detect depression or other psychiatric problems they may experience, (c) promptly offered counseling and psychiatric treatment, (d) provided social and emotional support, and (e) offered respite care of patients.

Institutional (professional) caregivers, along with family caregivers, need to be trained in supporting and interacting with the patient. Some research suggests that nursing home staff refrain from talking to or touching older patients with dementia (Kaplan & Hoffman, 1998), while there is evidence that therapeutic touch can reduce restlessness, random vocalizations, and possibly other undesirable behaviors in patients with dementia (Woods, Craven, & Whitney, 2005).

Before the caregivers are expected to use adaptive strategies, they need to be trained in managing patients with dementia. Such training should be offered to both family members and professional caregivers and should consist of the following:

- Educate caregivers about dementia, its causes, and consequences in general. Give the caregivers information on specific type of neurological disease and the dementia it causes. Educate the caregivers about the long-term rehabilitative needs and the patient's prognosis.

- Offer caregivers information on community resources available to them. The resources may include agencies that offer financial help, volunteer support, self-help groups, and social and professional organizations.

- Provide counseling to the caregivers to cope with the demands of caring for a patient with a degenerative neurological disease.

- Make respite care available to the caregivers. Respite care gives family members a break from the unrelenting demands of care and gives them an opportunity to relax or attend to other aspects of their lives.

An additional and important area of caregiver support involves training them in managing the patient's communicative, cognitive, and behavioral deficits. Such strategies are summarized in the sections that follow.

Management of General Behavioral Problems

Management of behavioral problems of patients with dementia is a serious concern to all caregivers. Prudent management of those problems also helps secure the patient's safety, health, and comfort.

Behaviors that the caregivers find most distressing include emotional outbursts, agitation, depression, hallucinations, egression (leaving the house), memory problems, and related difficulties. Such psychiatric problems as hallucinations and depressions may be medically treated, as noted earlier. Nonmedical behavioral management strategies include the following tactics:

- Teach family members and other caregivers to analyze the antecedents of disruptive behaviors. Note that most disruptive behaviors, including agitation and emotional outbursts, are triggered by such environmental events as too little or too much sensory stimulation. Too much noise, too many tightly scheduled activities, too hard task demands, general fatigue, uncontrolled physical symptoms, and lack of sleep may trigger agitation and outbursts. Lack of sensory stimulation the patient is used to (e.g., lack of soothing music, a quiet place to relax, a game or activity the patient enjoys) also may trigger disruptive behaviors.

- Teach family members and other caregivers to minimize or eliminate antecedents that trigger disruptive behaviors. For example, ask the caregivers to stop making impossible demands on the patient. Teach caregivers to maximize conditions that seem to promote more desirable behaviors or actions the patients enjoy. For example, ask the caregivers to provide for a favorite game or music. Teach the caregivers to positively reinforce all desirable behaviors.

- Teach caregivers to offer limited choices to avoid confusion or chaos. For example, caregivers may give a choice of only two food items at a time (e.g., "do you want orange juice or milk?") or two clothing items (e.g., "do you want to wear this blue shirt or this green shirt?").

- Teach caregivers to lay out the clothes in the order in which they are worn.

- Teach caregivers to offer the needed help instead of confronting the patient.

- Teach caregivers to carefully observe depressed patients to identify activities and sensory stimulations they enjoy. Ask the caregivers to increase the frequency of such stimulation (e.g., music) and activities (e.g., watching TV).

- Teach caregivers to reduce the frequency of situations that tend to provoke anxiety in patients. The caregivers may find that reducing task demands, simplifying daily routines, and following a predictable schedule of activities may reduce the patient's anxiety.

- Teach caregivers to positively reinforce desirable behaviors and withhold praise, attention, and other forms of reinforcers for undesirable behaviors.

Management of Cognitive and Communicative Deficits

Successful behavioral and medical treatment programs tend to affect both cognition and communication, as the two sets of skills are closely interrelated. There are grounds to question the usefulness of this distinction. Improvement in some cognitive functions may or may not result in improved communication skills. For instance, a patient who performs better on a block design test of intelligence may or may not communicate better. Improvement in other cognitive functions may have an effect on some communication skills. For instance, a patient whose memory improves may recall names more readily and thus show improvement in discourse.

On the other hand, improvement in communication may almost always imply some improvement in cognition as well. For instance, a patient who is directly taught to name pictures of family members may be said to have improved his or her memory—a cognitive function. For the speech-language pathologist, it is more significant that the patient's naming skills and discourse have improved. As this example shows, cognitive treatment may target noncommunicative intellectual skills or communicative skills. When the latter is targeted, the distinction between cognitive and communicative treatment is not critical.

Speech-language pathologists work with a team of specialists. Management of communication problems, cognitive deficits, psychiatric symptoms, and behavioral deviations is interrelated. During the early stages of dementia, speech-language pathologists teach the skills that are most crucial in maintaining communication. Steps taken to improve memory skills will help a great deal. The clinician targets functional memory skills for each client. The methods of teaching them are not necessarily unique.

Stabilizing or improving communication between the patient and others is the main concern of the speech-language pathologist. Although the speech-language pathologist may take the lead role in designing and implementing strategies that enhance communication to and from the patient, all caregivers, including family and professional, are involved in the process. The patient in the early stages who understands that his or her skills are deteriorating is open to treatment strategies. In such cases, some direct treatment procedures may be productive. In the later stages, when the patient loses insight into his or her deteriorating skills and behaviors, such direct intervention is not effective. Therefore, in the latter stages, the concern is to maintain communication to the extent possible by helping caregivers to adapt to the rapidly declining patient skills and behavior.

As noted in the previous two chapters, decline in cognitive and communication skill is progressive. Nonetheless, attempts to minimize this decline are worthwhile, especially in the earlier and intermediate stages of the disease. Several studies have shown that cognitive decline may be checked, even if temporarily through behavioral interventions. Chapman et al. (2004) demonstrated that cognitive-communication stimulation, when combined with the drug donepezil, an acetylcholinesterase inhibitor, may be beneficial. A cognitive-communication group received training in producing relevant verbal content through discussion and describing life events, promoting involvement in hobbies and activities at home, and educating participants and their families on Alzheimer's disease. The authors report improved discourse and emotion and reduced behavioral problems in patients with Alzheimer's disease, but the precise methods of treatment were not described in operational terms.

A series of studies by Quayhagen and associates (Quayhagen & Quayhagen, 1989, 2001; Quayhagen et al., 2000) on cognitive stimulation and early-stage day care for Alzheimer's patients and counseling for caregivers have generally reported positive results in improved cognition, emotional responses, and general behavior. Caregivers tended to experience less depression.

Another series of studies by Arkin (1998, 2001), Arkin and Mahendra (2001), and Mahendra and Arkin (2003, 2004) have shown that a comprehensive program of language stimulation, physical exercise (fitness and strength training sessions), and social interactions (service at social agencies and recreational activities) can produce positive changes in patients with dementia. Language stimulation activities covered an extensive list of skills, including picture and object description, story recall with quiz, category naming, generative naming, problem solving, proverb interpretation, word association, and famous name recall. Reporting on a 4-year program of exercise, language, and social interventions, Mahendra and Arkin (2003) showed that patients with dementia improved their discourse skills. That the program could be implemented with the help of trained undergraduate students is a significant aspect of this program.

Another line of investigations has shown that a variety of external memory aids are effective in triggering appropriate behaviors at right times. Generally, making the patient rehearse the information in the form of memory drills is not effective. A more effective strategy to improve memory skills is to teach patients to use external memory aids (see Turkstra, 2001, for a review). For instance, Bourgeois (1990) and Bourgeois and Mason (1996) demonstrated that patients with dementia whose reading skills were still intact effectively used *memory wallets*—index cards on which personal and factual information was written. The patients used the cards to produce more appropriate and more elaborate verbal expressions than without the cards.

Studies also have shown that repeated questions and demands of patients with dementia may be reduced by directing them to memory books, index cards, or information posted on a bulletin board (see Bourgeois et al., 2003, for a review). Caregivers could be easily trained to redirect patients to such devices.

Many forms of external memory aids have been shown to prompt timely and correct responses from patients with dementia. These include various forms of calendars, cue cards, diaries, written to-do lists, weekly planners, written daily reminders, watch alarms, timers, vibrating signals, prominently displayed written signs and orientation boards; and many other forms of cues have been helpful to many patients. These devices, however, are effective only to the extent that patients remember to use them; in many cases, they may need constant prompts from caregivers to use the memory aids (Bourgeois et al., 2003).

A few studies on a procedure called *spaced retrieval* have produced impressive results in promoting the use of external memory aids. The method has been shown to be effective in improving the use of memory aids in patients with different kinds of dementia (see Camp et al., 2000, and Bourgeois et al., 2003, for reviews). **Spaced retrieval** is a procedure in which the patient is taught to recall a piece of information with progressively longer intervals; it is essentially a behavioral shaping method in which the duration between recalls of specific information is gradually increased. Because of the shaping procedure, few or no errors are made; such errorless learning is thought to promote better retention (Bourgeois et al., 2003).

The spaced retrieval training may begin with a question such as, " When you want to know what you should do today, you look at your list of daily activities. What do you do when you want to know about what you should do today?" If the patient replies, "I look at my list of daily activities," the clinician reinforces the client for the correct responses and proceeds to talk about extraneous topics for a predetermined duration (1 minutes, 2 minutes, etc). At the end of an interval, the clinician asks the question again. If the response is wrong, the clinician models the correct response, the patient imitates and gets reinforced. The interval between the prompts (questions) is increased gradually until the patient gives correct responses with a 24-hour interval between prompts. When the intervals reach several minutes, the clinician may train other skills during that interval (e.g., having the patient sort objects instead of simply talking about extraneous topics).

With a few exceptions, studies on cognitive stimulation and communication training have generally failed to give specific details on procedures. Reports specify well what they trained, but not how they did it. Treatment reports would be more helpful to clinicians if they described the treatment procedures in greater detail and with operational specificity.

Clinical experience and research of the kind summarized so far suggest that clinicians can implement several procedures to improve or sustain memory skills and reduce the effects of other cognitive deficits in patients with dementia. The procedures summarized here include direct cognitive or communication training in the patient and training patients to seek help from others (see also Bayles & Kaszniak, 1987; Bayles & Kim, 2003; Brookshire, 2003; Lubinski, 1995; Shadden & Toner, 1997):

- Use one or more of the direct intervention procedures that have been researched in case studies and controlled experimental evaluations (e.g., previously described spaced retrieval method, memory wallets, cognitive stimulation combined with physical exercise and social activities, cognitive stimulation in conjunction with pharmacological treatment).

- Get caregivers involved in all treatment programs so that they, too, are able to provide the needed support for patients' activities and communication skills.

- Design various reminders for tasks and activities: memory wallets, daily planners, alarms, written instructions, to-do lists, staff reminders, self-monitoring devices, vibrating electronic devices to remind of appointments or activities, written signs that remind of activities and their times, orientation signs in living quarters, answers on bulletin boards to frequently asked questions, and large digital watches the patient wears and consults.

- Use tangible stimuli whenever possible during treatment; train caregivers to use tangible stimuli whenever practical during conversation.

- Teach the patient to write down a list of what to do each day.

- Teach the client to write down instructions and directions when memory begins to fade.

- Teach the patient to keep phone numbers and possessions in a particular, invariable place.

- Teach the patient to keep a checklist of things to do before leaving the house.

- Teach the patient to carry a card with the names, addresses, and phone numbers of caregivers.

- Have the patient wear a bracelet that contains identifying information and names, addresses, and phone numbers of caregivers.

- Place a large calendar in the patient's living room and bedroom and cross off the current date every night; this might help maintain orientation to day and time.
- Have the patient keep a map to frequently visited places (e.g., homes of relatives or friends, shops, and restaurants).
- Teach the patient to request that messages, especially more complex directions and instructions, be given orally as well as in writing.
- Teach the patient to consult written messages and instructions frequently enough to follow through.
- Teach the patient to request more time to speak or respond to questions. This might be especially useful to patients who have word-finding problems or unusually long reaction times.
- Teach the patient to express or gesture his or her inability to understand a message when such is the case. This will prompt the speaker to alter the message to make it more easily understandable.
- Teach the patient to ask the speaker to repeat a spoken message when it is not understood.
- Teach the patient who forgets the topic of conversation to request conversational partners to remind him or her of the topic.
- Teach the patient to give descriptions of objects and persons or nonverbally indicate the use of objects when attempts at naming fail.
- Teach the patient to use gestures, signs, facial expressions, and any other form of nonverbal communication when words fail.
- Emphasize effective communication, not grammatical or phonological accuracy of expressions.
- Use effective behavioral principles in teaching both the patients and their caregivers; teach them to prompt, shape, model, and positively reinforce verbal or nonverbal communicative attempts.

Caregiver strategies to help improve or maintain communication are as important as direct intervention with the patients. Because of the progressive nature of the disease, caregivers need to continuously modify their behavior to achieve as much success as possible in meaningful communication.

Several communication strategies have been described involving patients with dementia and their family members or professional caregivers. Clinicians have generally recommended such strategies; some of the strategies are based on common sense and social etiquette (see Small, Gutman, Makela, & Hillhouse, 2003, for a review and a study result; see also Bayles & Kim, 2003; Doody et al., 2001; Kaplan & Hoffman, 1998; Orange, 2001; Rabins, Lyketsos, & Steele, 1999; Shekim, 1997; Weiner, 1996). Not all strategies have been shown to be equally effective or commonly used by caregivers. In fact, few strategies have been subjected to experimental analysis. Therefore the clinician needs to evaluate the usefulness of each suggested strategy with the individual patient, his or her family members, and professional caregivers. With caution and with a view to evaluate their usefulness, the clinician may train caregivers to:

- Ask questions and immediately prompt for correct actions (e.g., "What do you do today at 10? *Look at your list and then tell me.*")

- Give a cue to a correct response (similar to cues provided to patients with aphasia; see Chapter 9).

- Approach patients slowly, as they become apprehensive about sudden events.

- Establish eye contact before speaking; place yourself in the patient's visual field before speaking.

- Have the patient wear eyeglasses and hearing aids before speaking to him or her.

- Secure the patient's attention before speaking; call out the patient's name, repeatedly if necessary, until the patient attends to you.

- Find out if the patient responds better to first name or last name. Avoid terms of endearment (e.g., "honey" or "sweetheart"). Use your first name if the patient responds better to his or her first name.

- Bend down or kneel to speak to a seated patient.

- Listen carefully to the patient's communicative attempts; do not interrupt the patient.

Even with impaired language expression, the patient may communicate with a few key words.

- Encourage circumlocution; let the patient talk in indirect and roundabout ways when word retrieval hinders specific expressions.

- Supplement verbal expression with gestures, smile, posture, and other cues. When necessary, first give a nonverbal cue before the verbal command. For instance, gesture the patient to stand up before telling the patient, "It is time to go to the dining room for breakfast."

- Model the requested behavior along with verbal instructions. For instance, while asking the patient to wipe the dining table, demonstrate the action, and then give the cloth to the patient.

- Speak clearly, directly, and in simple, short sentences, but not necessarily slowly as a slower rate may not help.

- Repeat complex sentences when such sentences are necessary for communication as repetition may help comprehension.

- Within the limitations of the patient's hearing acuity, speak softly, rather than loudly.

- Avoid complex conversational material.

- Specify referents when they speak, and minimize the use of pronouns. For example, when referring to other persons, the caregiver should avoid the use of *he* and *she;* instead, the caregiver should use the names of those persons. Similarly, when referring to objects, the names should be preferred to the pronoun *it.*

- Ask yes/no questions when factual responses are needed (e.g., "would you like cereal for breakfast?" instead of "what would you like to eat for breakfast?").

- Ask open-ended questions to encourage free expression of narratives, feelings, and opinions.

- Ask only one question at a time; wait for a response as the patient may need more time, and give cues and prompts as needed.

- Minimize task complexity and ask the patient to do one thing at a time.

- Give single-step directions; supplement directions with gestures or modeling of actions required.

- Give manual guidance or physical support for actions requested. For example, physically help the patient stand up as the request to stand up is made.

- Be redundant, and restate important information. Repeat instructions with different words as verbatim repetitions may not be useful.

- Keep topics familiar and objects of conversation observable.

- Ask questions during the patient's narrative attempts to keep the patient on the same topic and to help maintain the story sequence. Ask such questions as "How does the story begin?" "What happened next?" "Who did it?" "What did she say?" "How did the story end?"

- Respond directly and in a matter-of-fact manner when the patient asks the same question repeatedly. If possible, direct the patient's attention to a message board, a memory aid, a printed list, and such other sources of information. Also, try to distract the patient with an activity or a new topic of conversation.

- Use touch to comfort, to draw attention, to reassure, and to strengthen verbal contact.

- Pay close attention to the patient's nonverbal behaviors, especially when communication skills deteriorate. The caregiver may try to decipher meaning in the patient's facial expressions, body postures, gestures, and other nonverbal behaviors.

- Attend to the patient's prosodic features, which may be intact up to a point and be effective in communication, even though the words used may not be appropriate.

- Speak to the patient with normal prosodic features; avoid monotonous tone or exaggerated articulation.

- Positively reinforce appropriate verbal and nonverbal behaviors. Offer verbal praise for compliant behaviors.

- Watch for first language expressions that may emerge in a bilingual patient. Get help in interpreting such expressions.
- Always say *good-bye* or give other departing signals.

Environmental Modifications

Environmental modifications refer to changes in the structure of living conditions to help maintain communication and interaction, reduce undesirable behaviors, and sustain the general health and safety of the patient (Calkins & Chafetz, 1996). Such environmental modifications need to be implemented in patients' living environments, which may be their homes or professional settings such as nursing homes. Few experimental studies have been done to evaluate the effectiveness of environmental modifications, although there is some evidence that caregivers may be trained to redesign their home environment and that they can sustain the training effects 12 months post-training (Gitlin, Hauck, Dennis, & Winter, 2005).

To modify the patients' environment, caregivers and professionals need to work as a team to accomplish some or all of the following:

- Establish a simple routine for the patient, and structure the patient's living environment. The patient's schedule of activity should be fairly constant across days, although providing some variety may enhance the quality of the patient's life. Also, consider individual differences; some do well with little structure.
- Generally, structure the professional settings more like home settings.
- Reduce sensory stimuli that lead to agitation, disruptive actions, aggressive behaviors, and discomfort. Minimize noise that tends to distress patients with dementia. Eliminate loud buzzers and minimize the use of loud public address systems. Carpet the living areas and drape windows to minimize sound and noise that bounce off hard surfaces. When talking to the patient, turn off televisions and radios.
- Use sounds associated with living conditions to cue and calm patients. For instance, main-

tain kitchen sounds that announce dinner time (such as the sounds of setting a dinner table) or bird sounds and music that soothe patients.

- Avoid stimuli that interfere with vision in patients who have reduced visual capacity due to aging and dementia. Minimize direct and glaring sunlight. Arrange for even lighting in the living areas to avoid dark corners that some patients may find frightening.

- Use contrast to enhance visual discrimination and prompt appropriate actions. For instance, use tableware that contrasts with the dining table and carpets that contrast with the walls.

- Avoid using a single room for multiple purposes. Use different rooms for specific activities.

- Limit access to hazardous materials. Keep knives, scissors, hammers, screwdrivers, and such other tools out of reach. In the kitchen, install devices that automatically switch off stoves or induction cooktops that do not burn people.

- Do not impoverish the patients' environment. Let the patients retain access to non-hazardous items that they would like to pick up, explore, or use (e.g., a soft ball, books or magazines, games).

- Use various cuing strategies to improve awareness and orientation. Use multiple cues that use both words and pictures to orient patients to their bedrooms, bathrooms, dining rooms, and other spaces. In a professional setting, have some personal items at the entrance of patients' bedrooms or bathrooms.

- Serve food at predictable times in specific and relatively constant places. Use such stimuli as music or some activity that signals other activities, such as eating.

- Let patients use their family pictures, games, and other belongings and religious or culturally significant items in their bedrooms in professional settings.

- Let patients maintain some of the routines or activities they enjoyed in their home setting. For instance, instead of forcing an unfamiliar task (e.g., basket weaving or painting) on some residents, let them maintain their usual activities or hobbies (card playing or knitting).

- Provide for security while not overly curtailing freedom. Use one or more of a variety of methods to control egression (going out of homes): door locks that may be out of reach of patients or hidden; fabric attached through Velcro across door handles and locks; and electronic security devices that require a code entry to unlock the doors.

- Provide for freedom of movement, which is known to decrease agitation, while ensuring the patients' security and safety. For instance, design a secured courtyard or a garden into which the doors open for the patient to walk about.

- Minimize changes in floor levels; if this is not possible, increase contrast between levels by attaching colored tapes at critical levels.

- Install sturdy furniture with rounded edges to minimize injury.

Terminal Care

Patients in the terminal stage require assistance in all aspects of their living. Terminal-stage patients are unable to walk, talk, dress, and bathe. They are likely to experience urinary and fecal incontinence. They tend to experience such comorbid medical conditions as dysphagia, aspiration pneumonia, urinary tract infections, septicemia (a systemic disease of the blood), decubitus ulcers (bedsores or pressure ulcers), fever when administered antibiotics, and many other diseases and complications (Rabins, Lyketsos, & Steele, 1999).

Terminal-stage care involves management of medical problems. Dysphagia, for example, can be managed with such typical measures as offering lukewarm and relatively thick liquids, raising the head of the bed while feeding, and slow feeding of small quantities of food. Good skin care (such as frequent repositioning of the patient in bed) will help minimize decubitus ulcers. Such measures as dressing patients in their own clothes, grooming in their own fashion, maintaining oral hygiene, and frequently changing products designed to control incontinence will help maintain the patients' dignity and comfort. Most families and medical personnel find it unacceptable to use heroic measures to save the life of patients in their terminal stage of dementia (Rabins, Lyketsos, & Steele, 1999).

Dementia treatment efficacy research is limited. Clinicians should watch for studies that report on new treatment options and effectiveness for techniques commonly described in sources such as these. Experts generally believe that clinical management of patients will produce notable changes in patients' behaviors, although as dementia progresses, the returns diminish. Working with families and other caregivers at all stages of a patient's dementia is essential.

Suggested Readings

Read the following for additional information on assessment and clinical management of patients with dementia:

Bayles, K. A., & Kim, E. S. (2003). Improving the functioning of individuals with Alzheimer's disease: Emergence of behavioral interventions. *Journal of Communication Disorders, 36,* 327–343.

Bourgeois, M., Camp, C., Rose, M., White, B., Malone, M., Carr, J., & Rovine, M. (2003). A comparison of training strategies to enhance use of external aids by persons with dementia. *Journal of Communication Disorders, 36,* 361–378.

Ferris, S. F., & Mohs, R. C. (2001). Measuring treatment efficacy in Alzheimer's disease. In C. M. Clark & J. Q. Trojanowski (Eds.), *Neurodegenerative dementias: Clinical features and pathological mechanisms* (pp. 395–404). New York: McGraw-Hill.

Kaplan, M., & Hoffman, S. B. (1998). *Behavior in dementia: Best practice for successful management.* Baltimore, MD: Health Professions Press.

Mahendra, N., & Arkin, S. M. (2003). Effects of four years of exercise, language, and social interventions on Alzheimer discourse. *Journal of Communication Disorders, 36,* 395–422.

Ogrocki, P. K., & Welsh-Bohmer, K. A. (2000). Assessment of cognitive and functional impairment in the elderly. In C. M. Clark & J. Q. Trojanowski (Eds.), *Neurodegenerative dementias: Clinical features and pathological mechanisms* (pp. 15–32). New York: McGraw-Hill.

Rabins, P. V., Lyketsos, C. G., & Steele, C. D. (1999). *Practical dementia care.* New York: Oxford University Press.

Shadden, B. B., & Toner, M. A. (Eds.) (1997). *Aging and communication.* Austin, TX: PRO-ED.

Tomoeda, C. K. (2001). Comprehensive assessment for dementia: A necessity for differential diagnosis and management. *Seminars in Speech and Language, 22*(4), 275–289.

Appendix A

The Coursebook Method of Teaching and Learning

Effective teaching is a concern of all teachers. Instructors look for teaching devices that are effective, easy to teach from, and current. They also look for teaching devices that are easily updated. Students, too, look for easy-to-use devices that help them learn without unnecessary effort and frustration. Instructors and students alike look for devices that help integrate lectures and textbook information.

A persistent problem of teaching and learning is that lectures and printed information are not integrated. The two sources of information often are nonparallel, sometimes even contradictory. A frustrating problem for all but a few speed-writing students is taking accurate notes in the classroom. But this is mostly an unnecessary problem dictated by the lecture method of instruction and unintegrated printed (textbooks and other sources) and handwritten (class notes) materials. There should be no need for students to write down in the classroom the definition of terms, outline of topics, major steps of assessment or treatment procedures, arguments, or issues. Such important information should be available in printed form to reduce the pressure of rapid writing.

In spite of their best efforts, the notes most students take are incomplete and can even be inaccurate. Moreover, students who are furiously taking notes on technical and unfamiliar topics cannot fully listen, understand, reflect, and discuss. When the basic terms, concepts, steps, procedures, and summaries are printed in a textbook that also permits the students to take class notes on the pages of that text itself, the students may find the classroom a more inviting place to discuss, offer comments, and ask questions.

The traditional textbooks, although containing most of the information students need, are not easily integrated with lecture notes. That is why students feel compelled to write down everything an instructor says, including what might be found in their textbooks. Therefore, textbooks do not offer solutions to classroom problems of writing, listening, and discussing. Students end up with two sources of unintegrated information: the textbook and their class notes. A *coursebook* is designed to solve these classroom problems students face. At the end of each lecture period, they have the text and the class notes integrated into a single source because they take notes on the textbook pages themselves. It is a teaching tool that helps both the student and the instructor who also may make notations in the textbook that serve as lecture notes.

What Is a Coursebook?

A coursebook may be designed either as a lecture outline printed on the left half of each page or a textbook that gives sufficiently detailed information on topics discussed. This coursebook is designed as a textbook on which students can take notes because the textual information is printed only on the left half of each page. The empty space on the right half of the book pages is designed to take additional class notes. Therefore, a coursebook is a multipurpose book.

A coursebook that is also designed as a textbook:

- has printed text while providing space for taking lecture notes
- offers information just like any textbook, but in a format that helps both instructors and students
- gives an opportunity for students to take notes that are parallel to textbook information
- offers information needed to make clinical decisions in the easy-to-use tables that are integrated with the text (no stand-alone tables)
- describes steps, procedures, methods, and techniques in bulleted list format for easy understanding and application
- reduces the pressure of note taking
- provides the instructor a means to teach with supplied textbook information as well as space to organize his or her own unique presentations to the class
- provides the student a means to learn and integrate information from different sources, including the instructor's perspectives

What This Book Does for the Student

- The left half of each page offers information on the topic.
- The student can think of this book as a textbook presenting information in a format that is the easiest to integrate with class notes. The student does not need to write as much while listening to the lectures. All textbook information is already printed for the student in the left-hand column.
- The right half of all pages are empty so that students can write notes on them. Students need to write only new information, additional examples, and expansions that the instructor offers in the class. The handwritten notes are more likely to be unique and newer information and perspectives the individual instructors offer.
- The empty portions of each page also may be used out of classrooms. For instance, the student can take notes from journal articles or newer books read at home or at the library.
- When used properly, a coursebook makes a single, integrated, updated source of information on a topic.
- Properly completed coursebooks can be a valuable reference for clinical work and for studying for master's degree comprehensive examinations and the PRAXIS examination for ASHA certification and state licensure where applicable.

What This Book Does for the Instructor

- Foremost, a coursebook is a textbook unconventionally designed as an instructional package, already prepared for the instructor.
- The instructors may use the printed information as lecture notes and outlines, saving much time and effort preparing for the class.
- The book provides selected information printed so that it may be directly copied on transparencies for overhead projection.
- On the blank right side of each page, the instructor may write additional notes, examples, reminders, and other devices used during the lecture. Recent research studies published in journals and other references also may be written on the right-hand side. In addition, the empty space may be used to write down student assignments. In essence, both the instructor and the student will use the blank portions of pages in much the same way: to write additional information.
- The book reduces the need to repeat or dictate information, especially technical terms and their definitions. Instructors know that much classroom time is wasted in this unnecessary activity.
- The book will help instructors reduce the unwanted variability in student note taking.

Appendix B

Glossary of Medical Abbreviations and Symbols

Speech-language pathologists working with patients who have aphasia and other neurogenic language and speech disorders need to know the commonly used medical abbreviations and symbols they are likely to find in patients' medical records. In planning assessment and treatment for these patients, the clinician needs to have a clear understanding of their medical status, including the prescription drugs they are taking. What follows is a list of commonly used medical abbreviations and symbols; but other acronyms, abbreviations, and symbols may be unique to a given setting. A speech-language pathologist or a student clinician who is not familiar with an abbreviation or symbol should consult a nursing or medical staff member instead of guessing its meaning.

a.c.	before meals
ACU	ambulatory care unit or acute care unit
ACVD	atherosclerotic cardiovascular disease
Al	allergy
A.M	morning
Amb	ambulatory
A&O	alert and oriented
Asp	aspirate
ATC	around the clock
AW.	atomic weight
A&W.	alive and well
BADL	basic activities of daily life
BAER	brainstem auditory evoked response
BALB	binaural alternate loudness balance (test)
BBB	blood brain barrier
b.i.d.	twice a day
b.i.n.	twice a night
b.p.	blood pressure
BSER	brainstem evoked response (audiometry)
c̄	with
c-a	cardioarterial
Ca	calcium; cathodal, cathode
CA	cancer
caps.	capsule

CAT	computerized axial tomography
C.C.	cardiac catheterization or chief complaint
cc	cubic centimeter
CCU	coronary care unit or critical care unit
CDC	Centers for Disease Control
CHF	congestive heart failure
CHI	closed-head injury
CN	cranial nerve
CNS	central nervous system
C/O	complains of
comp.	compound
CP	cerebral palsy
CPD	cardiopulmonary disease
CPR	cardiopulmonary resuscitation
CSF	cerebrospinal fluid
CVA	cerebrovascular accident
CXR	chest X-ray
d.	day
DC (D/C)	discontinue or discharge
dil	dilute
div.	divide
DNR	do not resuscitate
DNT	did not test
DOA	dead on arrival
DSA	digital subtraction angiography
DU	diagnosis unknown
Dx	diagnosis
ECG	electrocardiogram
ECHO	echocardiogram
ECU	emergency care unit
e.m.p.	as directed
FH	family history
FIM	functional independence measure
Fx	fracture
Gm., g.	gram
h.	hour
h.s., hor. som.	hour of sleep or bedtime
HUC	hospital unit clerk
Hx.	history
IAO	immediately after onset
ICU	intensive care unit
i.m.	intramuscular
i.v.	intravenous
LOS	length of stay
Lt. (L)	left
LTM	long-term memory
mcg.	microgram

m.dict.	as directed	SLP	speech-language pathologist
mg.	milligram	sol.	solution
ml.	milliliter	ss, sss.	one half
M.	mix	Stat.	immediately
MRI	magnetic resonance imaging	STM	short-term memory
MS	mental status or multiple sclerosis	Sx	symptom
MVA	motor vehicle accident	tab.	tablet
N.F.	National Formulary	tal.	such
NGT.	nasogastric tube	tal. dos.	such doses
NKA	no known allergies	TAR	therapy authorization request
no.	number	TBI	traumatic brain injury
non.rep.	do not repeat (no refills)	t.i.d.	three times a day
n.p.o.	nothing by mouth	t.i.n.	three times a night
OG	oralgastric tube	TM	tympanic membrane or transport maximum
OTC	over the counter (nonprescription drug)	TMJ	temporomandibular joint
p.c.	after meals	TPR	temperature, pulse, respiration
P.M.	afternoon (evening)	tsp.	teaspoonful
p.o.	by mouth	Tx	therapy (treatment)
ppm	parts per million	w.a.	while awake
p.r.n.	as necessary	WBC	white blood cell
Px	physical exam	WFL	within functional limits
pt.	patient	Wk	week
q.	every	WNL	within normal limits
q.a.d.	every other day	y.o.	year old
q.d.	every day	yr.	year
q.h.	every hour	♀	**female**
q.i.d.	four times a day	♂	**male**
q.o.d.	every other day (q.a.d.)	↑	above or increase
q.v.	as much as you wish	↓	below or decrease
rep	let it be repeated	O	absent or no response
RO	renew order	**O**	**no or none**
R/O	rule-out	?	doubtful or unknown
Rt. (R)	right	—	negative
Rx	prescription or therapy (treatment)	+	positive
s	without		

Appendix C

The World Health Organization (2001) International Classification of Functioning, Disability, and Health (ICF)

The World Health Organization in 1980 had published a system for classifying impairments, disabilities, and handicaps that result from various diseases (WHO, 1980). Called the International Classification of Impairments, Disabilities, and Handicaps (ICIDH), the classification system provided a common language to not only describe but distinguish different kinds of consequences that follow a disease or a disorder. For instance, diseases and disorders may lead to:

- Impairment: Loss of abnormality of psychological, physiological, or anatomical structure or function
- Disability: Restriction or lack of ability to perform an activity in the manner or within the range considered normal for a human being
- Handicap: A disadvantage for a given individual that limits or prevents the fulfillment of a role that is normal for that individual

The important consequence for diverse health care professionals, including speech-language pathologists, of this classification is that diseases have different kinds of consequences and a careful analysis and distinction is necessary to fully understand the client and design an assessment and treatment model. For example, it became clear that it is no longer sufficient to just describe just the symptoms of aphasia and try to assess and remediate them. It became necessary to understand the personal, social, occupational, and family consequences of strokes and aphasia to design an effective treatment program. One thrust of the WHO classification was to expand the restricted medical model of diseases and symptoms to include the social and personal philosophies and approaches to understanding and remediating health and diseases that produce varied consequences for the individual, family, and society.

In 2001, the WHO revised its 1980 classification system and called it the Classification of Functioning, Disability, and Health, or ICF. The revision was a response to criticism that the earlier version placed too much emphasis on the medical model of diseases, impairment, and disability instead of overall health status. Additional criticism was that the role of the environmental and social factors that affect the health status of individuals was not emphasized. The revision avoids these implications and emphasizes the quality of life—not only the limitations, but also the strengths of individuals (what someone can do); and environmental factors, social conditions, family structure and support, and communication patterns that need to be considered in evaluating a person's overall health. Instead of emphasizing the consequences of diseases, the revision emphasizes the various components of health. The revision also avoids the term *handicap* and uses the term *disability* to include various kinds of impairments, restrictions, and limitations individuals experience (Eadie, 2003; Yarus, 2003; WHO, 2001).

The 2001 revision is organized in terms of (1) body functions, (2) body structures, (3) activities and participation, and (4) contextual factors (environmental and personal) that affect health and well-being of individuals. *Body functions* include sensory, mental, voice and speech, and the functions of various physiological and neural systems of the body. Among others, the *mental functions* include consciousness, orientation, and intellectual functions. Among others, the *voice and speech functions* include speech, voice, and fluency. The *body structure* section is an overview of various neurophysiological structures and systems that support functions.

The *activities and participation section* of the ICF explicitly avoids the *handicap* concept of the earlier version and describes such activities as learning and applying knowledge, general task demands, communication, mobility, self-care, domestic life, interpersonal interactions and relationships, major life areas, and community, social, and civic life as important components in evaluating an individual's health experiences and status. An important distinction made in this section is what a person does (*performance*) versus what a person could do (*capacity*) but is not doing because of *limitations* or *restrictions* (instead of handicap).

The *contextual factors* include environmental factors that negatively or positively affect an individual's health and functioning. The *environmental factors* refer to all external variables (physical and social conditions) that affect the health experiences of individuals and include such factors as work, home, and school situations; social environment; cultural context; social and other support systems and policies; and products and technology that affect health and performance. The *personal factors* include such "internal" variables as an individual's background, coping strategies an individual uses, psychological assets, and other strengths.

The clinician implications of the ICF for the speech-language pathologist are explored by Eadie (2001, 2003) and Yarus (2003). Generally speaking, to design effective assessment and intervention procedures, it is more important to consider the entire personal, family, and social milieu of a client than to list symptoms and disabilities. The client's social and cultural background, the person's abilities and limitations, and the overall quality of life the person has led and is still capable of leading are also equally important considerations. A client-specific approach in which an individual and his or her personal, family, and social variables are assessed before planning a rehabilitation or treatment program is advocated in this book and is consistent with the basic tenets of ICF.

In trying to be comprehensive, the ICF has described various aspects of health and well-being, some of which are quite vague and nonoperational. Such variables as "capacity" of an individual in contrast to performance, "psychological assets," "background of an individual's life," "coping styles," and "overall behavior patterns and character style" are difficult to quantify or even observe systematically. Nonetheless, the ICF can help redirect the clinician's efforts to understand the client in broader personal, family, and social contexts instead of concentrating on symptoms and their reductions.

Interested readers can access the ICF on WHO's Web site: *http://www.who.int/en/*.

Appendix D

Internet Resources for Clinicians and Consumers

Clinicians can get much useful information on strokes, dementia, and traumatic brain injury that they can share with patients and their families. The following sites have patient (and family) education materials, information on early signs, timely treatment, research and advances in diagnosis and treatment, and prevention measures that people can take.

Strokes and Aphasia

1. National Stroke Association: *http://www.stroke.org*
2. American Stroke Association: *http://www.strokeassociation.org*
3. Mayo Clinic: *http://www.mayoclinic.com*
4. National Aphasia Association: *http://www.aphasia.org*
5. National Institute of Neurological Diseases and Stroke: *http://www.ninds.nih.gov*
6. Centers for Disease Control and Prevention (CDC): *http://www.cdc.gov/*

Dementia

1. National Institute of Neurological Diseases and Stroke: *http://www.ninds.nih.gov/disorders/alzheimersdisease*

2. Alzheimer's Association: *http://www.alz.org*
3. National Institute on Aging, Alzheimer's Disease Education & Referral Center (ADEAR): *http://www.alzheimers.org/*
4. Center for Disease Control and Prevention (CDC): *http://www.cdc.gov/*

Traumatic Brain Injury

1. National Institute of Neurological Diseases and Stroke: *http://www.ninds.nih.gov/disorders/tbi*
2. Mayo Clinic: *http://www.mayoclinic.com*
3. Brain Injury Association of America: *http://www.biausa.org/Pages/types_of_brain_injury.html*
4. Centers for Disease Control and Prevention (CDC): *http://www.cdc.gov/*

A Comprehensive Source from the National Library of Medicine, Maintained By the National Institutes of Health

For a variety of health and disease-related information, visit: *http://www.nlm.nih.gov/medlineplus*

References

Abbot, R. D., White, L. R., Ross, G. W., Masaki, K. H., Curb, J. D., & Petrovitch, H. (2004). Walking and dementia in physically capable elderly men. *Journal of the American Medical Association, 22; 292* (12), 1447–1453.

Abrahams, J., & Camp, C. (1993). Maintenance and generalization of object naming training associated with degenerative dementia. *Clinical Gerontologist, 12* (3), 57–71.

Adamovich, B. L. (1997). Traumatic brain injury. In L. L. LaPointe (Ed.), *Aphasia and related neurogenic language disorders* (2nd ed., pp. 226–237). New York: Thieme Medical Publishers.

Adamovich, B. B., & Henderson, J. (1992). *Scales of cognitive ability for traumatic brain injury.* Chicago: Riverside.

Ad Hoc Dementia Assessment Task Force. (1991). Meeting report: Antidementia drug assessment symposium. *Neurobiology of Aging, 12,* 379–382.

Albert, M. L. (1973). A simple test of visual neglect. *Neurology, 23,* 658–664.

American Heart Association. (2005). *Heart disease and stroke statistics: 2005 update.* Dallas, TX: Author. Available online at: http://www.strokeassociation.org.

American Psychiatric Association. (2000). *Diagnostic and statistical manual of mental disorders* (4th ed, text revision). Washington, DC: Author.

Andrews, B. T. (2000). Prognosis in severe head injury. In P. R. Cooper & J. G. Golfinos (Eds.), *Head injury* (4th ed., pp. 555–563). New York: McGraw-Hill.

Appell, J., Kertesz, A., & Fishman, M. (1982). A study of language functioning in Alzheimer's patients. *Brain and Language, 17,* 73–81.

Arkin, S. (1998). Alzheimer memory training; previous success replicated. *American Journal of Alzheimer's Disease, 13,* 102–104.

Arkin, S. (2001). Alzheimer rehabilitation by students: Intervention and outcomes. *Neuropsychological Rehabilitation, 11,* 273–317.

Arkin, S., & Mahendra, N. (2001). Discourse analysis of Alzheimer's patients before and after interventions: Methodology and outcome. *Aphasiology, 15* (6), 533–569.

Aten, J. L., Caliguri, M. P., & Holland, A. (1982). The efficacy of functional communication therapy for chronic aphasic patients. *Journal of Speech and Hearing Disorders, 47,* 93–96.

Aten, J., Wertz, R. T., Simpson, M., Vogel, D., & Garner, D. (1991). A long-term follow-up of aphasic patients after intensive treatment. In T. E. Prescott (Ed.), *Clinical aphasiology, Vol. 20* (pp. 299–306). Austin, TX: Pro-Ed.

Avent, J. R. (1997). Group treatment in aphasia using cooperative learning methods. *Journal of Medical Speech-Language Pathology, 5* (1), 9–26.

Basso, A. (2003). *Aphasia and its therapy.* New York: Oxford University Press.

Basso, A., Capitani, E., & Vignolo, L. A. (1979). Influence of rehabilitation on language skills in aphasic patients: A controlled study. *Archives of Neurology, 36,* 190–196.

Basso, A., & Rusconi, M. L. (1998). Aphasia in left-handers. In P. Coppens, Y. Lebrun, & A. Basso (Eds.), *Aphasia in atypical populations* (pp. 1–34). Mahwah, NJ: Lawrence Erlbaum.

Battle, D. (Ed.). (2002). *Communication disorders in multicultural populations* (2nd ed.). Boston: Butterworth-Heinemann.

Bayles, K. A., & Kaszniak, A. W. (1987). *Communication and cognition in normal aging and dementia.* Austin, TX: Pro-Ed.

Bayles, K. A., & Kim, E. S. (2003). Improving the functioning of individuals with Alzheimer's disease: Emergence of behavioral interventions. *Journal of Communication Disorders, 36,* 327–343.

Bayles, K. A., & Tomoeda, C. (1991). *Arizona Battery for Communication Disorders of Dementia* (Research Edition). Tucson, AZ: Canyonlands Publishing.

Bear, M. F., Connors, B. W., & Paradiso, M. A. (2001). *Neuroscience: Exploring the brain* (2nd ed.). Baltimore, MD: Lippincott Williams & Wilkins.

Bennett, D. A., Beckett, L. A., Wilson, R. S., Murray, A. M., & Evans, D. A. (1998). Parkinsonian signs and mortality from Alzheimer's disease. *Lancet, 351,* 1631.

Benson, D. F. (1979a). *Aphasia, alexia, and agraphia.* New York: Churchill Livingstone.

Benson, D. F. (1979b). Aphasia rehabilitation. *Archives of Neurology, 36,* 187–189.

Benson, D. F. (1985). Aphasia. In H. K. Valenstein (Ed.), *Clinical neurophysiology.* New York: Oxford University Press.

Benson, D. F., & Ardila, A. (1996). *Aphasia: A clinical perspective.* New York: Oxford University Press.

Benton, A. L. (1992). *The revised visual retention test* (5th ed.). San Antonio, TX: Psychological Corporation.

Benton, A., & Anderson, S. W. (1998). Aphasia: Historical perspectives. In M. T. Sarno (Ed.), *Acquired aphasia* (3rd ed., pp. 1–24). New York: Academic Press.

Benton, A. L., & Hamsher, K. (1978). *Multilingual aphasia examination* (Rev. ed.). Iowa City: University of Iowa.

Benton, A. L., & Joynt, R. J. (1960). Early descriptions of aphasia. *Archives of Neurology (Chicago), 3,* 205–221.

Berker, E. A., Berker, A. H., & Smith, A. (1986). Translation of Broca's 1865 report: Localization of speech in the third frontal convolution. *Archives of Neurology (Chicago), 43,* 1065–1072.

Beukelman, D. B., Burke, R., & Yorkston, K. M. (2003). Dysarthria and traumatic brain injury. In K. Hux (Ed.), *Assisting survivors of traumatic brain injury* (135–168). Austin, TX: Pro-Ed.

Beukelman, D., & Mirenda, M. (1989). *Augmentative communication: Management of children and adults with severe communication disorders* (2nd ed.). Baltimore: Paul H. Brookes.

Beukelman, D. R., & Yorkston, K. M. (1991). *Communication disorders following traumatic brain injury: Management of cognitive, language, and motor impairments.* Austin, TX: Pro-Ed.

Beukelman, D. R., Yorkston, K. M., & Reichle, J. (2000). *Augmentative and alternative communication for adults with acquired neurologic disorders.* Baltimore, MD: Paul H. Brookes.

Bhatnagar, S. C. (2002). *Neuroscience for the study of communicative disorders* (2nd ed.). Baltimore: Williams & Wilkins.

Bhogal, S. K., Teasell, R., Foley, N. C., & Speechley, M. (2003). Rehabilitation of aphasia: More is better. *Top Stroke Rehabilitation, 10* (2), 66–76.

Bhogal, S. K., Teasell, R., & Speechley, M. (2003). Intensity of aphasia therapy, Impact on recovery. *Stroke, 34,* 987–993.

Bigler, E. D. (Ed.) (1990). *Traumatic brain injury.* Austin, TX: Pro-Ed.

Bigler, E. D., Clark, E., & Farmer, J. E. (Eds.). (1997). *Childhood traumatic brain injury: Diagnosis, assessment, and injury.* Austin, TX: Pro-Ed.

Blessed, G., Tomlinson, B. E., & Roth, M. (1968). The association between quantitative measures of dementia and of senile changes in the cerebral gray matter of elderly subjects. *British Journal of Psychiatry, 114,* 797–811.

Blomert, L., Kean, M. L., Koster, C., & Schokker, J. (1994). Amsterdam-Nijmegen Everyday Language Test: Construction, reliability, and validity. *Aphasiology, 8* (4), 381–407.

Bloodstein, O. (1995). *A handbook on stuttering* (5th ed.). Clifton Park, NY: Thomson Delmar Learning.

Blosser, J. L., & DePompei, R. (1994). *Pediatric traumatic brain injury.* San Diego, CA: Singular Publishing Group.

Bourgeois, M. (1990). Enhancing conversation skills in Alzheimer's disease using a prosthetic memory aid. *Journal of Applied Behavior Analysis, 23,* 29–42.

Bourgeois, M. (2005). Dementia. In L. L. LaPointe (Ed.), *Aphasia and related neurogenic language disorders* (3rd ed., pp. 199–213). New York: Thieme.

Bourgeois, M., Camp, C., Rose, M., White, B., Malone, M., Carr, J., & Rovine, M. (2003). A comparison of training strategies to enhance use of external aids by persons with dementia. *Journal of Communication Disorders, 36,* 361–378.

Bourgeois, M., & Mason, L. (1996). Memory wallet intervention in an adult day care setting. *Behavioral Interventions, 11,* 3–18.

Boyle, M. (2004). Semantic feature analysis treatment for anomia in two fluent aphasia syndromes. *American Journal of Speech-Language Pathology, 13* (3), 236–249.

Brookshire, R. (2003). *An introduction to neurogenic communication disorders* (6th ed.). St. Louis: Mosby Year Book.

Brookshire, R., & Nicholas, L. E. (1993). *The discourse comprehension test.* Minneapolis, MN: BRK Publishers.

Brookshire, R., & Nicholas, L. E. (1997). *The discourse comprehension test: Test manual* (Rev. ed). Minneapolis, MN: BRK Publishers.

Brown, J. I., Fischco, V. V., & Hanna, G. (1993). *The Nelson-Denny reading skills test.* Chicago: Riverside.

Bryan, L. L. (1995). *The right hemisphere language battery* (2nd ed.). London: Whur Publishers.

Burns, M. (1997). *The Burns brief inventory of communication and cognition.* San Antonio, TX: Psychological Corporation.

Burns, M. S., Halper, A. S., & Mogil, S. I. (1985). *Clinical management of right hemisphere dysfunction.* Rcokville, MD: Aspen.

Butcher, J. (2000). Alzheimer's amyloid hypothesis gains support. *Lancet, 356,* 2161.

Calkins, M. P., & Chafetz, P. K. (1996). Structuring environment for patients with dementia. In M. F. Weiner (Ed.), *The dementias: Diagnosis, management, and research* (2nd ed., pp. 297–311). Washington, DC: American Psychiatric Press.

Calvin, W. H., & Ojemann, G. A. (1980). *Inside the brain.* New York: New American Library.

Camp, C., Bird, M. J., & Cherry, K. C. (2000). Retrieval strategies as a rehabilitation aid for cognitive loss in pathological aging. In R. D. Hill, L. Backman, & A. S. Neely (Eds.), *Cognitive rehabilitation in old age* (pp. 224–248). New York: Oxford University Press.

Camp, C., Foss, J., O'Hanlon, A., & Stevens, A. (1996). Memory interventions for persons with dementia. *Applied Cognitive Psychology, 10,* 193–210.

Carrow-Woodfolk, E. (1999). *Test for auditory comprehension of language* (3rd ed.). Austin, TX: Pro-Ed.

Caspari, I. (2005. Wernicke's asphasia. In L. L. LaPointe (Ed.), *Aphasia and related neurogenic language disorders* (3rd ed), pp. 142–154). New York: Thieme.

Castro, A. J., Merchut, M. P., Neafsey, E. J., & Wurster, R. D. (2002). *Neuroscience: An outline approach.* St. Louis: Mosby.

Chapey, R. (1981). Assessment of language disorders in adults. In R. Chapey (Ed.), *Language intervention strategies in adult aphasia* (pp. 31–84). Baltimore, MD: Williams & Wilkins.

Chapey, R. (Ed.). (2001) *Language intervention strategies in adult aphasia and related neurogenic disorders* (4th ed.). Baltimore: Lippincott Williams & Wilkins.

Chapey, R., Duchan, J. F., Elman, R. J., Garcia, L. J., Kagan, A., Lyon, J. G., & Simmons-Mackie, N. (2001). Life participation approach to aphasia: A statement of values for the future. In R. Chapey (Ed.), *Language intervention strategies in aphasia and related neurogenic communication disorders* (4th ed., pp. 235–245). Philadelphia: Lippincott Williams & Wilkins.

Chapman, S. B., Weiner, M. F., Rackley, A., Hynan, L. S., Zientz, J. (2004). Effects of cognitive-communication stimulation for Alzheimer's disease patients treated with donepezil. *Journal of Speech, Language, and Hearing Research, 47* (5), 1149–1163.

Cimino-Knight, A. M., Hollingsworth, A. L., & Gonzalez Rothi, L. J. (2005). The transcortical aphasias. In L. L. LaPointe (Ed.), *Aphasia and related neurogenic language disorders* (3rd ed., pp. 169–185). New York: Thieme Medical Publishers.

Clark, C. M. (2000). Clinical manifestations and diagnostic evaluation of patients with Alzheimer's disease. In C. M. Clark & J. Q. Trojunowski (Eds.), *Neurodegenerative dementias* (pp. 95–111). New York: McGraw-Hill.

Clark, C. M., & Trojunowski, J. Q. (Eds.). (2000). *Neurodegenerative dementias.* New York: McGraw-Hill.

Colcher, A., & Stern, M. B. (2001). Treatment of Parkinson's disease. In C. M. Clark & J. Q. Trojunowski (Eds.), *Neurodegenerative dementias* (pp. 205–217). New York: McGraw-Hill.

Cole, M. F., & Cole, M. (1971). *Pierre Marie's papers on speech disorders.* New York: Hafner Press.

Collins, M. J. (1991). *Diagnosis and treatment of global aphasia.* San Diego, CA: Singular Publishing Group.

Collins, M. J. (2005). Global aphasia. In L. L. LaPointe (Ed.), *Aphasia and related neurogenic language disorders* (3rd ed., pp. 186–198). New York: Thieme Medical Publishers.

Collins, M. J., Wertz, T. (1981). Coping with success. The maintenance of therapeutic effect in aphasia. In R. H. Brookshire (Ed.), *Clinical aphasiology* (Vol. 14, pp. 156–163). Minneapolis, MN: BRK Publishers.

CoolSpring Software (n.d.). *The Test of Visual Field Attention.* Walkersville, MD: Author.

Cooper, P. R., & Golfinos, J. G. (Eds.). (2000). *Head injury* (4th ed.). New York: McGraw-Hill.

Coppens, P., & Hungerford, S. (1998). Crossed aphasia. In P. Coppens, Y. Lebrun, & A. Basso (Eds.), *Aphasia in atypical populations* (pp. 203–260). Mahwah, NJ: Lawrence Erlbaum.

Coppens, P., Lebrun, Y., & Basso, A. (Eds.). (1998). *Aphasia in atypical populations.* Mahwah, NJ: Lawrence Erlbaum.

Corina, D. (1998). Aphasia in users of signed languages. In P. Coppens, Y. Lebrun, & A. Basso (Eds.), *Aphasia in atypical populations* (pp. 261–309). Mahwah, NJ: Lawrence Erlbaum.

Coulson, I., Strang, V., Marino, R., & Minichiello, V. (2004). Knowledge and lifestyle of healthy older adults related to modifying the onset of vascular dementia. *Archives of Gerontology and Geriatrics, 39* (1), 43–58.

Crary, M. A., Haak, N. J., & Malinsky, A. E. (1989). Preliminary psychometric evaluation of an acute aphasia screening protocol. *Aphasiology, 3,* 611–618.

Cummings, J. L., & Benson, F. D. (1992). *Dementia: A clinical approach.* Newton, MA: Butterworth-Heinemann.

Damasio, A. (1981). The nature of aphasia: Signs and syndromes. In M. T. Sarno (Ed.), *Acquired aphasia* (pp. 51–65). New York: Academic Press.

Damasio, A. (2001). Neural basis of language disorders. In R. Chapey (Ed.), *Language intervention strategies in aphasia and related neurogenic communication disorders* (4th ed., pp. 18–36). Philadelphia: Lippincott Williams & Wilkins.

Darley, F. L. (1982). *Aphasia.* Philadelphia: W. B. Saunders.

David, R., Enderby, P., & Bainton, D. (1982). Treatment of acquired aphasia: Speech therapists and volunteers compared. *Journal of Neurology, Neurosurgery, and Psychiatry, 45,* 957–961.

Davis, G. A. (1992). A survey of adult aphasia. Englewood Cliffs, NJ: PrenticeHall.

Davis, G. A. (2000). *Aphasiology: Disorders and clinical practice.* Needham Heights, MA: Allyn & Bacon.

Davis, G. A., & Wilcox, J. (1981). Incorporating parameters of natural conversation in aphasia. In R. Chapey (Ed.), *Language intervention strategies in adult aphasia* (pp. 169–194). Baltimore, MD: Williams & Wilkins.

Deaton, A. V. (1990). Behavioral change strategies for children and adolescents with traumatic brain injury. In E. D. Bigler (Ed.), *Traumatic brain injury* (pp. 231–249). Austin, TX: Pro-Ed.

Dejong, R., Osterlund, O. W., & Roy, G. W. (1989). Measurement of quality-of-life changes in patients with Alzheimer's disease. *Clinical Therapeutics, 11,* 545–554.

DeRenzi, E., & Faglioni, P. (1978). Normative data and screening power of a shortened version of the Token Test. *Cortex, 14,* 41–49.

DeRenzi, E., & Vignolo, L. A. (1962). The token test: A sensitive test to detect receptive disturbances in aphasics. *Brain, 85,* 665–678.

Dickson, D. W. (2001). Neuropathology of Pick's disease. *Neurology, 56* (Suppl 4), S16–S18.

Doesborgh, S. J., van de Sandt-Koenderman, M. W., Dippel, D. W., van Harskamp, F., Koudstaal, P. J., & Visch-Brink, E. G. (2004). Effects of semantic treatment on verbal communication and linguistic processing in aphasia after stroke: A randomized controlled trial. *Stroke, 35* (1), 141–146.

Donnan, G. A., Carey, L., & Saling, M. M. (1999). More (or less) on Broca. *Lancet, 353* (9158), 1061–1062.

Doody, R. S. (2000). Treatment strategies in Alzheimer's disease. In C. M. Clark & J. Q. Trojunowski (Eds.), *Neurodegenerative dementias* (pp. 115–116). New York: McGraw-Hill.

Doody, R. S., Stevens, J. C., Beck, C., Dubinsky, R. M., Kaye, J. A., Gwyther, L., Mohs, R. C., Thal, L. J., Whitehouse, P. J., Dekosky, S. T., & Cummings, J. L. (2001). Practice parameter: Management of dementia (an evidence based review): Report of the Quality Standards Subcommittee of the American Academy of Neurology. *Neurology, 56,* 1154–1166.

Dorland's illustrated medical dictionary (28th ed.) (1994). Philadelphia: W. B. Saunders.

Doyle, P. J., Goldstein, H., & Bourgeois, M. S. (1987). Experimental analysis of syntax training in Broca's aphasia: A generalization and social validation study. *Journal of Speech and Hearing Disorders, 52* (2), 143–155.

Duffy, J. R. (1995). *Motor speech disorders.* St. Louis: Mosby.

Dunn, L. M., & Dunn L. M. (1981). *Peabody picture vocabulary test* (Rev. ed.). Circle Pines, MN: American Guidance Service.

Eggert, G. H. (1977). *Wernicke's work on aphasia.* The Hague: Mouton.

Eisenson, J. (1954). *Examining for aphasia.* New York: Psychological Corporation.

Elman, R. J. (Ed.). (1999). *Group treatment for neurogenic communication disorders: The expert clinician's approach.* Woburn, MA: Butterworth-Heinemann.

Elman, R. J. (2005). Social and life participation approaches to aphasia intervention. In L. L. La-Pointe (Ed.), *Aphasia and related neurogenic language disorders* (3rd ed., pp. 39–50). New York: Thieme Medical Publishers.

Elman, R. J., & Bernstein-Ellis, E. (1999). The efficacy of group communication treatment in adults with chronic aphasia. *Journal of Speech, Language, and Hearing Research, 42,* 411–419.

Enderby, P. M. (1983). *Frenchay Dysarthria Assessment.* San Diego, CA: College-Hill Press.

Erkinjuntti, T., Kurz, A., Gauthier, S., Bullock, R., Lilienfeld, S., Rao, C., & Damaraju, V. (2002). Efficacy of galantamine in probable vascular dementia and Alzheimer's disease combined with cerebrovascular disease: A randomised trial. *Lancet, 359,* 1283–1290.

Ferris, S. F., & Mohs, R. C. (2000). Measuring treatment efficacy in Alzheimer's disease. In C. M. Clark & J. Q. Trojanowski (Eds.), *Neurodegenerative dementias: Clinical features and pathological mechanisms* (pp. 395–404). New York: McGraw-Hill.

Fitch-West, J., & Sands, E. S. (1998). *The bedside evaluation screening* (2nd ed.) (BEST2). Austin, TX: Pro-Ed.

Folstein, M. F., Folstein, S. E., & McHugh, P. R. (1975). Mini-Mental State: A practical method for grading the cognitive state of patients for the clinician. *Journal of Psychiatric Research, 12,* 189–198.

Fordyce, D. J. (1991). Conceptual issues in cognitive rehabilitation. In D. R. Beukelman & K. M. Yorkston (Eds), *Communication disorders following traumatic brain injury: Management of cognitive, language, and motor impairments* (pp. 57–73). Austin, TX: Pro-Ed.

Fox, N. C., Crum, W. R., Scahill, R. I., Stevens, J. M., Janssen, J. C., & Rosser, M. N. (2001).

Imaging of onset and progression of Alzheimer's disease with voxel-compression mapping of serial magnetic resonance images. *Lancet, 358,* 201–205.

Frankish, H. (2001). Genetic locus increases susceptibility to Alzheimer's disease. *Lancet, 357,* 2031

Frattali, C. M. (Ed.). (1998). *Measuring outcomes in speech-language pathology.* New York: Thieme.

Frattali, C. M., Thompson, C. K., Holland, A. L., Wohl, C. B., & Ferketic, M. M. (1995). *Functional assessment of communication skills for adults* (ASHA FACS). Rockville, MD: American Speech-Language-Hearing Association.

Freed, D. (2000). *Motor speech disorders: Diagnosis and treatment.* Clifton Park, NY: Thomson Delmar Learning.

Freed, D., Celery, K., & Marshall, R. C. (2004). Effectiveness of personalized and phonological cueing on long-term naming performance by aphasic subjects: A clinical investigation. *Aphasiology, 18* (8), 743–757.

Friedland, R. (1993). Epidemiology, education, and the etiology of Alzheimer's disease. *Neurology, 43,* 246–249.

Fromm, D., & Holland, A. L. (1989). Functional communication in Alzheimer's disease. *Journal of Speech and Hearing Disorders, 54,* 535–540.

Gates, W. H., MacGinitie, R. K., Maria, K., et al. (2000). *Gates-MacGinitie reading test.* Chicago: Riverside.

Gauthier, L., Dehaut, F., & Joanette, Y. (1989). The Bells test: a quantitative and qualitative test for visual neglect. *International Journal of Clinical Neuropsychology, 11,* 49–54.

Geshwind, N. (1965). Disconnexion syndromes in animals and man. *Brain, 88,* 237–294, 585–644.

Geshwind, N. (1967). Wernicke's contributions to the study of aphasia. *Cortex, 3,* 449–463.

Giasson, B. I., Galvin, J. E., Lee, V. M.-Y., & Trojanowski, J. Q. (2001). The cellular and molecular pathology of Parkinson's disease. In

C. M. Clark & J. Q. Trojunowski (Eds.), *Neurodegenerative dementias* (pp. 219–228). New York: McGraw-Hill.

Giles, G. M., & Clark-Wilson, J. (1993). *Brain injury rehabilitation: A neurofunctional approach.* London: Chapman & Hall.

Gillette, Y. (2003). *Achieving communication independence: A comprehensive guide to assessment and intervention.* Eau Claire, WI: Thinking Publications.

Gillis, R. J. (1996). *Traumatic brain injury: Rehabilitation for speech-language pathologists.* Boston: Butterworth-Heinemann.

Gitlin, L. N., Hauck, W. W., Dennis, M. P., & Winter, L. (2005). Maintenance of effects of the home environmental skill-building program for family caregivers and individuals with Alzheimer's disease and related disorders. *Journal of Gerontology, 60* (3), 368–374.

Goldstein, K. (1948). *Language and language disturbances. New York: Grune & Stratton.*

Golper, L. A. (1996). Language assessment. In G. L. Wallace (Ed.), *Adult aphasia rehabilitation* (pp. 57–86). Boston: Butterworth-Heinemann.

Goodglass, H. (1988). Historical perspectives on concepts of aphasia. In F. Boller & J. Grafman (Eds.), *Handbook of neuropsychology* (Vol. 1, pp. 51–63). Amsterdam: Elsevier.

Goodglass, H. (1993). *Understanding aphasia.* San Diego, CA: Academic Press.

Goodglass, H., & Kaplan, E. (1983). *The assessment of aphasia and related disorders* (2nd ed.). Philadelphia: Lee & Febiger.

Goodglass, H., Kaplan, E., & Barresi, B. (2001). *The Boston diagnostic aphasia examination* (3rd ed.). Austin, TX: Pro-Ed.

Goodglass, H., Kaplan, E., & Barresi, B. (2001). *The assessment of aphasia and related disorders* (3rd ed.). Philadelphia: Lippincott Williams & Wilkins.

Gordon, W. A., & Associates (1984). *Evaluation of the deficits associated with right-brain damage: Normative data on the Institute of Rehabilitation*

Medicine test battery. New York: Department of Behavioral Sciences, NYU Medical Center.

Graham, D. I., & Gennarelli, T. A. (2000). Pathology of brain damage after head injury. In P. R. Cooper & J. G. Golfinos (Eds.), *Head injury* (4th ed., pp. 133–153). New York: McGraw-Hill.

Graham-Kegan, L., & Caspari, I. (1997). Wernicke's aphasia. In L. L. LaPointe (Ed.), *Aphasia and related neurogenic language disorders* (2nd ed., pp. 42–62). New York: Thieme Medical Publishers.

Grant, D. A., & Berg, E. A. (1948). A behavioral analysis of degree of reinforcement and ease of shifting to new responses in Weight-type card sorting problem. *Journal of Experimental Psychology, 38,* 403–411.

Greener, J., Enderby, P., & Whurr, R. (2001). Pharmacological treatment of aphasia following stroke. Cochrane Database Systematic Review, 4, CD000424.

Greenberg, D. A., Aminoff, M. J., & Simon, R. P. (2002). *Clinical neurology* (5th ed.). New York: Lange Medical Books/McGraw-Hill.

Hachinsky, V. F., Illiff, L. D., Zilhka, E., & Associates (1975). Cerebral blood flow in dementia. *Archives of Neurology, 32,* 632–637.

Hagen, C. (2000, February). *Ranchos Los Amigos Levels of Cognitive Functioning—Revised.* Downey, CA: Comunication Disorders Services: Ranchos Los Amigos National Rehabilitation Center.

Hagen, C., & Malkamus, D. (1979). Interaction strategies for language disorders secondary to head trauma. Paper presented at the annual convention of the American Speech-Language-Hearing Association, Atlanta, GA.

Haines, D. E. (2004). *Neuroanatomy: An atlas of structures, sections, and systems* (6th ed.). Philadelphia: Lippincott Williams & Wilkins.

Haines, D. E., & Lancon, J. A. (2003). *A review of neuroscience.* New York: Churchill Livingstone.

Hake, A. M., & Farlow, M. R. (2001). Huntington's disease. In C. M. Clark & J. Q. Tro-junowski (Eds.), *Neurodegenerative dementias* (pp. 301–310). New York: McGraw-Hill.

Halper, A., Cherney, L. R., & Burns, M. S. (1996). *Clinical management of right hemisphere dysfunction (2nd ed.).* Gaithersburg, MD: Aspen.

Hamdy, R. C., Turnbull, J. M., Edwards, J., & Lancaster, M. M. (1998). *Alzheimer's disease: A handbook for caregivers* (3rd ed.). St. Louis: Mosby.

Hanna, G., Schell, L. M., & Schreiner, R. (1977). *The Nelson reading skills test.* Chicago: Riverside.

Harper, P. S. (Ed.). (1996). *Huntington's disease.* London: W. B. Saunders.

Harrington, T., & Apostolides, P. (2000). Penetrating brain injury. In P. R. Cooper & J. G. Golfinos (Eds.), *Head injury* (4th ed., pp. 349–359). New York: McGraw-Hill.

Hartley, L. L. (1995). *Cognitive-communicative abilities following brain injury. San Diego, CA: Singular Publishing Group.*

Haskins, S. (1976). A treatment procedure for writing disorders. In R. H. Brookshire (Ed.), *Clinical aphasiology conference proceedings* (pp. 192–199). Minneapolis, MN: BRK.

Head, H. (1926). *Aphasia and kindred disorders.* London: Cambridge University Press.

Hegde, M. N. (1998). *Treatment procedures in communicative disorders* (3rd ed.). Austin, TX: Pro-Ed.

Hegde, M. N. (2001). *Hegde's pocketguide to assessment in speech-language pathology* (2nd ed.). Clifton Park, NY: Thomson Delmar Learning.

Hegde, M. N. (2003). *Clinical research in communicative disorders: Principles and strategies* (3rd ed.). Austin, TX: Pro-Ed.

Hegde, M. N., & Davis, D. (2005). *Clinical methods and practicum in speech-language pathology* (4th ed.). Clifton Park, NY: Thomson Delmar Learning.

Helm-Estabrooks, N. (1981). *Helm Elicited Language program for Syntax Stimulation.* Austin, TX: Pro-Ed.

Helm-Estabrooks, N. (1986). Diagnosis and management of neurogenic stuttering in adults. In K. O. St. Louis (Ed.), *The atypical stutterer* (pp. 193–218). New York: Academic Press.

Helm-Estabrooks, N., & Albert, M. L. (2004). *A manual of aphasia therapy* (2nd ed.). Austin, TX: Pro-Ed.

Helm-Estabrooks, N., Fitzpatrick, P. M., & Barresi, B. (1982). Response of an agrammatic patient to a syntax stimulation program for aphasia. *Journal of Speech and Hearing Disorders, 46,* 422–427.

Helm-Estabrooks, N., & Holland, A. (Eds.). (1998). *Approaches to the treatment of aphasia.* San Diego, CA: Singular Publishing Group.

Helm-Estabrooks, N., & Hotz, G., (1991). *Brief test of head injury.* Chicago: Riverside.

Helm-Estabrooks, N., Ramsberger, G., Nicholas, M., & Morgan, A. (1989). *Boston assessment of severe aphasia.* Austin, TX: Pro-Ed.

Hering-Hanit, R., Achiron, R., Lipitz, S., & Achiron, A. (2001). Asymmetry of fetal cerebral hemispheres: In utero ultrasound study. *Archives of Disease in Childhood-Fetal and Neonatal Edition, 85* (3), F194–F196.

Heyn, P., Abreu, B. C., & Ottenbacher, K. J. (2004). The effects of exercise training on elderly persons with cognitive impairment and dementia: A meta-analysis. *Archives of Physical Medicine and Rehabilitation, 85* (10), 1694–1704.

Hick, J., Zornberg, G. L., Jick, S. S., Seshadri, S., & Drachman, D. A. (2000). Statins and the risk of dementia. *Lancet, 356,* 1627–1631.

Hickin, J., Herbert, R., Best, W., Howard, D., & Osborne, F. (2002). Phonological therapy for word finding difficulties: A re-evaluation. *Aphasiology, 16,* 981–999.

Hodges, J. R. (2001). Frontotemporal dementia (Pick's disease): Clinical features and assessment. *Neurology, 56* (Suppl 4), S6–S9.

Holland, A. L. (1980). *Communicative abilities in daily living.* Baltimore, MD: University Park Press.

Holland, A. (1996). Pragmatic assessment and treatment for aphasia. In G. L. Wallace (Ed.), *Adult aphasia rehabilitation* (pp. 161–173). Boston: Butterworth-Heinemann.

Holland, A. L., & Beeson, P. (1999). Aphasia groups: The Arizona experience. In R. Elman (Ed.), *Group treatment for neurogenic communication disorders: The expert clinician's approach* (pp. 77–84). Woburn, MA: Butterworth-Heinemann.

Holland, A. L., Frattali, C. M., & Fromm, D. (1998). *Communication activities in daily living* (2nd ed.). Austin, TX: Pro-Ed.

Holland, A. L., Fromm, D. S., DeRuyter, F., & Stein, M. (1996). Treatment efficacy: Aphasia. *Journal of Speech and Hearing Research, 39* (5), S27–S36.

Hopper, T. L. (2003). "They are just going to get worse anyway": Perspective on rehabilitation for nursing home residents with dementia. *Journal of Communication Disorders, 36,* 345–359.

Horner, R. D., Swanson, J. W., Bosworth, H. B., & Matchar, D. B. (2003). Effects of race and poverty on the process and outcome of inpatient rehabilitation services among stroke patients. *Stroke, 43* (4), 1027–1031.

Huber, W. (1999). The role of piracetam in the treatment of acute and chronic aphasia. *Pharmacopsychiatry, 32* (Suppl) 1, 38–43.

Hux, K., Manasse, N., Weiss, A., & Beukelman, D. R. (2001). Augmentative and alternative communication for persons with aphasia. In R. Chapey (Ed.), *Language intervention strategies in adult aphasia and related neurogenic disorders* 4th ed., (pp. 675–687). Baltimore, MD: Lippincott Williams & Wilkins.

Jackson, J. H. (1874). On affections of speech from diseases of the brain. *Brain, 1,* 304–330.

Jacobs, B. S., Boden-Albala, B., Lin, I. F., & Sacco, R. L. (2002). Stroke in the young in the Northern Manhattan Stroke Study. *Stroke, 33* (12), 2789–2793.

Jakobson, R. (1956). Two aspects of language and two types of aphasic disturbances. In R. Jakobson & M. Halle (Eds.), *Fundamentals of language* (pp. 55–87). The Hague: Mouton.

Jacques, A., & Jackson, G. A. (2000). *Understanding dementia* (3rd ed.). New York: Churchill Livingstone.

Jagust, W. (2001). Understanding vascular dementia. *Lancet, 358,* 2097–2098.

Jennett, B., & Teasdale, G. (1981). *Management of head injuries.* Philadelphia: FA Davis Company.

Jeremitsky, E., Omert, L., Dunham, C. M., Protetch, J., & Rodriguez, A. (2003). Harbingers of poor outcome the day after severe brain injury: hypothermia, hypoxia, and hypoperfusion. *Journal of Trauma, 54* (2), 312–319.

Johnson, N., Barion, A., Rademaker, A., Rehkemper, G., & Weintraub, S. (2004). The Activities of Daily Living Questionnaire: A validation study in patients with dementia. *Alzheimer's Disease and Associated Disorders, 18* (4), 223–230.

Jones, R. W. (2001). Inflammation and Alzheimer's disease. *Lancet, 358,* 436–437.

Kagan, A. (1995). Revealing the competence of aphasic adults through conversation: Challenge to health professions. *Topics in Stroke Rehabilitation, 2,* 15–28.

Kagan, A., Black, S. E., Duchan, J. F., Simmons-Mackie, N., & Square, P. (2001). Training volunteers as conversation partners using supported conversational for adults with aphasia (SCA): A controlled trial. *Journal of Speech, Language, and Hearing Research, 44,* 624–638.

Kagan, A., & Gailey, G. F. (1993). Function is not enough: Training conversation partners for aphasic adults. In A. L. Holland & M. M. Forbes (Eds.), *Aphasia treatment: World perspectives* (pp. 199–225). San Diego, CA: Singular Publishing Group.

Kaiser, H. (Ed.). (1995). *Bilingual speech-language pathology: An Hispanic focus.* San Diego, CA: Singular Publishing Group.

Kaplan, E., Goodglass, H., & Weintraub, S. (2001). *The Boston naming test.* Philadelphia: Lippincott Williams & Wilkins.

Kaplan, M., & Hoffman, S. B. (1998). *Behavior in dementia: Best practice for successful management.* Baltimore, MD: Health Professions Press.

Kapp, M. B. (2002). Legal standards for the medical diagnosis and treatment of dementia. *Journal of Legal Medicine, 23* (3), 25–32.

Kearns, K. P. (2005). Broca's aphasia. In L. L. La-Pointe (Ed.), *Aphasia and related neurogenic language disorders* (3rd ed., pp. 117–141). New York: Thieme Medical Publishers.

Kearns, K. P., & Elman, R. J. (2001). Group therapy for aphasia: Theoretical and practical considerations. In R. Chapey (Ed.), *Language intervention strategies in aphasia and related neurogenic communication disorders* (4th ed., pp. 315–337). Philadelphia: Lippincott Williams & Wilkins.

Kearns, K. P., & Potechin-Scher, G. (1989). The generalization of response elaboration training effects. In T. E. Prescott (Ed.), *Clinical aphasiology* (Vol. 18, pp. 223–246). San Diego, CA: College-Hill Press.

Keenan, J. S., & Brassell, E. G. (1975). *Aphasia language performance scales.* Murphresboro, TN: Pinnacle Press.

Kempler, D. (1995). Language changes in dementia of the Alzheimer type. In R. Lubinski (Ed.), *Dementia and communication* (pp. 98–114). San Diego, CA: Singular Publishing Group.

Kertesz, A. (1982). *Western aphasia battery.* New York: Grune & Stratton.

Kessler, J., Thiel, A., Karbe, H., & Heiss, W. D. (2000). Piracetam improves activated blood flow and facilitates rehabilitation of post-stroke aphasic patients. *Stroke, 31,* 2112–2116.

Kiernan, J. A. (2005). *Barr's the human nervous system: An anatomical viewpoint* (8th ed.). Philadelphia: J. B. Lippincott.

King, W. J., MacKay, M., & Sirnick, A. (2003). Shaken baby syndrome in Canada: Clinical characteristics and outcomes of hospital cases. *Canadian Medical Association Journal, 168* (2), 155–159.

Klein, A. M., Ferrante, R. J., & Ball, M. F. (2001). Cellular and molecular pathology of Huntington's disease. In C. M. Clark &

J. Q. Trojunowski (Eds.), *Neurodegenerative dementias* (pp. 311–328). New York: McGraw-Hill.

Korczyn, A. D. (2001). Hallucinations in Parkinson's disease. *Lancet, 358* (9287), 1031–1032.

Kraus, J. K., & McArthur, D. L. (2000). Epidemiology of brain injury. In P. R. Cooper & J. G. Golfinos (Eds.), *Head injury* (4th ed., pp. 1–26). New York: McGraw-Hill.

LaPointe, L. L. (1977). Base-10 programmed stimulation. Task specification, scoring and plotting performance in aphasia therapy. *Journal of Speech and Hearing Disorders, 42,* 90–105.

LaPointe, L. L. (Ed.) (2005). *Aphasia and related neurogenic language disorders* (3rd ed.). New York: Thieme Medical Publishers.

LaPointe, L. L., & Horner, J. (1978). The functional auditory comprehension task (FACT): Protocol and test format. *FLASHA Journal,* 27–33.

LaPointe, L. L., & Horner, J. (1998). *Reading comprehension battery for aphasia* (Rev. ed.). Austin, TX: Pro-Ed.

Larkin, M. (1998). Alzheimer's disease prevalence may quadruple. *Lancet, 352,* 965.

Larsen, C. (1998). *HIV and communication disorders.* Clifton Park, NY: Thomson Delmar Learning.

Lee, L. (1971). *Northwestern syntax screening test.* Evanston, IL: Northwestern University Press.

Le Roux, P. D. (2000). Prevention and management of seizures in the head injured patient. In P. R. Cooper & J. G. Golfinos (Eds.), *Head injury* (4th ed., pp. 499–516). New York: McGraw-Hill.

Levin, H. S., O'Donnell, V. N., & Grossman, R. G. (1979). The Galveston orientation and amnesia test: A practical scale to assess cognition after head injury. *Journal of Nervous Mental Disorders, 167,* 675–684.

Lincoln, N. B., Mulley, G. P., Jones, A. C., & Associates. (1984). Effectiveness of speech therapy for aphasic stroke patients: A randomized controlled trial. *Lancet, 2,* 1197–1200.

Lindvall, O. (2001). Stem cell transplantation. *Lancet, 358* (Supplement), S47.

Lindvall, O., & Bjorklund, A. (2000). First step towards cell therapy for Huntington's disease. *Lancet, 456* (9246), 1945–1946.

Linebaugh, C. W. (1997). Lexical retrieval problems. In L. L. LaPointe (Ed.), *Aphasia and related neurogenic language disorders* (2nd ed., pp. 112–132). New York: Thieme Medical Publishers.

Litvan, I. (2001). Therapy and management of frontal lobe dementia patients. *Neurology, 56* (Suppl 4), S41–S44.

Logemann, J. A. (1998). *Evaluation and treatment of swallowing disorders* (2nd ed.). Austin, TX: Pro-Ed.

Lomas, J., Pickard, L., Bester, S., & Associates. (1989). The communicative effectiveness index: Clinical and research assessment of head injury outcome. *International Rehabilitation Medicine, 7,* 145–149.

Love, R. J., & Webb, W. G. (2001). *Neurology for the speech-language pathologist* (4th ed.). Boston: Butterworth.

Lubinski, R. (1981). Speech, language, and audiology programs in home health care agencies and nursing homes. In D. S. Beasley & G. A. Davis (Eds.), *Aging: Communication processes and disorders* (pp. 339–356). New York: Grune & Stratton.

Lubinski, R. (Ed.). (1995). *Dementia and communication.* San Diego, CA: Singular Publishing Group.

Lubinski, R., & Frattali, C. (Eds.). (1994). *Professional issues in speech-language pathology.* San Diego, CA: Singular Publishing Group.

Luria, A. R. (1963). *Restoration of function after brain injury.* Oxford, England: Pergamon Press.

Luria, A. R. (1970). *Traumatic aphasia.* The Hague: Mouton.

Lyon, J. (1997). Volunteers as partners: Moving intervention outside the treatment room. In B. B. Shadden & M. A. Toner (Eds.), *Aging and communication* (pp. 299–323). Austin, TX: Pro-Ed.

Lyon, J. (1998). Treating real-life functionality in a couple coping with severe aphasia. In N. Helm-

Estabrooks & A. Holland (Eds.), *Approaches to the treatment of aphasia* (pp. 203–240). San Diego, CA: Singular Publishing Group.

Mahendra, N. (2001). Direct interventions for improving the performance of individuals with Alzheimer's disease. *Seminars-in-Speech-and-Language, 22* (4), 291–304.

Mahendra, N., & Arkin, S. M. (2003). Effects of four years of exercise, language, and social interventions on Alzheimer discourse. *Journal of Communication Disorders, 36,* 395–422.

Mahendra, N., & Arkin, S. M. (2004). Exercise and volunteer work: Context for AD language and memory interventions. *Seminars-in-Speech-and-Language, 25* (2), 151–167.

Martin, A. D. (1981). The role of theory in therapy: A rationale. *Topics in Language Disorders, 1,* 63–72.

Marshall, R. C. (1999). *Introduction to group treatment for aphasia: Design and management.* Boston: Butterworth-Heinemann

Marquardt, T. P., Stoll, J., & Sussman, H. (1990). Disorders of communication in traumatic brain injury. In E. D. Bigler (Ed.), *Traumatic brain injury* (pp. 181–205). Austin, TX: Pro-Ed.

McMurray, C. T. (2001). Huntington's disease: Expanding horizons for treatment. *Lancet, 358* (Suppl), s37.

McNeil, M. R., Doyle, P. J., Spencer, K., Goda, A. J., Flores, D., & Smith, S. (1997). A double-blind, placebo controlled, pharmacological and behavioral treatment of lexical-semantic deficits in aphasia. *Aphasiology, 11,* 385–400.

McNeil, M. R., & Prescott, T. E. (1978). *The revised token test.* Baltimore, MD: University Park Press.

Mentis, M., Briggs-Whittaker, J., & Gramigna, G. D. (1995). Discourse topic management in senile dementia of the Alzheimer's type. *Journal of Speech and Hearing Research, 38,* 1054–1066.

Mlcoch, A. G., & Metter, E. J. (2001). Medical aspects of stroke rehabilitation. In R. Chapey (Ed.), *Language intervention strategies in adult*

aphasia (pp. 37–54). Baltimore, MD: Williams & Wilkins.

Mohr, J. P. (1980). Revision of Broca's aphasia and the syndrome of Broca's area infarction and its implication in aphasia theory. *Clinical Aphasiology Conference Proceedings* (pp. 1–16). Minneapolis, MN: BRK Publishers.

Molloy, D. W., & Lubinski, R. (1995). Dementia: Impact and clinical perspectives. In R. Lubinski (Ed.), *Dementia and communication* (pp. 2–21). Philadelphia: B. C. Decker.

Morris, J. C. (1993). The Clinical Dementia Rating Scale (CDR): Current version and scoring rules. *Neurology, 43,* 2412–2414.

Morris, J. C. (2001). Frontotemporal dementias. In C. M. Clark & J. Q. Trojunowski (Eds.), *Neurodegenerative dementias* (pp. 279–290). New York: McGraw-Hill.

Murdoch, B. E., & Theodoros, D. G. (2001). *Traumatic brain injury: Associated speech, language and swallowing disorders.* Albany, NY: Singular Thomson Learning.

Murray, L. L. (2000). Spoken language production in Huntington's and Parkinson's disease. *Journal of Speech, Language, and Hearing Research, 43* (6), 1350–1366.

Murray, L. L., & Chapey, R. (2001). Assessment of language disorders in adults. In R. Chapey (Ed.), *Language intervention strategies in adult aphasia* (pp. 55–118). Baltimore, MD: Williams & Wilkins.

Murray, L. L., & Stout, J. (1999). Discourse comprehension in Huntington's and Parkinson's diseases. *American Journal of Speech-Language Pathology, 8* (2), 137–148.

Mychack, P., Kramer, J. H., Boone, K. B., & Miller, B. L. (2001). *Neurology, 56* (Suppl 4), S11–S14.

Myers, P. S. (1997). Right hemisphere syndrome. In L. L. LaPointe (Ed.), *Aphasia and related neurogenic language disorders* (2nd ed., pp. 201–225). New York: Thieme Medical Publishers.

Myers, P. S. (1999). *Right hemisphere damage.* Clifton Park, NY: Thomson Delmar Learning.

Nickels, L. (2002). Therapy for naming disorders: Revisiting, revising, and reviewing. *Aphasiology, 16* (10/11), 935–979.

Nickels, L., & Best, W. (1996a). Therapy for naming disorders (Part I): Principles, puzzles and progress. *Aphasiology, 10* (1), 21–47.

Nickels, L., & Best, W. (1996b). Therapy for naming disorders (Part II): Specifics, surprises and suggestions. *Aphasiology, 10* (2), 109–136.

Nielsen, J. M. (1936). *Agnosia, apraxia and aphasia: Their value in cerebral localization.* New York: Hafner.

Nolte, J. (2002). *The human brain: An introduction to its functional anatomy* (5th ed.). St. Louis: Mosby Year Book.

Ogrocki, P. K., & Welsh-Bohmer, K. A. (2000). Assessment of cognitive and functional impairment in the elderly. In C. M. Clark & J. Q. Trojanowski (Eds.), *Neurodegenerative dementias: Clinical features and pathological mechanisms* (pp. 15–32). New York: McGraw-Hill.

Olanow, C. W., Watts, R. L., & Koller, W. (2001). An algorithm (decision tree) for the management of Parkinson's disease. *Neurology, 2001, 56* (Suppl 5):S1–S88.

Orange, J. B. (2001). Family caregivers, communication, and Alzheimer's disease. In M. L. Hummert & J. F. Nussbaum (Eds.), *Aging, communication, and health* (pp. 225–248). Mahwah, NJ: Erlbaum.

Orange, J. B., Lubinski, R., & Higginbotham, D. J. (1996). Conversational repair by individuals with dementia of the Alzheimer's disease. *Journal of Speech and Hearing Research, 39,* 881–895.

Paradis, M. (1987). *The assessment of bilingual aphasia.* Hillsdale, NJ: Lawrence Erlbaum.

Paradis, M. (1998). Aphasia in bilinguals: How atypical is it? In P. Coppens, Y. Lebrun, & A. Basso (Eds.), *Aphasia in atypical populations* (pp. 35–66). Mahwah, NJ: Lawrence Erlbaum.

Payne, J. C. (1994). *Communication profile: A functional skills survey.* San Antonio, TX: Communication Skill Builders.

Payne, J. C. (1997). *Adult neurogenic language disorders: Assessment and treatment.* San Diego, CA: Singular Publishing Group.

Peach, R. K. (2001). Clinical intervention for global aphasia. In R. Chapey (Ed.), *Language intervention strategies in aphasia and related neurogenic communication disorders* (4th ed., pp. 487–512). Philadelphia: Lippincott Williams & Wilkins

Penfield, W., & Roberts, L. (1959). *Speech and brain mechanisms.* Princeton, NJ: Princeton University Press.

Perry, R. J., & Miller, B. L. (2001). Behavior and treatment in frontotemporal dementia. *Neurology, 56* (Suppl 4), S46–S50.

Pimental, P. A., & Kingsbury, N. A. (1989). *Neuropsychological aspects of right brain injury.* Austin, TX: Pro-Ed.

Porch, B. E. (2001). *Porch index of communicative ability* (4th ed.). Palo Alto, CA: Consulting Psychologists Press.

Prutting. C. A., & Kircher, D. M. (1987). A clinical appraisal of the pragmatic aspects of language. *Journal of Speech and Hearing Disorders, 52,* 105–119.

Pulvermuller, F., Neininger, B., Elbert, T., Mohr, B., Rockstroh, B., Koebbel, P., & Taub, E. (2001). Constrained-induced therapy of chronic aphasia after stroke. *Stroke, 32* (7), 1621–1626.

Quayhagen, M, & Quayhagen, M. (1989). Differential effects of family-based strategies on Alzheimer's disease. *The Gerontologist, 49,* 150–155.

Quayhagen, M., & Quayhagen, M. (2001). Testing of cognitive stimulation intervention for dementia caregiving dyads. *Neuropsychological Rehabilitation, 11,* 319–332.

Quayhagen, M., Quayhagen, M., Carbeil, R., Hendrix, R., Jackson, J., & Snyder, L. (2000). Coping with dementia: Evaluation of four non-pharmacological interventions. *International Psychogeriatrics, 12,* 249–265.

Rabins, P. V., Lyketsos, C. G., & Steele, C. D. (1999). *Practical dementia care.* New York: Oxford University Press.

Radonjic, V., & Rakuscek, N. (1991). Group therapy to encourage communication ability in aphasic patients. *Aphasiology, 5* (4–5), 451–455.

Rajput, A. H. (2001). Epidemiology and clinical genetics of Parkinson's disease. In C. M. Clark & J. Q. Trojunowski (Eds.), *Neurodegenerative dementias* (pp. 177–192). New York: McGraw-Hill.

Rappoport, M., Hall, K. M., Hopkins, K., & Associates. (1982). Disability rating scale for severe head trauma: Coma to community. *Archives of Physical Medicine and Rehabilitation, 63,* 118–123.

Rascol, O., Goetz, C., Koller, W., Poewe, W., & Sampaio, C. (2002). Treatment interventions for Parkinson's disease: An evidence based assessment. *Lancet, 359* (9317), 1589–1598.

Raven, J. C. (1960). *The standard progressive matrices.* New York: Psychological Corporation.

Raymer, A. (2005). Naming and word retrieval problems. In L. L. LaPointe (Ed.), *Aphasia and related neurogenic language disorders* (3rd ed., pp. 68–82). New York: Thieme Medical Publishers.

Rayner, H., & Marshall, J. (2003). Training volunteers as conversation partners for people with aphasia. *International Journal of Language and Communication Disorders, 38* (2), 149–64.

Reisberg, B., Ferris, S. H., DeLeon, M. J., & Crook, T. (1982). The global deterioration scale for assessment of primary degenerative dementia. *American Journal of Psychiatry, 139,* 1136–1139.

Reitan, R. M. (1991). *Aphasia Screening Test* (2nd ed.). Tucson, AZ: Reitan Neuropsychology Laboratory.

Ritchie, K., & Lovestone, S. (2002). The dementias. *The Lancet, 360* (9347), 1759–1766.

Ripich, D. N. (1995). Differential diagnosis and assessment. In R. Lubinski (Ed.), *Dementia and communication* (pp. 188–222). San Diego, CA: Singular Publishing Group.

Robey, R. R. (1994). Efficacy of treatment for aphasic persons: A meta-analysis. *Brain and Language, 47,* 585–608.

Robey, R. R. (1998). A meta-analysis of clinical outcomes in the treatment of aphasia *Journal of Speech, Language, and Hearing Research, 41,* 172–187.

Robey, R. R., Schultz, M. C., Crawford, A. B., & Sinner, C. A. (1999). Single-subject clinical-outcome research: designs, data, effect sizes, and analyses. *Aphasiology, 13* (6), 445–473.

Rosen, W. G., Mohs, R. C., & Davis, K. L. (1984). A new rating scale for Alzheimer's disease. *American Journal of Psychiatry, 141,* 1356–1364.

Rosenbek, J. C., LaPointe, L. L., & Wertz, R. T. (1989). *Aphasia: A clinical approach.* Austin: TX: Pro-Ed.

Ross, D. G. (1996). Ross information processing assessment (2nd ed.). Austin, TX: Pro-Ed.

Rossor, M. N. (2001). Pick's disease: A clinical overview. *Neurology, 56* (Suppl 4), S3–S5.

Rothi, L. J. G. (1997). Transcortical aphasias. In L. L. LaPointe (Ed.), *Aphasia and related neurogenic language disorders* (2nd ed., pp. 91–111). New York: Thieme Medical Publishers.

Sacktor, N. (2002). The epidemiology of human immunodeficiency virus-associated neurological disease in the era of highly active antiretroviral therapy. *Journal of Neurovirology, 8* (Suppl 2), 115–121.

Sarno, M. T. (1969). *The functional communication profile: Manual of directions.* New York: New York University Medical Center, Institute of Rehabilitaion Medicine.

Sarno, M. T. (Ed.). (1998). *Acquired aphasia* (3rd ed.). New York: Academic Press.

Schoenberg, B. S., Anderson, D. W., & Haerer A. F. (1985). Severe dementia: Prevalence and clinical features in a biracial US population. *Archives of Neurology, 42,* 740–743.

Schuell, H. M. (1955). *The Minnesota Test for the Differential Diagnosis of Aphasia.* Minneapolis: University of Minnesota Press.

Schuell, H. M. (1973). *Differential diagnosis of aphasia with the Minnesota test* (2nd ed., revised by Sefer, J. W.). Minneapolis: University of Minnesota Press.

Schuell, H., Jenkins, J. J., & Carroll, J. B. (1962). A factor analysis of the Minnesota Test for Differential Diagnosis of Aphasia. *Journal of Speech and Hearing Research, 5,* 349–369.

Schuell, H. M., Jenkins, J. J., & Jimenez-Pabon, E. (1964). *Aphasia in adults: Diagnosis, prognosis and treatment.* New York: Hoeber Medical Division, Harper & Row.

Screen, R. M., & Anderson, N. B. (1994). *Multicultural perspectives in communication disorders.* San Diego, CA: Singular Publishing Group.

Seikel, J. A., King, D. W., & Drumright, D. G. (2005). *Anatomy and physiology for speech, language, and hearing* (3rd ed.). Clifton Park, NY: Thomson Delmar Learning.

Shadden, B. B., & Toner, M. A. (Eds.). (1997). *Aging and communication.* Austin, TX: Pro-Ed.

Shekim, L. O. (1997). Dementia. In L. L. La-Pointe (Ed.), *Aphasia and related neurogenic language disorders* (2nd ed., pp. 238–249). New York: Thieme Medical Publishers.

Shewan, C. M. (1981). *Auditory comprehension test for sentences.* Chicago: Biolinguistics Clinical Institutes.

Shimomura, T., & Mori, E. (1998). Obstinate imitation behaviour in differentiation of frontotemporal dementia from Alzheimer's disease. *Lancet, 352,* 623–624.

Shipley, K. G., & McAfee, J. G. (2004). *Assessment in speech-language pathology: A resource manual* (3rd ed.). Clifton Park, NY: Thomson Delmar Learning.

Simon, R. P., Aminoff, M. J., & Greenberg, D. A. (1999). *Clinical neurology* (4th ed.). Stamford, CT: Appleton & Lange.

Simmons-Mackie, N. (1997). Conduction aphasia. In L. L. LaPointe (Ed.), *Aphasia and related neurogenic language disorders* (2nd ed., pp. 63–90). New York: Thieme Medical Publishers.

Simmons-Mackie, N. (2001). Social approaches to aphasia treatment. In R. Chapey (Ed.), *Language intervention strategies in aphasia and related neurogenic communication disorders* (4th ed., pp. 246–268). Philadelphia: Lippincott Williams & Wilkins.

Simmons-Mackie, N. (2005). Conduction aphasia. In L. L. LaPointe (Ed.), *Aphasia and related neurogenic language disorders* (3rd ed., pp. 155–168). New York: Thieme Medical Publishers.

Simuni, T., & Hurtig, H. I. (2001). Parkinson's disease: Clinical picture. In C. M. Clark & J. Q. Trojunowski (Eds.), *Neurodegenerative dementias* (pp. 193–203). New York: McGraw-Hill.

Skelly, M. (1979). *Amerind gestural code based on universal American Indian hand talk.* New York: Elsevier-North Holland.

Sklar, M. (1983). *Sklar aphasia scale.* Los Angeles: Western Psychological Services.

Small, J. A., Gutman, G., Makela, S., & Hillhouse, B. (2003). Effectiveness of communication strategy used by caregivers of persons with Alzheimer's disease during activities of daily living. *Journal of Speech, Language, Hearing Research, 46,* 353–367.

Snow, A. L., Norris, M. P., Doody, R., Molinari, V. A., Orengo, C. A., & Kunik, M. E. (2004). Dementia Deficits Scale: Rating self-awareness of deficits. *Alzheimer's Disease and Associated Disorders, 18* (1), 22–31.

Solfrizzi, V., D'Introno, A., Colacicco, A. M., Capurso, C., Del Parigi, A., Capurso, S., Gadaleta, A., Caourso, A., & Panza, F. (2005). Dietary fatty acids intake: Possible role in cognitive decline and dementia. *Experimental Gerontology, 40* (4), 257–270.

Solfrizzi, V., Panza, F., & Capurso, A. (2003). The role of diet in cognitive decline. *Journal of Neural Transmission, 10* (1), 95–110.

Spencer, K. A., Doyle, P. J., McNeil, M. R., Wambaugh, J. L., Park, G., & Carroll, B. (2000). Examining the facilitative effects of rhyme in a patient with output lexicon damage. *Aphasiology, 14,* 567–584.

Sperry, R. W. (1964). The great cerebral commissure. *Scientific American, 246,* 124–135.

Spreen, O., & Benton, A. L. (1977). *Neurosensory Center Comprehensive Examination for Aphasia.* Victoria, BC: University of Victoria.

Spreen, O., & Risser, A. (1998). Assessment of aphasia. In M. T. Sarno (Ed.), *Acquired aphasia* (3rd ed., pp. 71–156). New York: Academic Press.

Stanczak, D. E., et al. (1984). Assessment of level of consciousness following severe neurological insult. *Journal of Neurosurgery, 60,* 955–960.

Stanton, K., Yorkston, K. M., Talley-Kenyon, V., & Associates. (1981). Language utilization in teaching reading to left neglect patients. In R. H. Brookshire (Ed.), *Clinical Aphasiology Conference Proceedings* (pp. 262–271). Minneapolis, MN: BRK Publishers.

Subramanian, T. (2001). Cell transplantation for the treatment of Parkinson's disease. *Seminars in Neurology, 21* (1), 103–115.

Sys-Eur Investigators. (1998). Prevention of dementia in randomized double-blind placebo-controlled Systolic Hypertension in Europe (Sys-Eur) trial. *Lancet, 352,* 1347–1351.

Tanner, D. C., & Culbertson, W. (1999). *Quick assessment for aphasia.* Oceanside, CA: Academic Communication Associates.

Teasdale, G., & Jennett, B. (1976). Assessment and prognosis of coma after head injury. *Acta Neurochirargica (Wien), 34,* 45–55.

Teng, E. L., & Chui, K. (1987). The modified Mini-Mental State (3MS) Examination. *Journal of Clinical Psychiatry, 48,* 314–318.

Terrell, B. & Ripich, D. (1989). Discourse competence as a variable in intervention. *Seminars in Speech and Language: Aphasia and Pragmatics, 10,* 282–297.

Thomas, R. G. (2000). Biostatistical issues in neurodegenerative disease. In C. M. Clark & J. Q. Trojunowski (Eds.), *Neurodegenerative dementias* (pp. 411–414). New York: McGraw-Hill.

Tien, R., & Chesnut, R. M. (2000). Medical management of the traumatic brain injured patient. In P. R. Cooper & J. G. Golfinos (Eds.), *Head injury* (4th ed., pp. 457–482). New York: McGraw-Hill.

Tomoeda. C. K. (2001). Comprehensive assessment for dementia: A necessity for differential diagnosis and management. *Seminars in Speech and Language, 22* (4), 275–289.

Tompkins, C. A. (1995). *Right hemisphere communication disorders: Theory and practice.* Clifton Park, NY: Thomson Delmar Learning.

Tonkovich, J. D. (2002). Multicultural issues in the management of neurogenic communication and swallowing disorders. In D. E. Battle (Ed.), *Communication disorders in multicultural populations* (3rd ed., pp. 233–265). Boston: Butterworth-Heinemann.

Tseng, C., & McNeil, M. (1997). Nature and management of acquired neurogenic dysgraphias. In L. L. LaPointe (Ed.), *Aphasia and related neurogenic language disorders* (2nd ed., pp. 172–200). New York: Thieme Medical Publishers.

Turkstra, L. S. (2001). Treating memory problems in adults with neurogenic communication disorders. *Seminars in Speech and Language, 22* (2), 147–155.

Walker-Baston, D., Curtis, S., Nagarajan, R., Ford, J., Dronkers, N., Salmeron, E., Lai, J., & Urwin, D. H. (2001). A double-blind, placebo controlled study of the effects of amphetamine in the treatment of aphasia. *Stroke, 32* (9), 2093–2098.

Wallace, G. L. (1996). Management of aphasic individuals from culturally and linguistically diverse populations. In G. L. Wallace (Ed.), *Adult aphasia rehabilitation* (pp. 103–119). Boston: Butterworth-Heinemann.

Webb, W. (1997). Acquired dyslexias. In L. L. LaPointe (Ed.), *Aphasia and related neurogenic language disorders* (2nd ed., pp. 151–171). New York: Thieme.

Webster, D. B. (1999). *Neuroscience of communication* (2nd ed.). Albany, NY: Singular Thomson.

Wechsler, D. (1987). *Wechsler Memory Scale—Revised: Manual.* New York: Psychological Corporation.

Wechsler, D. (1997). *Wechsler Adult Intelligence Scale–III: Manual.* New York: Psychological Corporation.

Weiner, M. F. (1996). *The dementias: Diagnosis, management, and research* (2nd ed.). Washington, DC: American Psychiatric Press.

Weisenburg, T. S., & McBride, K. L. (1964). *Aphasia.* New York: Hafner.

Wepman, J. M. (1951). *Recovery from aphasia.* New York: Ronald Press.

Wertz, R. T., Collins, M. J., Weiss, D., Kurtzke, J. F., Friden, T., Brookshire, R. H., Pierce, J., Holtzapple, P., Hubbard, D. J., Porch, B. E., West, J. A., Davis, L., Matovich, V., Morley, G. K., & Resurreccion, E. (1981). Veterans administration cooperative study on aphasia: A comparison of individual and group treatment. *Journal of Speech and Hearing Research, 24,* 580–594.

Wertz, T. (1996). Clinical descriptions. In G. L. Wallace (Ed.), *Adult aphasia rehabilitation* (pp. 39–56). Boston: Butterworth-Heinemann.

Wertz, R. T., LaPointe, L. L., & Rosenbek, J. C. (1984). *Apraxia of speech in adults: The disorder and its management.* San Diego, CA: Singular Publishing Group.

Whurr, R. (1996). *The aphasia screening test* (2nd ed.). San Diego, CA: Singular.

Wilberger, J. E., Jr. (2000). Emergency care and initial evaluation. In P. R. Cooper & J. G. Golfinos (Eds.), *Head injury* (4th ed., pp. 27–40). New York: McGraw-Hill.

Williams, J. M. (1991). *Memory assessment scales professional manual.* New York: Psychological Corporation.

Wilson, B. A., Cockburn, J., & Halligan, P. (1987). *Behavioral inattention test.* Suffolk, England: Thames Valley Test Compnay.

Wirz, S., Skinner, C., & Dean, E. (1990). *Revised Edinburgh functional communication profile.* Tuscon, AZ: Communication Skill Builders.

Woodcock, R. W., & Johnson, M. B. (1989). *Woodcock-Johnson psycho-educational battery—* Revised. Allen, TX: DLM Teaching Resources.

Woods, D. L., Craven, R. F., & Whitney, J. (2005). The effects of therapeutic touch on behavioral symptoms of persons with dementia. *Alternative Therapeutic Health and Medicine, 11* (1), 66–74.

World Health Organization. (2001). *International classification of functioning, disability and health, ICF.* Geneva, Switzerland: WHO.

Yeo, G., & Gallagher-Thompson, D. (1996). *Ethnicity and the dementias.* Washington, DC: Taylor & Francis.

Yorkston, K. M., & Beukelman, D. R. (1981). *Assessment of intelligibility of dysarthric speech.* Austin, TX: Pro-Ed.

Yorkston, K. M., Beukelman, D. R., & Bell, K. R. (1988). *Clinical management of dysarthric speakers.* San Diego, CA: College-Hill Press.

Yorkston, K. M., Beukelman, D. R., Strand, E. A., & Bell, K. R. (1999). *Management of motor speech disorders in children and adults* (2nd ed.). Austin, TX: Pro-Ed.

Yorkston, K. M., Miller, R. M., & Strand, E. A. (2003). *Management of speech and swallowing in degenerative diseases* (2nd ed.). Austin, TX: Pro- Ed.

Zemlin, W. (1998). *Speech and hearing science: Anatomy & physiology* (4th ed.). Englewood Cliffs, NJ: PrenticeHall.

Glossary

Acceleration/deceleration injuries. Brain injuries caused by an accelerating and then decelerating movement of the head and the brain inside the skull.

Acetylcholine (Ach). A neurotransmitter that helps improve cognitive function and psychiatric and behavioral symptoms; offered as medical treatment for dementia.

Acute stage. The initial and often medically most serious stage of an injury (including brain injury) or a sudden attack such as stroke.

Afferent nerves. Also known as *sensory nerves;* those that carry sensory impulses from the peripheral sense organs toward the brain.

Amines. Neurotransmitters that include *acetylcholine (Ach), dopamine, epinephrine, histamine, norepinephrine,* and *serotonin.*

Agnosia. Difficulty grasping the meaning of certain stimuli in the absence of sensory impairment.

Agrammatic speech. Characteristic of nonfluent aphasias; speech with missing grammatical elements.

Agraphia. Writing problems associated with recent brain injury.

AIDS dementia complex. A form of progressive dementia caused by the human immunodeficiency virus (HIV) infection; also known as *HIV encephalopathy.*

Alexia. Reading problems due to recent neurological impairment; loss of previously acquired reading skills; contrasted with **dyslexia.**

Alexia with agraphia. Reading and writing problems due to recent neurological impairment.

Alexia without agraphia. Reading problems due to recent brain injury with intact writing skills.

Alternative communication. Nonverbal means of expression for persons who are extremely limited in functional verbal communication; this means may replace verbal communication.

Ambilingual (perfect bilingual). A person who speaks each of the two languages with the same, native proficiency.

Amines. A group of neurotransmitters that include acetylcholine (Ach), dopamine, serotonin, and other chemicals.

Amino acids. Neurotransmitters that include gamma-aminobutyric acid (GABA), glutamate (Glu), and glycine (Gly).

Amnesia. Total or near total loss of memory.

Aneurysm. A balloonlike swelling of a weak and thin portion of an artery that eventually ruptures.

Angular acceleration. Movement of the head at an angle (nonlinear), causing brain injury; movement caused by an angular force.

Angular gyrus. A gyrus that lies posterior to the supramarginal gyrus; damage to the angular gyrus is associated with naming, reading, and writing difficulties and, in some cases, *transcortical sensory aphasia.*

Anomia. Difficulty naming objects or persons; difficulty recalling nouns during conversation; a problem found in most types of aphasia.

Anomic aphasia. An aphasic syndrome whose overriding feature is a persistent and severe naming problem in the context of relatively intact language skills.

Anosagnosia. Denial of illness as in a patient who refuses to believe that his or her arms are paralyzed.

Anoxia. Oxygen deprivation or deficiency.

Anterior cerebral artery. Supplies blood to mostly the middle portion of the frontal and parietal lobes, including the basal ganglia and corpus callosum.

Anterior (rostral). An anatomical part in the frontal part of the reference structure; in case of the brain, it is the frontal part of the brain.

Anterograde amnesia. Difficulty remembering events following traumatic brain injury; the same as posttraumatic amnesia.

Anticoagulation agents. A group of drugs that helps prevent blood clotting in patients whose stroke is due to cardiac embolus.

Antiplatelet agents. Drugs that prevent the formation of blood platelets that play a role in coagulation (clotting) of the blood.

Antipsychotic (neuroleptic) drugs. Drugs that help control such psychiatric symptoms as delusions, hallucinations, and depression.

Aorta. The main artery of the heart; carries the blood from the left ventricle to all parts of the body, except the lungs.

Aphasia. Language disorder based on recent brain trauma or pathology.

Aphemia. Broca's term to describe language disorders associated with brain lesions, now called **Broca's aphasia.**

Aphonia. Lack of voice; a voice disorder.

Apraxia. A movement disorder; difficulty executing sequenced and volitional movements in the absence of sensory or neuromuscular problems.

Apraxia of speech. A neurogenic speech disorder caused by difficulty in motor planning of speech and characterized by a difficulty in initiating articulation, effortful articulation, groping articulatory movements, and articulatory inconsistency in the absence of speech muscle weakness or paralysis.

Apraxic agraphia. Writing problems associated with apraxia.

Arachnoid. A thin, semitransparent, nonvascular, delicate, and weblike membrane with the dura mater above and the pia mater below; part of the meninges that cover the brain.

Arterial lines. Tubes inserted into arteries to continuously monitor blood pressure of patients.

Arterioles. Smaller branches of larger arteries.

Association fibers. Short or long fibers that connect areas *within* a hemisphere.

Associationist. A view of aphasia that holds that words and verbal concepts are associated with objects and events and that this association is broken in patients with aphasia.

Astrocytes. A variety of glial cells of the central nervous system; small cells with varied branches that occupy the space between neurons.

Astrocytomas. Malignant tumors that arise from astrocytes.

Atherosclerosis. A slowly developing arterial disease process in which the arteries are hardened and narrowed from an accumulation of lipids and other particles.

Auditory agnosia. An inability to recognize or understand the meaning of auditory stimuli, although the peripheral hearing is normal.

Auditory verbal agnosia or pure word deafness. A disorder in which the patients cannot understand the meaning of spoken words though they can hear them.

Augmentative communication. Modes of nonverbal communication that enhance, expand, or augment the limited verbal communication skills of a person.

Automated speech. Such routine and overlearned speech production as reciting the days of the week, the alphabet, or the seasons in an year.

Autonomic nervous system. System that regulates the internal environment of the body; mobilizes under stress.

Axon. A nerve fiber that is longer than dendrites.

Bacterial meningitis. Infection of the meninges and cerebrospinal fluid.

Basal ganglia. Structures found deep within the brain; include caudate nucleus, putamen, and globus pallidus; modulates movement.

Basilar artery. The conjoined vertebral arteries.

Binswanger's disease. Also called *subcortical arteriosclerotic encephalopathy;* associated with *leukoareosis,* which is atrophy of the subcortical white matter that produces a variety of subcortical vascular dementia.

Blood-brain barrier. A mechanism that prevents the cerebral penetration of harmful chemical substances and infectious microorganisms.

Bradykinesia. A movement disorder; difficulty initiating movement and generally slow movement.

Brainstem. A structure that includes the **medulla, pons,** and **midbrain.**

Broca's aphasia. A type of aphasia characterized by nonfluent, effortful, and agrammatic but generally meaningful language production with relatively better auditory comprehension; may be associated with dysarthria.

Broca's area. The left, lower, and posterior portion of the frontal lobe on the inferior frontal gyrus at the juncture of the lateral and central fissures; concerned with speech production.

Buccofacial apraxia. Difficulty in performing buccofacial movements when requested.

Carotid endarterectomy. A surgical procedure in which thrombus formed in the common or internal carotid artery is removed to improve blood flow to the brain.

Carotid phonoangiography. A method of assessing the health of the carotid arteries by the characteristics of the sound generated by the blood gushing through the arteries.

Caudal. The portion that refers to the lower or tail section of the spinal cord; it may also refer to the back part of the brain.

Central nervous system. Includes the brain and the spinal cord, both encased in bone.

Cerebellum. A major portion of the hindbrain; regulates motor movements.

Cerebral angiography. A radiographic procedure in which radiopaque contrast material is injected into selected arteries, typically the femoral artery in the groin.

Cerebral toxemia. Poisoning of the brain.

Cerebral vasospasm. Constriction of the muscular layer surrounding blood vessels.

Cerebral ventricles. A system of interconnected cavities deep within the brain; contains the cerebrospinal fluid.

Cerebrospinal fluid (CSF). Fluid within the ventricles of the brain.

Cerebrovascular accidents (CVAs). Strokes; frequent and immediate cause of aphasia.

Cerebrum. The cerebral cortex; the final integrative and executive structure of the nervous system.

Chorea. The major neurologic symptom of Huntington's disease; irregular, spasmodic, involuntary movement of the limbs, neck, head, and facial muscles.

Circle of Willis. The anastomosed form of the two carotid and the two vertebral arteries; a common (redundant) blood supply to various cerebral arterial branches.

Circumlocution. Talking in a round-about manner; "beating around the bush" instead of expressing directly.

Client-specific measures. Measures of skills or target behaviors that are specific to an individual client.

Cluttering. A disorder of fluency characterized by excessively fast rate and increased number of dysfluencies.

Coagulation. Clotting of the blood.

Cognition. Complex of intellectual functions, including knowledge, memory, and the presumed modes of information processing in the brain.

Coma. A state in which the patient is unconscious and unresponsive to most or all external stimulation.

Commissural fibers. Band of fibers that connect the corresponding areas of the two hemispheres.

Commissurotomy. Surgical severance of the corpus callosum.

Computed tomography. A noninvasive radiological procedure for scanning sections of body structures; popularly known as CT scan.

Conduction aphasia. A type of aphasia characterized by paraphasic fluency, good comprehension, and impaired repetition.

Confrontation naming. Naming objects or persons when asked to; difficult for patients with aphasia.

Constructional impairment. A form of visuospatial (perceptual) impairment in which the patient is unable to perform such tasks as copying a block design.

Contrecoup. Injury to the brain at the site opposite of the initial impact; caused by a moving brain that hits the inside portion of the skull.

Coronal plane. A vertical cut, resulting in two halves of the brain or other anatomic structure.

Corpus callosum. A broad band of fibers at the base of the hemispheres; connects the two hemispheres.

Coup injury. Brain injury at the point of impact trauma, caused by the compression of the skull at that point.

Cranial nerves. Twelve pairs of nerves that are attached to the base of the brain and emerge from the brainstem; they innervate larynx, tongue, pharynx, and muscles of face, neck, and head.

Craniocerebral trauma. Also known as **traumatic brain injury.**

Creutzfeldt-Jakob disease. A neurological disease associated with diffuse and varied loss of neurons in many cortical areas, the basal ganglia, the thalamus, the brainstem, and the spinal cord; may lead to dementia.

Crossed aphasia. A rare form of aphasia in right-handed individuals who sustain a single right hemisphere lesion.

Cues. A variety of prompting stimuli used to teach naming responses; see **phonetic cues** and **semantic cues.**

Delirium. Impaired consciousness associated with cognitive deficits.

Delusions of persecution. False but stubborn belief that one's own family members and others are conspiring to harm self.

Dementia. An acquired neurological syndrome often associated with progressive deterioration in intellectual skills and general behavior.

Dementia pugilistica (punch drunk). A variation of posttraumatic dementia seen in professional boxers who sustain repeated head injuries.

Dendrites. Short, unmyelinated nerve fibers that extend from the cell body.

Diencephalon. A structure between the brainstem and the cerebral hemispheres.

Diffuse axonal injury. Twisting and tearing damage to cerebral axons; due to angular movement of the head.

Diffuse vascular injury. Small and widespread ruptures in the brain's blood vessels.

Diffusion-weighted MRI. A magnetic resonance imaging procedure that constructs pictures of structures based on its detection of microscopic motion of water protons in the brain tissue.

Disconnection syndromes. Problems in movement, reading, and naming due to damage to the corpus callosum that disconnects the two cerebral hemispheres.

Discriminative stimuli. Special stimuli that help evoke target skills (e.g., a colored border on the left margin of a printed page to force attention to the left side of the page).

Disorientation. Confusion about time, space, other persons, and self; a symptom of brain injury.

Distal. Structures that are farther from a reference structure.

Dominant bilingual. A persons who speaks two languages, but one with a greater proficiency than the other.

Dopamine. An inhibitory neurotransmitter, produced especially by the neuronal cells in substantia negra of basal ganglia; reduced dopamine is a suspected cause of several symptoms found in Parkinson's disease.

Doppler ultrasonography. Also called *ultrasound;* helps assess arterial health by measuring the velocity of blood flow.

Dorsal. Refers to the back portion, but refers specifically to the portion that lies between the superior and posterior portions of the brain (or other structures).

Dura mater. A tough, thick membrane with one side adhering to the skull and the other side to the arachnoid; part of the meninges that protect the brain.

Dysarthria. A neurogenic speech disorder caused by muscular weakness that affects respiratory, phonatory, articulatory, resonance, and prosodic features of speech.

Dyslexia. Children's difficulty in learning to read, even though instruction was adequate.

Dysphagia. Disorders of swallowing.

Echolalia. Repeating what is heard; a parrotlike imitative response.

Edema. Swelling of tissue.

Efferent nerves. Also known as *motor nerves;* those that transmit impulses away from the central nervous system.

Electromyography. A method of studying muscle functions by recording the electrical potential the nerves generate when they contract.

Embolism. An arterial disease in which a moving or traveling fragment of arterial debris blocks a small artery through which it cannot pass.

Embolus. A traveling mass that may have been formed farther away from the place where it occludes a vessel.

Empty speech. Generally fluent and grammatically correct speech that does not make sense because of extensive paraphasias.

Encephalopathy. Diseases of the brain, often degenerative.

Environmental modifications. Changes made in the structure of living conditions of patients with dementia and other disabilities to help maintain daily living skills, including communication and social interaction.

Epidural (extradural) hematoma. Accumulation of blood between the dura mater and the skull.

Epileptic focus. The damaged or pathological brain area that triggers epileptic attacks.

Equilingual (balanced). A persons who speaks two languages with equal proficiency, regardless of the mastery level.

External carotid artery. A branch of the common carotid artery; supplies blood to muscles of the face and neck, nasal and oral cavities, and sides of the head, skull, and dura matter.

Fissure of Rolando (central sulcus). A major fissure that runs laterally (from one side of the brain to the other), downward, and forward.

Fissures. Furrows in the brain.

Frontal alexia. Reading skills in patients who have suffered damage to areas in the frontal cortex.

Frontotemporal dementia (syndrome). A form of dementia associated with degeneration in the right and left frontal lobe, temporal lobe, or both the lobes; Pick's disease is a part of this syndrome.

Functional assessment tools. Assessment instruments that sample communication skills exhibited under natural and social communication contexts.

Functional magnetic resonance imaging (fMRI). A procedure in which a contrast material is intravenously administered to the patient before MRI to detect changes in cerebral blood flow as the patient experiences different states or performs different activities.

GABA (gamma-amino butyric acid). An inhibitory neurotransmitter that is reduced in some neurodegenerative diseases, including Huntington's disease.

Geographic disorientation. Confusion about one's own geographic location.

Glial cells. Nonneuronal cells, also known as *glia* for *glue* or *neuroglia;* provide a structural framework for the neural cells.

Glioblastoma multiforme. The most malignant of tumors in the glia; associated with a high death rate.

Gliosis. An excess accumulation of astrocytes (a neuroglia cell) in the atrophied regions of the brain in patients who have variants of frontotemporal dementia.

Global aphasia. The most severe form of aphasia which has a generalized (global) effect on communication skills

Gyri. Elevated masses on the surface of the brain.

Hemineglect. Tendency to neglect one side of his or her body; common in patients with right hemisphere syndrome.

Hemorrhagic strokes. Strokes that result from ruptured cerebral blood vessels causing cerebral bleeding.

High-frequency deep brain stimulation (DBS). Implantation of electrodes in target brain cells; the electrodes connected to an externally controllable pulse generator placed over the chest wall, just below the skin; a treatment procedure for patients with Parkinson's disease.

High-velocity injuries. Brain injuries caused by military weapons, rifles, and other automatic assault weapons.

Holistic approach. The view that the brain functions as an integrated unit and that a lesion in one area affects functions of most if not all areas; contrasts with the **localizationist** view.

Horizontal plane. Sectioning brain (or other anatomic structures) into two halves.

Human immunodeficiency virus encephalopathy. Also known as *AIDS dementia complex.*

Huntington's disease. A neurodegenerative disease associated with loss of neurons primarily in the basal ganglia (especially in the caudate nucleus and the putamen).

Hydrocephalus. Accumulation of the cerebrospinal fluid that causes a dilation of the cerebral ventricles; in children, may be associated with mental retardation.

Hyperfluency. Extremely fluent and flowing speech that may be more or less meaningless.

Hyperkinetic agraphia. A disorder of writing associated with tremors, tics, chorea, and dystonia.

Hypokinetic agraphia (micrographia). A motor disorder of writing with unusually small letters or letters that get progressively smaller in a piece of writing.

Hypotension. Reduced blood pressure.

Impression (impact) trauma. Trauma to a structure (such as the head) at the point of initial contact with a striking object.

Incontinence. Lack of control on urinary function.

Internal carotid artery. A branch of the common carotid artery; the major blood supplier to the brain.

Intracerebral hematoma. Accumulation of blood within the brain.

Intracranial hematoma. Accumulation of blood from hemorrhage within the skull or the brain.

Intracranial neoplasms (tumors). Pathological growths within the cranial structures.

Intravenous thrombolytic therapy. A form of drug treatment for stroke patients with stroke; known as recombinant tissue plasminogen activator (t-PA).

Ischemia. Interrupted blood supply and the resulting deprivation of oxygen.

Ischemic penumbra. A tissue region surrounding the major locus of infarction.

Ischemic strokes. Cerebrovascular accidents caused by occlusive vascular disorders that block or interrupt arterial blood flow to a region of the brain resulting in oxygen deprivation that causes infarction.

Lacuna. A hollow space, cavity, or gap in an anatomic structure.

Lacunar states. Hollow spaces in the brain associated with a variety of vascular dementia.

Language of confusion. Confabulated and confused language associated with traumatic brain injury, intoxication, metabolic and chemical imbalances, and brain diseases; to be distinguished from aphasia.

Lateral cerebral fissure (sulcus). A deep fissure that starts at the lower (inferior) frontal lobe at the base of the brain and moves laterally and upward; also known as the *sylvian fissure.*

Lateral plane. Structures that lie away from the median plane.

Left neglect. A condition in which the patient is unaware of objects and persons on the left side; often associated with right hemisphere injury.

Levodopa. A neurotransmitter that is the most commonly prescribed drug treatment for patients with Parkinson's disease; helps movement disorders.

Lewy bodies. Intraneural inclusion granules; found in the basal ganglia, brainstem, spinal cord, and sympathetic ganglia of patients with Parkinson's disease and those diagnosed with Lewy body dementia.

Lewy body dementia. A form of dementia caused by Lewy bodies and characterized by visual and auditory hallucinations, paranoid thoughts, and mild features of Parkinson's disease.

Linear acceleration. The straight-line movement of the head when a force strikes the head midline.

Localizationist. One who holds the view that particular behavioral functions are strictly controlled by specific structures within the brain.

Logoclonia. Repeating the final syllable of words.

Longitudinal cerebral fissure. A fissure that separates the left and the right hemisphere of the cerebrum.

Low-velocity injuries. Brain injury produced by such agents as an arrow, nail gun, knife, and such other projectiles.

Lumbar puncture. A method of diagnosing infections or hemorrhages in the central nervous system by an analysis of a sample of cerebrospinal fluid.

Magnetic resonance angiography (MRA). A procedure in which the rate and velocity of blood supply to the selected cerebral structures are measured.

Magnetic resonance imaging (MRI). A method of generating pictures of brain structures with the help of a powerful magnetic field that alters the electrical activity of the brain.

Median plane. A longitudinal (vertical) section that divides the brain (or other anatomic structures) into a right half and a left half.

Medulla. Also known as *medulla oblongata* and *myelencephalon;* the upward extension of the spinal cord.

Meningiomas. Tumors that grow within the cerebral meninges.

Metastatic intracranial tumors. Tumors that have grown elsewhere in the body, but have migrated into the brain where they begin to grow.

Microglia. A type of CNS glial cells that are elongated and dark staining, with long and branched cytoplasmic processes (thin projections).

Midbrain. Also called **mesencephalon;** lies above the pons.

Middle cerebral artery. The biggest branch of the internal carotid artery; supplies the entire lateral surface of the cortex, including the major regions of the frontal lobe.

Mixed transcortical aphasia. A type that combines symptoms of transcortical motor aphasia and transcortical sensory aphasia (a fluent form of aphasia) with language impairment with retained repetition skills.

Modeling. A clinician's production of a correct response designed to encourage imitation by the client.

Motor agraphia. A group of writing disorders due to neuromotor problems.

Motor nerves. Neurons that cause muscle contractions (movement) or glandular secretions.

MRI spectroscopy. A scanning method to create images of brain structures by detecting biochemical composition of tissue.

Multi-infarct dementia (MID). A form of dementia caused by multiple strokes, often in bilateral regions of the brain; a form of vascular dementia.

Multiple bilateral cortical infarcts. Repeated strokes in both the hemispheres that produce a variety of mixed vascular type of dementia with both cortical and subcortical pathology.

Myelin. A white, protective, and fatty material that wraps around the nerve fibers.

Myelination. Electrochemical insulation around some axons of the white matter; normally missing in the gray matter.

Necrosis. Damaged cells.

Neglect. Reduced sensitivity to stimuli, reduced awareness of space, or absence of previously learned responses to stimuli in certain visual fields.

Nerves. Bundles of axons, dendrites, or both, specializing in certain functions.

Neuritic (senile) plaques. Minute areas of cortical and subcortical tissue degeneration; found in patients with Alzheimer's disease.

Neuroanatomy. The study of structures of the nervous system.

Neurodiagnostic methods. Mostly medical methods of diagnosing neural pathology and its various effects.

Neurofibrillary Tangles. Twisted and tangled neurofibrils; found in the brain of patients with Alzheimer's disease.

Neurofibrils. Filamentous structures in the nerve cell's body, dendrites, and axons.

Neurogenic stuttering. A fluency disorder found in some patients with cerebral diseases or trauma; may or may not be associated with aphasia.

Neurohistology. The study of the basic structures of neural cells, tissue, and organs in relation to their function.

Neurology. Medical study of neurological diseases and disorders and their diagnosis and treatment.

Neurons. Nerve cells.

Neurophysiology. A branch of neurology; study of the function of the nervous system.

Neurotransmitters. Chemical compounds within the axon terminal buttons that help transmit information across the synaptic space.

Nonacceleration injuries. Brain injury that occurs when a moving object hits a restrained (stationary) head.

Nonpenetrating injury. Closed-head brain injuries in which the skull may be fractured but the meninges remain intact.

Occupational therapists. Specialists concerned with daily living activities, including self-care (cooking, bathing, dressing, driving), safety, and such other functional skills.

Oligodendrocytes. A form of glial cells; found in both the gray and white matters of the central nervous system.

Oligodendrogliomas. Tumors found in the oligodendrocytes; typically found in the adult frontal lobes.

Oncologist. Cancer specialist.

Palilalia. Repeating one's own utterances.

Pallidotomy. Ablation of the internal segments of the globus pallidus; a form of surgical treatment for patients with Parkinson's disease.

Paraphasia. Errors of speech characterized by substitution of wrong sounds or words for target sounds or words.

Parkinson's disease. A neurological disease associated with nerve cell deterioration in basal ganglia and the brain stem; dopamine-producing cells are especially affected.

Penetrating brain injuries. An open wound in the head due to some crushing or penetrating agent, resulting in fractured or perforated skull, torn brain coverings (meninges), and various degrees of brain tissue damage.

Peptides. Neurotransmitters that include *cholecystokinin (CCK), dynorphin, neuropeptide y,* and *somatostatin.*

Peripheral nervous system. Includes all of the nervous system except for the brain and the spinal cord.

Phonetic cues. The clinician's production of the first letter or sound of the target word as a cue to the patient (e.g., "the word starts with a /b/" to prompt the production of *ball*).

Phrenology. A pseudoscience that correlated mental and intellectual skills with the shape and size of a person's skull.

Physical therapists. Specialists mostly concerned with improving the physical status of the patient by implementing various physical exercises and other programs to enhance physical strength, endurance, range of motion, and general mobility and balance.

Pia mater. A thin, delicate, and transparent membrane that adheres to the brain surface; part of the meninges that cover the brain.

Pick bodies. Dense intracellular formations in the neuronal cytoplasm, especially in nonpyramidal cells in the cerebral layers 2, 3, and 6; neuropathological feature found in frontotemporal dementia, including Pick's disease.

Pick cells. Ballooned, inflated, or enlarged neurons, especially in the lower and middle cortical layers; neuropathological feature found in frontotemporal dementia, including Pick's disease.

Pick's disease. A neurodegenerative disease associated with such neuropathological features as Pick cells and Pick bodies in the frontal and temporal lobes; now a part of the frontotemporal syndrome.

Platelets. A small disk-shaped structure in the blood that is mainly responsible for coagulation.

Pons. A part of *metencephalon,* which includes the cerebellum, not a part of the brainstem; a bridge to the hemispheres of the cerebellum.

Positron emission tomography (PET). A research tool to study activation of brain structures associated with various activities by measuring cerebral metabolic rates.

Postanoxic dementia. Dementia due to chronic anoxia (oxygen deficiency).

Posterior. The back portion of the brain or other structure.

Posterior cerebral arteries. Arteries that supply blood to the lower and lateral portions of the temporal lobes and the middle and lateral portions of the occipital lobes.

Posttraumatic memory loss. Difficulty remembering events following traumatic brain injury; the same as *anterograde amnesia.*

Pretraumatic memory loss. Difficulty remembering events that preceded traumatic brain injury; also known as *retrograde amnesia.*

Primary auditory cortex. A structure at the border of the superior temporal gyrus and the lateral fissure; concerned with hearing.

Primary focal lesions (injury). Localized brain lesions.

Primary intracranial tumors. Tumors that originate in the brain.

Primary motor cortex. Mostly the precentral gyrus in the frontal lobe that controls voluntary movements of skeletal muscles on the opposite (contralateral) side of the body.

Profusion-weighted magnetic resonance imaging. A scanning method that produces images based on blood flow variations.

Progressive supranuclear palsy (PSP). A degenerative neurological disorder whose symptoms are similar to those found in Parkinson's disease; associated with atrophy of cells in the basal ganglia.

Projection fibers. Band of fibers that transmit sensory information to the brain and motor information to the muscles and glands.

Propositional speech. Purposive, meaningful speech.

Prosopagnosia. Failure to recognize familiar faces; part of the right hemisphere syndrome.

Prospective memory. Remembering to do certain things at particular times.

Proximal. Structures that are relatively close to a reference structure.

Pseudodementias. Dementias associated with such psychiatric disorders as depression and schizophrenia.

Pulse oximeter. A small, clamplike instrument attached to a patient's toe, finger, or earlobe to measure the blood oxygen levels.

Pure agraphia. An isolated writing disorder, with all other language functions, including auditory comprehension, being normal or nearly so.

Random (unrelated) paraphasia. Substitution of words that are semantically or phonetically unrelated to target (intended) words; seen in patients with aphasia.

Recreation therapists. Specialists who manage the daily activities of patients in rehabilitation settings.

Reduplicative paramnesia. Belief in the existence of multiple and identical persons, places, and body parts; rarely found in patients with right hemisphere syndrome.

Regional cerebral blood flow (rCBF). A technique to assess the amount of blood flow in different areas of the brain.

Reliability. Consistency of repeated measures.

Reversible ischemic neurological deficit (RIND). Also known as minor strokes; symptoms may last more than 24 hours but the patient may recover completely or nearly so.

Rostral or anterior. Specific to brain, the portion that is in the frontal part of the head.

Retrograde amnesia. Difficulty remembering events that preceded traumatic brain injury; the same as *pretraumatic memory loss.*

Retrospective memory. Remembering past events.

Sagittal plane. Sectioning the brain with a longitudinal cut into unequal left and right portions.

Schizophrenia. A serious psychiatric disorder characterized by disorders of thought, affect, and behavior; speech may be inappropriate or confused.

Schwann cells. The myelin sheath of the peripheral nerves.

Secondary intracranial tumors. Also known as *metastatic intracranial tumors.*

Semantic cues. Clinician's production of a word that serves as a prompt for the target word in teaching naming (e.g., the clinician may say "it is the opposite of husband" to prompt the word *wife*).

Semantic paraphasia. Substitution of words that are similar in meaning; a language problem associated with aphasia.

Semilingual. A person who speaks two languages but neither is native-like and needs both to express himself or herself.

Sensory aphasia. Also known as *Wernicke's aphasia.*

Sensory nerves. Those that carry sensory impulses from the peripheral sense organs toward the brain; because they carry information toward the center, sensory nerves also are known as **afferent nerves.**

Shunt. A tube inserted in a structure of the body, such as an artery, to perform such functions as draining excessive fluid and keeping the structure open.

Sinuses. Channels through which the blood or other fluids flow.

Spaced retrieval. A procedure in which patients with dementia are taught to recall a piece of information with progressively longer intervals with few or no errors; essentially a behavioral shaping method.

Spinal cord. A cylindrical bundle of nerve fibers within the vertebral column; a caudal (lower) continuation of the medulla oblongata.

Spinal nerves. Thirty-one pairs of nerves that arise from the spinal cord.

Stem cells. Precursor cells that can differentiate into virtually any kind of body cell.

Stereotactic surgery. A surgical method aimed at subcortical structures used to map and treat subcortical abnormalities.

Stroke. A syndrome with acute onset, resulting in focal brain damage, caused by disturbed cerebral blood circulation; the same as cerebrovascular accidents.

Stupor. A state in which the patient is generally unresponsive but pain or other strong stimulus may arouse the patient for a brief period.

Stuttering. A disorder of fluency characterized by excessive amounts or durations of dysfluencies.

Subacute stage. A period following the acute stage when the patient is stabilized and is ready for various rehabilitation efforts; a period that facilitates functional recovery.

Subcortial aphasias are those that are associated with damage to structures below the cortex, often basal ganglia and the thalamus.

Subdural hematoma. Accumulation of blood between the dura and the arachnoid.

Subthalamic nucleotomy. Ablation of the subthalamic nucleus; a form of surgical treatment for patients with Parkinson's disease.

Sulci. The grooves and the valleys on the surface of the brain.

Superior. The top portion of the brain (or other structure).

Synapse. The point at which two neurons come in contact with each other; a neural junction.

Synaptic cleft. A physical, but not chemical, gap between neural junctions.

Tactile agnosia. A disorder in which patients cannot recognize objects they touch and feel when blindfolded (they do not see the objects) or hear the sounds the objects make.

Telodendria. Many small filaments of an axon.

Terminal Buttons. Small structures that cap the terminal points of an axon.

Thalamotomy. Surgical removal of the ventral intermediate nucleus of the thalamus; reduces the frequency and magnitude of tremors of patients with Parkinson's disease.

Thalamus. The largest of the diencephalon structures; integrates sensory experiences and relays them to cortical areas.

Thrombosis. A vascular disease involving the formation of a thrombus.

Thrombus. A blood clot that restricts blood supply to structures beyond.

Topic maintenance. Talking on the same topic for an extended and socially appropriate duration; a pragmatic language skill.

Topographic disorientation. Confusion about space; sometime found in patients with brain injury.

Transcortical motor aphasia. A variety of nonfluent aphasia characterized by agrammatic, effortful, telegraphic speech with preserved repetition skills.

Transcortical sensory aphasia. A type of aphasia characterized by fluent, well-articulated, paraphasic, somewhat echolalic, empty speech in the context of poor auditory comprehension.

Transient ischemic attack (TIA). "Ministrokes" whose symptoms last only a brief time (usually 30 minutes or less) without permanent effects; may be warning signs of more serious strokes that produce more lasting effects.

Traumatic brain injury. Injury to the brain sustained by physical trauma or external force (not a result of disease or stroke).

Trisomy 21. A genetic condition in which three free copies of chromosome 21 cause a type of mental retardation called Down Syndrome.

Tumors. Space-occupying lesions that cause swelling in, and increased pressure on, the surrounding tissue.

Turn taking. Appropriately playing the role of a listener and talker in conversation.

Unilingual. A person who speaks only one language.

Uremic encephalopathy. A form of dementia caused by chronic renal (kidney) failure.

Vascular dementia. A form of dementia caused by a variety of diseases that affect the cerebral vascular system.

Validity. Measures that reflect the skill intended to be measured.

Veins. A system that drains deoxygenated blood from organs and carries it back to the heart and lungs to reoxgenate the blood.

Ventilator. Also called a *respirator,* an instrument that maintains breathing for a patient who is unable breathe without external assistance.

Ventral. Lower portion of the brain.

Venues. Minute branches of veins.

Vertebral arteries. Branches of the two subclavian arteries that emerge from the aortic arch.

Videofluoroscopy. A radiological method of examining the physiological movements involved in swallowing to analyze swallowing disorders; especially useful in determining whether and why a patient aspirates (food moving into the airway); also known as *modified barium swallow study.*

Visual agnosia. A rare disorder in which the meaning of objects seen normally is not understood.

Watershed areas of the brain. A region of the brain that receives blood from the small end-branches (terminal branches) of all three primary arteries that supply blood to the brain—the anterior, middle, and posterior cerebral arteries; the blood supply could be somewhat inefficient because the region is farther away from the origins of the primary cerebral arteries.

Wernicke's aphasia. A type of aphasia characterized by fluent, paraphasic, empty, and grammatically correct verbal expressions associated with poor auditory comprehension.

Wernicke's area. The posterior two-thirds of the superior temporal gyrus in the left (or dominant) hemisphere; concerned with comprehension and formulation of speech.

Yaw. The tendency of moving objects to change their course; objects that penetrate the skull and change their course as they move inside the brain cause severe damage.